Advances in Gerontology Research

Advances in Gerontology Research

Edited by Riley Carter

AMERICAN
MEDICAL PUBLISHERS
www.americanmedicalpublishers.com

American Medical Publishers,
41 Flatbush Avenue,
1st Floor, New York,
NY 11217, USA

Visit us on the World Wide Web at:
www.americanmedicalpublishers.com

ISBN: 978-1-63927-000-2

Cataloging-in-Publication Data

Advances in gerontology research / edited by Riley Carter.
p. cm.
Includes bibliographical references and index.
ISBN 978-1-63927-000-2
1. Gerontology--Research. 2. Geriatrics. 3. Older people--Diseases.
4. Older people--Health and hygiene. I. Carter, Riley.

RC952.5 .A38 2022
618.97--dc23

Table of Contents

Preface

The world is advancing at a fast pace like never before. Therefore, the need is to keep up with the latest developments. This book was an idea that came to fruition when the specialists in the area realized the need to coordinate together and document essential themes in the subject. That's when I was requested to be the editor. Editing this book has been an honour as it brings together diverse authors researching on different streams of the field. The book collates essential materials contributed by veterans in the area which can be utilized by students and researchers alike.

The study of social, cultural, psychological, cognitive and biological aspects of aging is known as gerontology. It traces the progressive changes that take place in a cell, a tissue, an organ system and a total organism, with the passage of time. Geriatrics is a subset of gerontology that is concerned with the prevention and treatment of diseases in older people. Gerontology has various sub-fields such as biogerontology, social gerontology, environmental gerontology, and jurisprudential gerontology. Biogerontology deals with the biological aging process, its potential means and evolutionary origins. Social gerontology is concerned with working with older adults. Environmental gerontology falls under gerontology that seeks to improve the relationship between aging persons and their physical and social environments. Jurisprudential gerontology deals with the interaction of legal laws with the aging experience. The book aims to shed light on some of the unexplored aspects of gerontology and the recent researches in this field. It strives to provide a fair idea about this discipline and to help develop a better understanding of the latest advances within this field. Those in search of information to further their knowledge will be greatly assisted by this book.

Each chapter is a sole-standing publication that reflects each author's interpretation. Thus, the book displays a multi-facetted picture of our current understanding of application, resources and aspects of the field. I would like to thank the contributors of this book and my family for their endless support.

Editor

1

The Engagement in Physical Activity for Middle-Aged and Older Adults with Multiple Chronic Conditions: Findings from a Community Health Assessment

Wei-Chen Lee[1] **and Marcia G. Ory**[2]

[1] *Health Policy & Management, Program on Health Workforce Analysis and Policy, School of Rural Public Health, Texas A&M Health Science Center, College Station, TX 77843-1266, USA*
[2] *Health Promotion & Community Health Sciences, Program on Healthy Aging, School of Rural Public Health, Texas A&M Health Science Center, College Station, TX 77843-1266, USA*

Correspondence should be addressed to Wei-Chen Lee; wlee@srph.tamhsc.edu

Academic Editor: Astrid E. Fletcher

The current aging trends accompanying the increasing prevalence of multiple chronic conditions (MCCs) and decreasing participation in physical activity (PA) have swept the United States. In light of the magnitude of this phenomenon, this study seeks to identify the most common MCC combinations and their relationships with PA level. A cross-sectional study, *Brazos Valley Health Assessment*, was conducted between October 2009 and July 2010. All data analyses were performed by STATA 12.0. The overall sample which met the inclusion criteria is 2,603. Among people older than 45 years, chronic conditions of cardiovascular, endocrine, and musculoskeletal systems were the most prevalent. Participants with three chronic conditions were less likely to meet the PA standard than those with only two chronic conditions. Younger age, women, rural residence, and unsafe environments were related to the lower PA level. After adjusting for seven covariates, all MCCs combinations adversely affect the level of PA (OR < 1.0, $P < 0.05$). People with MCCs were among the least active subgroups despite the health benefits of doing exercise. Given the well-documented benefits of physical activity for delaying the onset or progression of MCCs, public health efforts to enhance regular PA in middle-aged and older adults are recommended.

1. Introduction

As seen globally [1], the population in the US is aging [2]. There were approximately 120.1 million adults aged 45 years or older (39.30% of the total US population) in 2011, and this number is expected to rise to 162.8 million (42.96% of the total US population) by 2030 [3]. The rapid escalation of the aging population has been accompanied by an increase in the prevalence of multiple chronic conditions (MCCs) [4, 5].

The recent national emphasis on MCCs (defined as two or more chronic conditions) can be attributed, in part, to studies documenting the association of MCC with increased risks of adverse health outcomes, higher health care use, and associated costs [6–8]. Recent national data reported that around 63 million Americans had MCCs, and this number is projected to grow to 81 million by 2020 [9, 10]. For people aged 45–64 years old, the percentage of adults with two or more of nine selected chronic conditions has increased 5 percent from 1999 to 2009 [11]. This number is more than 8 percent for the group of people older than 65 years of age. The prevalence of MCCs in Medicare or veteran populations has been further explored. Two-thirds of Medicare beneficiaries (around 21.4 million) had at least two or more chronic conditions which were associated with more hospitalizations, doctor visits, home health services, ER visits, and hospital readmissions [6]. Also their average Medicare spending is higher than the spending of beneficiaries with less than one chronic condition. The mean number of chronic conditions (out of 23 selected conditions) in veterans aged 65 and older was found to be 5.5 for men and 5.1 for women [12].

Both hypertension and hyperlipidemia were presented in the 9 of the 15 most prevalent triplets (i.e., a combination of three conditions).

Concurrently, the lack of physical activity (PA) is well recognized as a risk factor for chronic diseases [13]. It is likely that even more Americans will fail to meet national PA guidelines (e.g., being active for at least 30 minutes of moderate intensive activity for most days of the week) in the decades to come as the population ages [14, 15]. While PA is important for health promotion and disease prevention across individual's life course, older adults have less engagement in PA than younger age groups [16–18]. The percentages of adults participating in PA that met the national physical activity guidelines were 19.2% among people aged 45–54 years, 15.9% 55–64 years, 13.6% 65–74 years, and 7.3% 75–84 years, but only 4.0% among people aged 85 years and older [19]. Findings from these national statistics conclude that older people have lower levels of PA. The latest data from Behavioral Risk Factor Surveillance System (BRFSS) also noted that the percentage of no leisure-time physical activity (LTPA) is the highest in the oldest age group as compared to the younger age groups [20]. Multi-level policies are recommended to promote physical activity [7].

The provision of the new American health care reform law, the Patient Protection and Affordable Care Act (PPACA), supports the development and implementation of new approaches to help patients manage multiple chronic conditions [21]. Insufficient PA has been identified as a major risk factor for the onset and progression of multiple chronic conditions [22]. But the level of PA conducted by people with MCCs has not been specifically studied. The majority of prior studies focus on the relationship of single chronic condition such as diabetes or chronic obstructive pulmonary disease (COPD) and levels of PA in comparison to those without any chronic conditions [23, 24].

Only a few empirical studies address the relationships between MCCs and the engagement in or barriers to PA. For example, symptoms of one of chronic conditions or lifestyle behaviors that interfered with another condition/behavior often impede the population with MCCs from doing exercise [25]. One participant could not exercise for diabetes due to the difficult breathing, a syndrome of the asthma. One qualitative study suggests that long-term limitations on activity accompanying their MCC were the strongest barrier to PA participation [26]. These long-term physical symptoms consisted of pain/discomfort, fatigue/dizziness, weakness/lack of strength, shortness of breath, and poor balance. Other barriers found include poor-to-average self-rated general health, lack of social support, and transportation issues [27].

None of previous studies identify which combination of chronic conditions contributes the most to reduced engagement in PA. Further, there has been relatively little research conducted on MCCs which are grounded in a person-based perspective rather than a disease-based perspective. Previous studies primarily regard multiple chronic conditions or syndromes as a whole or a single concept. Nevertheless, different combinations of MCC should have different impacts on a person's quality of care and quality of life. Therefore, this study examines how the top three prevalent combinations affect the PA level of middle-aged and older adults.

There is a critical need to address the relationships between MCCs and involvement in PA and to identify whether there is a specific pattern of MCCs that is associated with different amounts PA involvement, controlling for other known correlates of PA. To address the current dearth of information in this area, three research objectives were proposed to (1) explore the prevalence of all types of MCC, (2) analyze the relationships between the top three prevalent combinations of MCC with the PA level and personal characteristics of middle-aged and older adults, and (3) examine the impacts of MCC on the PA level with controlling personal characteristics.

2. Methods

2.1. Data Source. This cross-sectional study draws on data from the 2010 Brazos Valley Health Status Assessment (BVHSA), a joint effort of the Brazos Valley Health Partnership (BVHP) and the Center for Community Health Development (CCHD) at the Texas A&M Health Science Center [28]. The survey was conducted between October 2009 and July 2010 in the Brazos Valley and one adjacent county, an area where more than 300,000 citizens live within 5,109 square miles [29]. The final version of the assessment also included other existing data collected by the Texas Department of State Health Services (DSHS), the 2000 Census, the CDC, the Texas Workforce Commission, and two projects *Healthy People 2010* as well as *Rural Healthy People 2010* [28].

2.2. Survey Design and Study Sample. From a comprehensive list of residential addresses, 15,000 households were randomly selected, and 10,501 were reached by phone [28]. Residents willing to participate in the survey received the survey instrument primarily in English, instructions, and a self-addressed stamped envelope. Overall, 5,362 agreed to complete a survey, and 3,360 households returned a complete survey (62.6%). For purpose of this study, we focused on participants who were at least 45 years old and who had at least one chronic condition. The data of 2,603 residents meeting the inclusion criteria was analyzed with the approval of Institutional Review Board at the Texas A&M University.

2.3. Dependent Variable: Level of Physical Activity (PA). In the survey, physical activities were categorized into moderate- and vigorous-intensity types. Descriptions of moderate activity (e.g., brisk walking) and vigorous activities (e.g., running) were provided to help respondents anchor their responses. The research participants were asked how many days per week they did moderate and/or vigorous activities for at least 10 minutes at a time. They were also asked how much total time per day they spent doing these activities. Through multiplying both answers (i.e., days per week and minutes per day), we obtained the total minutes of physical activities they participated in every week. The 2008 Physical Activity Guidelines for Americans recommends adults to have at least 150 minutes of moderate-intensity aerobic activity or at least

75 minutes of vigorous-intensity aerobic activity every week [22]. According to this guideline, the research participants were divided into two groups: one group who met the standard and another who failed to meet the PA national standard for adults.

2.4. Independent Variables: Combinations of Chronic Conditions. A chronic condition is a condition that requires ongoing medical services and is slow in its progress and long in its continuance [30, 31]. The survey participants were asked about whether they have been told by a medical care provider that they had any of the 21 selected conditions by circling *yes* or *no*. The 21 conditions could be classified into (1) central nervous system (e.g., depression, anxiety, developmental or learning disability, Parkinson's disease, and other mental health issues), (2) cardiovascular system (e.g., hypertension, congestive heart failure, high cholesterol, angina, heart attack, and stroke), (3) respiratory system (e.g., asthma and emphysema/chronic bronchitis/COPD), (4) endocrine system (e.g., obesity/overweight, diabetes, skin cancer, and nonskin cancer), (5) musculoskeletal disorders (e.g., arthritis/rheumatism), (6) genitourinary disorders (e.g., a disease of liver/cirrhosis/chronic hepatitis), and (7) gastro intestinal tract (e.g., inflammatory bowel disease/ulcerative colitis and stomach ulcer).

This study defines MCC as a health status in which patients experience symptoms of two or more systems of chronic systems (e.g., the combination of central nervous system and cardiovascular system) rather than counting up all the specific cardiovascular related conditions separately. In other words, this approach takes a system rather than a disease-specific approach. The numbers and percentages of all combinations were estimated among the research participants aged 45 years or older. Also this study addressed the characteristics and PA involvement of the top three combinations, including the combination of cardiovascular and endocrine system ($n = 293$), the combination of cardiovascular and musculoskeletal systems ($n = 143$), and the combination of cardiovascular, endocrine, and musculoskeletal systems ($n = 239$). These three combinations were defined to be exclusive to each other and hence reflect three different groups of participants.

2.5. Covariates. Characteristics of participants and environmental factors are covariates in the analysis model. Questions about personal characteristics and environmental factors were asked and employed as covariates in the regression models. Self-reported personal characteristics include age (i.e., 45~64 or above 65 years old), gender (i.e., male or female), the highest grade of education (i.e., less than high school, high school, or higher than high school), race/ethnicity (i.e., non-Hispanic White, African American, Hispanic, or other races such as Asian, Black, or Native American), and residence (i.e., rural or urban areas). Participants were also asked about the accessibility and safety to engage in PA in the neighborhood defined as the area all around their homes that they could walk to in 10–15 minutes. Accessibility refers to three questions about whether there were sidewalks, shops/stores, and recreation facilities in the neighborhood. Safety refers to three questions about whether participants themselves or their neighbors could feel free to do activities or walk outside. A scale was constructed giving one point for each "yes" response. A higher total score indicates more walkable and activity friendly neighborhood.

2.6. Analysis. Descriptive statistics were used to describe each study variable and reflect the first research objective. A correlation matrix was performed between two independent variables to test for multicollinearity. Bivariate analyses were conducted to respond to the second research objective, examining the associations between the PA level and personal characteristics, environmental factors, and combinations of chronic conditions. To achieve the third research objective, the logistic regression model was used to explore the associations between disease combinations and the PA level adjusting to seven covariates. Results were expressed as β coefficients with their P values and 95% confidence intervals. Two-tailed P values less than or equal to 0.05 were considered statistically significant. All statistical analyses were performed using the STATA version 12.

3. Results

3.1. Selection of Top 3 Prevalent MCCs. Overall, there were 2,603 adults aged 45 years or older. Multiple chronic conditions refer to a health status with chronic illnesses of two or more systems. Any two of 21 diseases selected in this survey could form 210 combinations, while any three of 21 diseases could form 1,330 combinations and so on. Among the combinations of two chronic conditions, the most prevalent one combined chronic problems is the cardiovascular and endocrine systems ($n = 293$, 11.26%, assigned as the group 1), followed by a combination of cardiovascular and musculoskeletal systems ($n = 143$, 5.49%, assigned as the group 2). Among the combinations of three chronic conditions, the most prevalent one is the combination of the cardiovascular, endocrine, and musculoskeletal systems ($n = 239$, 9.18%, assigned as the group 3). Other combinations do not account for more than 5% of the total participants, and so this study further analyzed participants' level of PA, demographics, and environmental factors only in those three groups.

3.2. Description of Participants in Total and in Different Type of MCC. A basic frequency distribution confirmed the completeness of our data with no variable having more than 5% of missing values (Table 1). The total number in Table 1 refers to all participants meeting the age inclusion criteria other than the three defined MCC groups. As indicated in Table 1, around half of our participants ($n = 1{,}300$) met the PA standard, but another half did not ($n = 1{,}303$). The group 3, representing those with three conditions, was least likely to meet the PA standard (46.44%). Overall, 45.02% of research sample are older than 65 years, 68.92% are women, 55.86% have received education more than the high school level, 80.95% are non-Hispanic White, 68.42% are living

TABLE 1: Distribution of physical activity, demographics, and environmental factors.

Number (%)	Total population (N = 2,603)	Cardiovascular + endocrine (N = 293)	Cardiovascular + musculoskeletal (N = 143)	Cardiovascular + endocrine + musculoskeletal (N = 239)
Physical activity				
Not met	1,303 (50.06)	142 (48.46)	68 (47.55)	128 (53.56)
Met the standard	1,300 (49.94)	151 (51.54)	75 (52.45)	111 (46.44)
Personal characteristics				
(1) Age				
45–64 years old	1,431 (54.98)	171 (58.36)	38 (26.57)	81 (33.89)
≥65	1,172 (45.02)	122 (41.64)	105 (73.43)	158 (66.11)
(2) Gender				
Female	1,794 (68.92)	175 (59.73)	104 (72.73)	137 (57.32)
Male	809 (31.08)	118 (40.27)	39 (27.27)	102 (42.68)
(3) Education				
Less than high school	130 (4.99)	8 (2.73)	6 (4.20)	14 (5.86)
High school	993 (38.15)	97 (33.11)	64 (44.76)	88 (36.82)
More than high school	1,454 (55.86)	187 (63.82)	71 (49.65)	134 (56.07)
Missing	26 (1.00)	1 (0.34)	2 (1.40)	3 (1.26)
(4) Race				
Non-Hispanic White	2,107 (80.95)	252 (86.01)	112 (78.32)	178 (74.48)
African American	252 (9.68)	14 (4.78)	25 (16.68)	39 (16.32)
Hispanic	172 (6.61)	22 (7.51)	5 (3.50)	13 (5.44)
Others	63 (2.42)	5 (1.73)	3 (2.10)	7 (2.93)
Missing	9 (0.35)	0 (0.00)	0 (0.00)	2 (0.68)
(5) Residence				
Urban	805 (30.93)	96 (32.77)	42 (29.37)	78 (32.64)
Rural	1,781 (68.42)	195 (66.56)	100 (69.93)	160 (66.95)
Missing	17 (0.65)	2 (0.68)	1 (0.70)	1 (0.42)
Environmental factors				
(6) Accessibility of PA location				
No access	1,269 (48.75)	142 (48.46)	69 (48.25)	117 (48.95)
Have access	1,334 (51.25)	151 (51.54)	74 (51.75)	122 (51.05)
(7) Safety of PA environment				
Not safe	747 (28.70)	88 (30.03)	37 (25.87)	62 (25.94)
Safe	1,856 (71.30)	208 (69.97)	106 (74.13)	177 (74.06)

in rural areas, 51.25% have accessibility to facilities such as a gym, and 71.30% reported that it is safe to engage in physical activity in their neighborhoods. Compared to the distributions of individual characteristics among three MCC groups, those in groups 2 and 3 had higher proportions of persons who were older than 65 (from group 1 to 3 are 41.64%, 73.43%, and 66.11%). Next, there were higher proportions of male participants in the groups 1 and 3 than those in the group 2 (40.27%, 27.27%, 42.68%). The percentages associated with education level, residence, accessibility, and safety are relatively similar across all groups. The majority of respondents across all categories were non-Hispanic White (86.01%, 78.32%, and 74.48%). Hispanic populations did not account for more than ten percent in any of three groups.

3.3. Description of Participants Met or Not Met the PA Standard. For the level of PA (i.e., met or not met the standard), statistically significant variation ($P < 0.05$) across personal characteristics, environmental factors, and combinations of chronic conditions were shown in Table 2. The level of physical activity tends to be lower (i.e., not met) among people who are 45 to 64 years old ($\chi^2 = 5.48$, $P = 0.019$), female ($\chi^2 = 53.02$, $P = 0.000$), perceived their

TABLE 2: Association between the level of physical activity and personal characteristics, environmental factors, and combinations of chronic conditions.

N (%)	Not met	Met the standard	χ^2 (P value)
Age			5.48 (0.019)
45–64	746 (52.13)	685 (47.87)	
65+	557 (47.53)	615 (52.47)	
Sex			53.02 (0.000)
Male	319 (39.43)	490 (60.57)	
Female	984 (54.85)	810 (45.15)	
Education			1.14 (0.566)
<High school	71 (54.62)	59 (45.38)	
High school	493 (49.65)	500 (50.35)	
>High school	729 (50.14)	725 (49.86)	
Race			0.87 (0.8333)
Non-Hispanic White	1,059 (50.26)	1,048 (49.74)	
African American	127 (50.40)	125 (49.60)	
Hispanic	85 (49.42)	87 (50.58)	
Others	28 (44.44)	35 (55.56)	
Residence			3.45 (0.063)
Rural	425 (52.80)	380 (47.20)	
Urban	870 (48.85)	911 (51.15)	
Accessibility			0.47 (0.492)
Unavailable	644 (50.75)	625 (49.25)	
Accessible	659 (49.40)	675 (50.60)	
Safety			4.00 (0.046)
Unsafe	397 (53.15)	350 (46.85)	
Safe	906 (48.81)	950 (51.19)	
MCC			10.34 (0.016)
0-1 disease	244 (41.85)	339 (58.15)	
Cardiovascular + endocrine	142 (48.46)	151 (51.54)	
Cardiovascular + musculoskeletal	68 (47.55)	75 (52.45)	
Cardiovascular + endocrine + musculoskeletal	128 (53.56)	111 (46.44)	

neighborhood to be unsafe ($\chi^2 = 4.00$, $P = 0.046$), and report chronic conditions in the three systems ($\chi^2 = 10.34$, $P = 0.016$).

3.4. Relationships between PA Level and Each Type of MCC. Table 3 shows the relationship between the level of PA and three MCC combinations (group 1: cardiovascular and endocrine systems; group 2: cardiovascular and musculoskeletal systems; group 3: cardiovascular, endocrine, and musculoskeletal systems) using people who had zero or only one chronic condition to be the reference group. Controlling for seven covariates, people with any type of MCC had lower level of PA involvement (Odds Ratio = 0.721 for the group 1, 0.664 for the group 2, and 0.515 for the group 3; $P < 0.05$). The odds of meeting the PA standard were 0.721 times for people in the group 1 compared to the odds for those having zero or only one chronic condition. Similarly, the odds of meeting the PA standard for the groups 2 and 3 were smaller than for the people without multiple chronic conditions.

4. Discussion

With age, the percentages of people ever diagnosed with chronic diseases are increasing [20]. As in previous studies [32], chronic problems with respect to the musculoskeletal system (e.g., arthritis), cardiovascular system (e.g., hypertension), and endocrine system (e.g., diabetes) are the most prevalent found in this community assessment of middle-aged and older adults. Conditions related to the cardiovascular system were part of all three MCC groupings reflecting their especially high rates among our survey respondents. Public awareness campaigns and lifestyle interventions for

TABLE 3: Logistic regression to identify relationships between PA level and disease combinations, adjusted by covariates.

(Met standard versus not met)	O.R. (95% C.I.)	P value
Independent variable		
0 or 1 chronic disease (reference group)	1.00	
Cardiovascular + endocrine	0.721 (0.536, 0.970)	0.031
Cardiovascular + musculoskeletal	0.664 (0.444, 0.993)	0.046
Cardiovascular + endocrine + musculoskeletal	0.515 (0.368, 0.721)	0.000
Covariates		
(1) Age (65 years or older)	1.820 (1.408, 2.352)	0.000
(2) Gender (female)	0.524 (0.409, 0.673)	0.000
(3) Education		
High school	1.652 (0.842, 3.240)	0.145
More than high school	1.462 (0.747, 2.861)	0.267
(4) Race		
Non-Hispanic White	0.987 (0.651, 1.496)	0.951
African American	1.448 (0.865, 2.423)	0.159
Hispanic	0.952 (0.441, 2.056)	0.901
(5) Residence (rural)	1.377 (1.047, 1.811)	0.022
(6) Accessibility of PA location (accessible)	1.274 (0.973, 1.669)	0.078
(7) Safety of PA environment (safe)	1.296 (0.963, 1.744)	0.087

lifetime risks of cardiovascular diseases such as smoking cessation, healthy diets, and active living are warranted to reduce the magnitude of cardiovascular conditions [33].

Simultaneously, the current aging process is accompanied by significant declines in the participation of physical activity [34]. This study finding is consistent with the report of a national survey, Behavioral Risk Factor Surveillance System (BRFSS), that only half of people older than 45 years have participated in 150 minutes or more of aerobic physical activity per week [20].

In this study, percentages of meeting the PA standard were lowest for people with a combination of conditions in three different systems. Warshaw in 2006 also reported that the activity limitations increase with the number of chronic conditions [35]. Not surprising, there are higher percentages of people older than 65 in the groups 2 and 3 which both include the chronic problem of musculoskeletal system confirming the well-cited age association with musculoskeletal problems [36]. On the other hand, there are higher percentages of male participants in the groups 1 and 3 which both have the chronic problem of the endocrine system. This finding is in line with another literature that male adults are more vulnerable to diabetes than their female counterparts [37]. Future research is recommended to explore how age and gender, interacting with over covariates, affect the onset and progression of musculoskeletal and endocrine conditions.

The policy implication (increase physical activity involvement) of this study is one of the focuses in the PPACA which encourages the development and implementation of interventions to care for older adults with MCC [5, 35]. Next, the findings of this study are consistent with the literature that female gender, rural residence, and no safe environments to do exercise were the risk factors of meeting the PA standard [14, 38–40]. However, people older than 65 years in this survey are more likely to meet the PA standard than middle-aged adults which is contrary to the findings of previous studies [19, 20, 41] but might be a reflection that older adults have more time for leisure activity. Education level, race, and accessibility do not show significant association with the level of PA. This might be due to the different demographic distribution of this Community Health Assessment from other national survey (e.g., this assessment represented more rural areas).

This research adds to the scant knowledge on the relationship between three MCC combinations and the PA participation among middle-aged and older adults. This study suggests that chronic conditions might impede people from participating in physical activity regardless of a person's age, gender, education, race, and residence, as well as accessibility and safety of the neighborhood. One study provides a good example that women with chronic diseases were less active despite the health benefits of doing exercise [38].

The research results related to a seven-county region in Central Texas and may not allow for generalizability to all US populations. Additionally, the self-reported responses on both physical activity and chronic conditions might be subject to bias relative to more objective measures such as physician reports. Given these limitations, longitudinal work must also be conducted to determine the causal association between the MCCs and PA level using more objective measures. More efforts are also needed to develop and tailor appropriate PA programs to people with multiple chronic conditions [42].

5. Conclusions

In the face of rapidly escalating aging populations along with age-related declines in physical, cognitive, and/or social functions, regular physical activity has been recognized as one of the most important factors impacting the aging process [14, 43]. Over the past two decades, medications prescribed to prevent the complications or treat the symptoms of chronic illnesses have increased rapidly [35]. Multiple chronic conditions that lead to the loss of independence, quality of life, and economic costs will continue to strain the US healthcare system [5, 9]. The findings of this Community Health Assessment reported the three most common MCC combinations and levels of physical activity for respondents in each of these groupings. To support the goal of successful aging [44, 45], endeavors to help middle-aged and older adults maintain regular physical activity are critical. Meanwhile, additional interdisciplinary research including medical, social, health behavioral, and environmental areas is needed to advance this field.

Acknowledgments

All authors have contributed substantially to the theoretical conception, the design of the research, the data analysis, and the writing and critical revision of the paper. The authors appreciate the Center for Community Health Development (CCHD) to provide the dataset of *Brazos Valley Health Assessment 2010* for this research. The authors declare that there is no conflict of interests.

References

[1] World Health Organization (WHO), "Health Topics: Aging," 2012, http://www.who.int/topics/ageing/en/.

[2] Administration on Aging (AOA), "Aging Statistics," 2011, http://www.aoa.gov/aoaroot/aging_statistics/index.aspx.

[3] US Census Bureau, "Age and Sex," 2012, http://www.census.gov/.

[4] T. Bodenheimer, E. Chen, and H. D. Bennett, "Confronting the growing burden of chronic disease: can the U.S. health care workforce do the job?" *Health Affairs*, vol. 28, no. 1, pp. 64–74, 2009.

[5] US Department of Health and Human Services (HHS), "HHS Initiative on Multiple Chronic Conditions," 2010, http://www.hhs.gov/ash/initiatives/mcc/.

[6] Center for Medicare and Medicaid (CMS), *Chronic Conditions Among Medicare Beneficiaries, Chartbook, 2012*, CMS Innovation, Baltimore, Md, USA, 2012.

[7] S. L. Norris, K. High, T. M. Gill et al., "Health care for older Americans with multiple chronic conditions: a research agenda," *Journal of the American Geriatrics Society*, vol. 56, no. 1, pp. 149–159, 2008.

[8] J. L. Wolff, B. Starfield, and G. Anderson, "Prevalence, expenditures, and complications of multiple chronic conditions in the elderly," *Archives of Internal Medicine*, vol. 162, no. 20, pp. 2269–2276, 2002.

[9] Partnership for Solutions, "Chronic Conditions: Making the Case for Ongoing Care," 2004, http://www.partnershipforsolutions.org/DMS/files/chronicbook2004.pdf.

[10] C. Vogeli, A. E. Shields, T. A. Lee et al., "Multiple chronic conditions: prevalence, health consequences, and implications for quality, care management, and costs," *Journal of General Internal Medicine*, vol. 22, supplement 3, pp. 391–395, 2007.

[11] V. M. Freid, A. B. Bernstein, and M. A. Bush, "Multiple chronic conditions among adults aged 45 and over: Trends over the past 10 years," 2012, http://www.cdc.gov/nchs/data/databriefs/db100.pdf.

[12] M. A. Steinman, S. J. Lee, W. J. Boscardin et al., "Patterns of multimorbidity in elderly veterans," *Journal of the American Geriatrics Society*, vol. 60, no. 10, pp. 1872–1880, 2012.

[13] Partnership to Fight Chronic Disease, "Need great, evidence lacking for people with multiple chronic conditions," 2012, http://www.fightchronicdisease.org/sites/fightchronicdisease.org/files/docs/MCC%20White%20paper%20October%202012%20-%20final%20draft.pdf.

[14] A. C. King and D. K. King, "Physical activity for an aging population," *Public Health Reviews*, vol. 32, no. 2, pp. 401–426, 2010.

[15] Federal Interagency Forum on Aging-Related Statistics, "Older Americans 2012: Key Indicators of Well-Being," 2012, http://agingstats.gov/agingstatsdotnet/Main_Site/Data/2012_Documents/Docs/EntireChartbook.pdf.

[16] B. Elsawy and K. E. Higgins, "Physical activity guidelines for older adults," *American Family Physician*, vol. 81, no. 1, pp. 55–59, 2010.

[17] D. H. Paterson, G. R. Jones, and C. L. Rice, "Ageing and physical activity: evidence to develop exercise recommendations for older adults," *Canadian Journal of Public Health*, vol. 98, pp. S69–108, 2007.

[18] B. L. Willis, A. Gao, D. Leonard, L. F. DeFina, and J. D. Berry, "Midlife fitness and the development of chronic conditions in later life," *Archives of Internal Medicine*, vol. 172, no. 17, pp. 1333–1340, 2012.

[19] Leading Health Indicators (LHIs), "Healthy People 2020: Nutrition, Physical Activity, and Obesity," 2011, http://www.healthypeople.gov/2020/LHI/nutrition.aspx?tab=data#PA_2_4.

[20] CDC, "Behavioral Risk Factor Surveillance System (BRFSS): Prevalence and Trends Data," 2011, http://apps.nccd.cdc.gov/brfss/page.asp?yr=2011&state=US&cat=CH#CH.

[21] A. K. Parekh, R. A. Goodman, C. Gordon, and H. K. Koh, "Managing multiple chronic conditions: a strategic framework for improving health outcomes and quality of life," *Public Health Reports*, vol. 126, no. 4, pp. 460–471, 2011.

[22] US Department of Health and Human Services (HHS), "2008 Physical Activity Guidelines for Americans," 2008, http://www.health.gov/PAGuidelines/pdf/paguide.pdf.

[23] M. C. Ashe, W. C. Miller, J. J. Eng, and L. Noreau, "Older adults, chronic disease and leisure-time physical activity," *Gerontology*, vol. 55, no. 1, pp. 64–72, 2009.

[24] T. Troosters, F. Sciurba, S. Battaglia et al., "Physical inactivity in patients with COPD, a controlled multi-center pilot-study," *Respiratory Medicine*, vol. 104, no. 7, pp. 1005–1011, 2010.

[25] E. A. Bayliss, J. F. Steiner, D. H. Fernald, L. A. Crane, and D. S. Main, "Descriptions of barriers to self-care by persons with comorbid chronic diseases," *Annals of Family Medicine*, vol. 1, no. 1, pp. 15–21, 2003.

[26] K. McFarlin, *Experiences of physical activity among older adults with multiple chronic conditions [M.S. thesis]*, The University of British Columbia, Vancouver, Canada, 2009.

[27] C. Hudon, H. Soubhi, and M. Fortin, "Relationship between multimorbidity and physical activity: secondary analysis from the Quebec health survey," *BMC Public Health*, vol. 8, p. 304, 2008.

[28] Center for Community Health Development (CCHD), "Brazos Valley Health Assessment: Executive Report," 2010, http://www.cchd.us/content/pdfs/assessmentreports/bvreport.pdf.

[29] Brazos Valley Council of Governments (BVCOG), "Welcome to BVCOG," 2012, http://www.bvcog.org/.

[30] T. Y. Liu-Ambrose, M. C. Ashe, and C. Marra, "Independent and inverse association of healthcare utilisation with physical activity in older adults with multiple chronic conditions," *British Journal of Sports Medicine*, vol. 44, no. 14, pp. 1024–1028, 2010.

[31] Partnership for Solutions, "Multiple Chronic Conditions: Complications in Care and Treatmen," 2002, http://www.partnershipforsolutions.org/DMS/files/multiplecoitions.pdf.

[32] Pfizer, "The health status of older adults: Findings from the National Health and Nutrition Examination Survey (NHANES) 1999–2004, the National Health Interview Survey (NHIS) 2005, and the Compressed Morality File (CMF) 2003," 2007, http://www.pfizer.com/files/products/The_Health_Status_of_Older_Adults_2007.pdf.

[33] National Heart Lung and Blood Institute (NHLBI), "Heart disease risk factors and lifetime risk of cardiovascular events," 2012, http://hp2010.nhlbihin.net/joinhin/news/professional/hdrisk.asp.

[34] CDC, "How much physical activity do older adults need?" 2012, http://www.cdc.gov/physicalactivity/everyone/guidelines/olderadults.html.

[35] G. Warshaw, "Introduction: advances and challenges in care of older people with chronic illness," *Generations*, vol. 30, no. 3, pp. 5–10, 2006.

[36] R. F. Loeser, "Age-related changes in the musculoskeletal system and the development of osteoarthritis," *Clinics in Geriatric Medicine*, vol. 26, no. 3, pp. 371–386, 2010.

[37] CDC, "2011 National Diabetes Fact Sheet," 2011, http://www.cdc.gov/DIABETES//pubs/estimates11.htm.

[38] R. C. Brownson, A. A. Eyler, A. C. King, D. R. Brown, Y. Shyu, and J. F. Sallis, "Patterns and correlates of physical activity among US women 40 years and older," *American Journal of Public Health*, vol. 90, no. 2, pp. 264–270, 2000.

[39] D. J. Frenk, "Environmental barriers to activity," 2013, http://www.hsph.harvard.edu/obesity-prevention-source/obesity-causes/physical-activity-environment/.

[40] S. L. Martin, G. J. Kirkner, K. Mayo, C. E. Matthews, J. L. Durstine, and J. R. Hebert, "Urban, rural, and regional variations in physical activity," *Journal of Rural Health*, vol. 21, no. 3, pp. 239–244, 2005.

[41] K. A. Cotter, "Health-related social control over physical activity: interactions with age and sex," *Journal of Aging Research*, vol. 2012, Article ID 321098, 10 pages, 2012.

[42] B. Resnick, M. G. Ory, K. Hora et al., "A proposal for a new screening paradigm and tool called Exercise Assessment and Screening for You (EASY)," *Journal of Aging and Physical Activity*, vol. 16, no. 2, pp. 215–233, 2008.

[43] US Department of Health and Human Services (HHS), "Healthy People 2020," 2012, http://www.healthypeople.gov/2020/topicsobjectives2020/overview.aspx?topicid=33.

[44] W. Chodzko-Zajko, A. Schwingel, and C. H. Park, "Successful Aging: the role of physical activity," *American Journal of Lifestyle Medicine*, vol. 3, no. 1, pp. 20–28, 2009.

[45] M. G. Ory, M. L. Smith, and B. Resnick, "Changing behavior throughout the life-course: translating the success of aging research," *Translational Behavioral Medicine*, vol. 2, no. 2, pp. 159–162, 2012.

2

Improving Quality of Life in Nursing Homes: The Structured Resident Interview Approach

Howard B. Degenholtz, Abby L. Resnick, Natalie Bulger, and Lichun Chia

University of Pittsburgh, 130 DeSoto Street, Pittsburgh, PA 15261, USA

Correspondence should be addressed to Howard B. Degenholtz; degen@pitt.edu

Academic Editor: Wojtek Chodzko-Zajko

The quality of life (QOL) of the approximately 1.5 million nursing facility (NF) residents in the US is undoubtedly lower than desired by residents, families, providers, and policy makers. Although there have been important advances in defining and measuring QOL for this population, there is a need for interventions that are tied to standardized measurement and quality improvement programs. This paper describes the development and testing of a structured, tailored assessment and care planning process for improving the QOL of nursing home residents. The Quality of Life Structured Resident Interview and Care Plan (QOL.SRI/CP) builds on a decade of research on measuring QOL and is designed to be easily implemented in any US nursing home. The approach was developed through extensive and iterative pilot testing and then tested in a randomized controlled trial in three nursing homes. Residents were randomly assigned to receive the assessment alone or both the assessment and an individualized QOL care plan task. The results show that residents assigned to the intervention group experienced improved QOL at 90- and 180-day follow-up, while QOL of residents in the control group was unchanged.

1. Background

This paper describes a novel assessment and care planning system for improving quality of life (QOL) in nursing homes. The Quality of Life Structured Resident Interview and Care Plan (QOL.SRI/CP) builds on a decade of research on measuring QOL and is designed to be easily implemented in any US nursing facility. The materials are compatible with the nursing home Minimum Data Set (MDS) 3.0. Instructions have been developed to allow for staged and iterative implementation.

QOL for people living in nursing facilities can be understood as a subjective assessment of the outcome of the clinical care, housing, and other services provided by the facility [1]. This concept of QOL is broader than that of health related quality of life (HRQOL), used in a lot of health care research [2, 3]. From the perspective of the individual resident, the concept of QOL refers to their perceptions of their own lives, as a function of their own personal preferences, personality, and life history as experienced in the daily environment of a nursing facility. Since nursing facilities structure not only the medical care but also the housing and social context, the definition of QOL for this population therefore incorporates the myriad ways that everyday life is facilitated and constrained by policies, procedures, and interactions with staff.

The QOL of the approximately 1.5 million nursing facility (NF) residents in the US is undoubtedly lower than desired by residents, families, providers, and policy makers [4]. Although the landmark Institute of Medicine report on nursing facility quality [5] and the subsequent 1987 legislative reforms placed high priority on QOL, much of the regulatory focus over the subsequent two decades was geared toward measuring and ensuring quality of care. One major outcome of those reforms was the development of the resident assessment instrument (also referred to as the MDS) which all NFs that accept Medicaid payment must use to collect data at regular intervals on all residents [6]. The RAI was designed primarily as a tool for *clinical* care planning and thus covers physical function, cognitive function, and other health care needs in detail [7]. The data derived from the RAI, known as the Minimum Data Set (MDS), are submitted to state licensure and certification agencies and subsequently to the Centers for Medicare and Medicaid Services (CMS) and serve as the main source of information for nursing home staff, policy makers, and researchers about the condition of nursing home residents. The data from the MDS have been used to develop indicators of quality of care for benchmarking and internal quality improvement and public reporting [8, 9]. The development of consumer friendly "report cards" is intended to use market forces to increase visibility and accountability for quality and further spur quality improvement efforts [10–12].

The recent revision of the MDS to version 3.0 has made major strides towards increasing attention paid to resident QOL [13]. Two changes are especially relevant. First, the designers have placed priority on resident self-report relative to observation and proxy report by incorporating "resident voice" in the assessment process. The general principle is that, for sections related to mood, pain, and preferences, the default expectation is to ask residents directly. Staff or family members can serve as a proxy only if the resident is unable to communicate or if an interpreter is not available [14, Appendix D]. The second is the inclusion of two sets of questions about "daily preferences (F0400)" and "activity preferences (F0500)" [14]. The inclusion of these items is designed to produce information about residents' preferences that can be used as a guide to create individualized care plans. All nursing homes are required to have multidisciplinary care plans for each resident which serves as the primary documentation of all daily care and services. Under the regulations, care plans are developed based on information collected with the RAI and are reviewed and updated on regular basis (typically 90 days unless there is a change in status).

The critical role of the assessment process as part of individualized care planning cannot be understated. The CMS State Operations Manual [15] provides interpretive guidance for the survey and certification process and specifically highlights residents' right to choose activities and schedules consistent with their interests and make choices about their lives. The guidance also identifies the expectation that facilities identify each resident's interests and needs and involve the resident in activities that appeal to his or her interests. To be in compliance, staff needs to recognize and assess preferences and define and implement activities (including but not limited to formal and scheduled group activities) in accordance with resident needs and goals.

It is therefore imperative that NFs have the "technology" to determine resident preferences and incorporate those preferences into the resident's care plan. The wording of the items in MDS 3.0 Section F is intended to identify issues that residents find "important" for their daily lives. The MDS 3.0 manual notes that these items are not meant to be all-inclusive [14]. In addition to breadth, what is missing from the MDS 3.0 items is an approach to eliciting two important factors crucial to care planning. First, there needs to be a way to elicit whether residents' appraisal of their daily experience meets their expectations, given that they find a particular issue important. Second, in order to develop a truly individualized plan of care, staff needs to have a way to learn the content of resident's preferences. In order to meet the regulatory and ethical expectations of respecting residents' rights of self-determination, staff need to consistently learn what, when, how, and with whom individual residents want to live their daily lives. The MDS 3.0 does not provide the detailed prompts or questions to address this expectation.

2. Methods

We developed a structured resident interview and care planning system for nursing home residents and tested it in a longitudinal randomized, controlled trial at three nursing homes. The following sections describe the quality of life assessment, care plan, and all evaluation procedures.

Every aspect of the assessment and care planning materials was extensively and iteratively pilot tested. The procedure was to develop a draft assessment and have two interviewers (a former director of social service and a recent social work graduate) conduct a series of interviews with a small sample of nursing residents from one facility. After each sample, the study team reviewed the results and made revisions to the approach. In this way, we were able to streamline the assessment process and simplify the scoring. The final version is described below.

The study was conducted at three not-for-profit nursing homes in the Pittsburgh area. One facility was part of a regional faith-based chain. Two were owned by a not-for-profit medical system: one in an urban setting and one on a suburban campus that also included personal care homes and independent living apartments. All three facilities had skilled units dedicated to postacute care; however residents living on those units were excluded from the study. The number of beds averaged 161 (range from 137 to 182). Each had relatively stable leadership during the study period.

2.1. QOL Structured Resident Interview. The QOL.SRI consists of two main components: the Domain Questionnaire (DQ) and the in-depth follow-up. The DQ contains 69 closed-ended items drawn from previous research to define and measure quality of life among nursing home residents [16]. The items are organized into 12 domains: comfort, security, food enjoyment, privacy, meaningful activities, religious practices, relationships, functional competence, dignity, individuality, autonomy, and spiritual well-being. Based on extensive pilot testing, items related to religious practices were separated from meaningful activities to create a new domain area that can be easily skipped for residents who report that they do not practice a religion. Each item was rated using an unfolded four-point scale. Residents were first asked a yes or no question, followed by a frequency question: "yes" was followed up with "always or often" and "no" was followed up with "rarely or never." This approach reduces the cognitive burden of using the full four-point scale [13] and improves participation rates [17].

Residents who provide a response that indicates "poor" quality of life (e.g., indicating they never find it easy to make friends) are asked to rate the importance of that issue. The importance rating follows the response categories used in the MDS 3.0 (very important, somewhat important, not very important, not important at all, and important but cannot do or no choice). This approach minimizes respondent burden by focusing on the information needed to make decisions about care planning around issues where there is a need for improvement.

A simple algorithm was developed to calculate a priority score by multiplying the QOL rating for each item by the importance rating for that item. If no importance rating was obtained, the priority score was blank. The numbers were arranged so that lower QOL received a lower score and higher importance received a lower score. Thus the product of the two numbers could be interpreted as a "rank" wherein priority is given to items in declining order (i.e., 1st, 2nd, 3rd, etc.). This information was then used as a guide for in-depth probing.

Each item on the DQ has a corresponding set of in-depth (ID) follow-up questions (see Table 2 for a sample item). These are open-ended probes designed to elicit the "what, where, when, and with whom" for each topic. To reduce respondent burden, the assessor selected only the top 5 ranking items for in-depth follow-up. Based on our pilot testing, we observed that occasionally residents might mention issues that are not covered in the DQ items or make other comments that indicate that an issue is very important to them. In these cases, the assessor was allowed to select one "wild-card" item to follow-up on an issue that might not have scored in the top 5 but nonetheless seemed especially important to the resident.

2.2. QOL Care Plan. The QOL care planning component can be considered a standardized "tailored" intervention. All residents received a standardized assessment; however the actual questions and the intervention they received were tailored to their own individual preferences based on their responses to the assessment questions. The approach is similar to an adaptive questionnaire.

The assessor used the residents' responses to the open ended component of the QOL.SRI to develop a draft QOL care plan task. These tasks were written on a simple form that identified the issue of concern, the goal in terms of resident QOL, the staff involved, and the frequency with which the task should be accomplished. The assessor used the responses to the ID questions to select one specific issue to address. Care was taken to develop tasks that were practical and feasible for staff to execute without requiring substantial amounts of additional time or resources. Impossible requests (e.g., visit with a deceased relative) were not addressed; however, roommate changes were considered. The draft care plan task was brought to the unit manager and the appropriate department head (i.e., if a task involved activities or dietary staff, the corresponding person was involved) for their review and approval. Afterwards, the task was placed into the appropriate order book for the department.

All three facilities used electronic point-of-care systems for nurse aides. In two of the facilities, a reminder was placed into a voice-activated system that informed the aide to check a project-specific order book placed at the nurses' station. In the third facility a detailed description of the task was placed onto the touch screen kiosk. Thus, in all three facilities, the QOL care plan task was placed at the same level of accountability as other orders.

2.3. Recruitment, Randomization, and Interview Process. We obtained a census of all residents living in each of the three participating facilities in order to screen for study eligibility. We excluded residents who were receiving hospice services and rehabilitation, were not elderly, did not speak English, were under infection quarantine, or lived in a dementia special care unit. Letters were sent by the facilities to all residents and, if available, community residing spouses or people with power of attorney informing them of the study and providing instructions on how to opt out. Research staff approached residents using a verbal informed consent script that included multiple check points for understanding. Residents were asked to repeat back key elements of the informed consent disclosure, and if their responses were not correct then the assessor terminated the interview. We anticipated heterogeneity in the types of care plans that residents in the treatment condition would receive; therefore residents were randomized to treatment and control conditions using a 60/40 allocation.

Residents were assessed at baseline. The complete assessment was repeated at 90 and 180 days. Residents who were randomized to the treatment group had a QOL care plan task provided to nursing home staff for implementation after the baseline interview. After the 180-day follow-up interview, QOL care plan tasks were written for all residents (treatment and control) and provided to staff.

2.4. Analysis. To assess the comparability of the treatment and control groups, we constructed physical function and cognitive function scores based on data drawn from the nursing home Minimum Data Set. Physical function was computed as the sum of level of difficulty with 10 activities of daily living (moving from lying position, transfer, walking in room, walking in corridor, moving between room and corridor, moving on and off the unit, dressing, eating, using the toilet, and grooming) (ranged from 0 to 40). Cognitive function was computed as the sum of items measuring short-term and long-term memory and ability to make daily decisions (ranged from 0 to 5).

We calculated QOL scores for each of the 12 QOL domains measured in the assessment. The change from baseline to 90 days was calculated and averaged across treatment and control groups. To display the 180-day findings, we calculated the average "difference in difference" between treatment and control groups. This yields a positive value if the QOL in the treatment group is higher than the QOL in the control group.

3. Findings

3.1. Sample. The results of subject recruitment are shown in Figure 1. Only 11 family members opted out on behalf of eligible residents. A total of 164 residents were approached (86

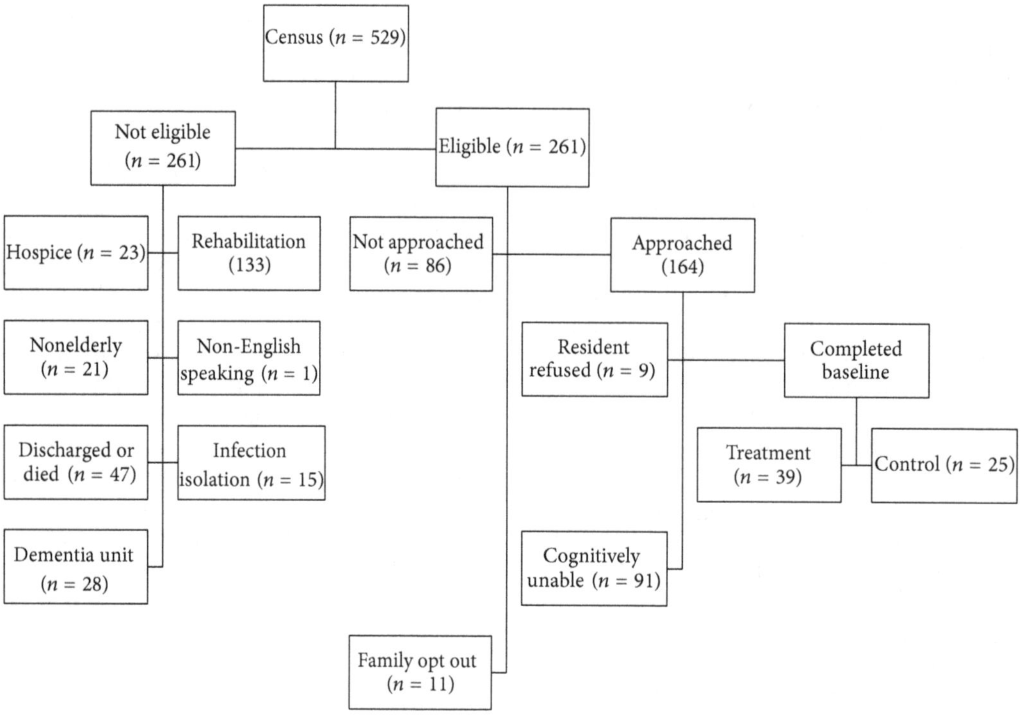

FIGURE 1: Sample recruitment.

additional residents were eligible but were not approached because we had reached our recruitment goal). A total of 64 residents were randomized using a 60/40 quota, yielding 39 in the treatment group and 25 in the control group. At the 90-day point, 12 residents from the treatment group were unavailable (3 were discharged, 4 had died, 2 were cognitively unable, 1 refused, 1 was quarantined, and 1 was physically unable to participate) and 6 from the control group were unavailable (2 were discharged, 2 had died, and 2 were cognitively unable). At the 180-day point, 5 residents from the treatment group were unavailable (1 was discharged, 3 were cognitively unable, and 1 was quarantined) and 4 from the control group were unavailable (1 had died, 1 was cognitively unable, and 2 refused). Our analysis is focused on those residents who were assessed at baseline and the 90-day assessment (a subset of whom were also assessed at 180 days).

At baseline, treatment and control groups were similar in terms of age (82.6 versus 82.4; $P = .923$), gender ($n = 6$; 15% male versus $n = 5$; 22% female; $P = .363$), and race ($n = 7$; 18% African American; $n = 3$; 13% African American; $P = .466$). Physical function scores were 22 and 24.0 in treatment and control ($P = .266$). Cognitive function scores were 1.5 and 1.6 in treatment and control ($P = .843$).

3.2. QOL Care Plans. Care plans were categorized based on the domain area of the issue that was being addressed. Table 1 lists the types of care plans and provides examples. The most common care plans addressed functional competence, followed by meaningful activities and comfort. Although none of the care plans were based on a topic elicited during the autonomy section of the assessment, all are written with an "autonomy" focus. All of the care plans direct staff to ask residents if, how, or when they would like things done. There is also some overlap. For example, the QOL care plan related to religious practices has an element of functional competence. The QOL care plan related to security focuses on relationships with staff because the resident indicated that staff is not responsive to her requests related to personal care that is physically painful. The decision was made to focus on improving her relationship with staff in order to reduce the tension and distrust.

3.3. Change in 90-Day QOL Scores. We calculated the change in QOL domain score for each resident and grouped QOL care plan target area. For example, the 5 residents whose care plans were focused on a comfort issue are grouped together. For comparison, we calculated the change in each of the 8 targeted QOL domains in the control group. Thus, in the comparison group, only those residents whose QOL care plan targeted a particular domain are included in the change score, whereas all of the control group members are used for all of the comparison domain scores. This is presented graphically in Figure 2. The average change in QOL across all domains in the treatment group was .25 (SD .40), compared to a slight decline of −.02 (SD .39) in the control group. This comparison was statistically significant using a one-sided t-test ($P = .014$).

3.4. Change in 180-Day QOL Scores. To examine the 180-day outcomes, we compared the change in the treatment group to the change in the control group on each domain score. This was calculated as the difference in difference; the

Table 1: Description of sample.

Care plan domain	N	Examples
Functional competence	7	(i) Ask resident if she would like her bathroom straightened up (ii) When in resident's room at same time as resident, ask her if she would like anything moved within her reach
Meaningful activities	6	(i) Ask resident about current reading materials and if she would like new books or other reading materials (ii) When there is an activity involving cards (blackjack, etc.) invite resident to join
Comfort	5	(i) Ask resident if she would like her pillows or bed height adjusted (ii) When assisting resident with getting dressed, ask resident if she would like to have any extra layers on or nearby (iii) Each night ask resident if the temperature of her room is acceptable
Food enjoyment	4	Ask resident if her food is warm enough and offer to microwave it if cold
Relationships	2	During one-on-one visits with resident ask if she would like materials for her in-room activities
Religious preferences	1	Twice a week, ask resident if she needs any of her religious materials moved within her reach
Individuality	1	(i) Once a week, visit with resident to talk about prior life experiences such as military service (ii) When giving care to resident take extra five minutes to engage resident in a conversation about talking points in his room
Security	1	Three days a week, stop in to see resident in her room and engage her in a short conversation

Table 2: Sample QOL.SRI item.

Domain	Item	Importance	How often?	How important?	In-depth probes
Relationships	In the past month, have people who work here stopped just to have a friendly conversation with you?	[1.5] Yes [3.8] No	[4] Always [3] Often [2] Rarely [1] Never	[1] Very [2] Somewhat [3] Not very [4] Not important [1.5] Important but cannot do (no choice)	Where do these conversations usually occur? When do these conversations occur? Who do you wish you could talk to more often?

resultant score is positive if the treatment group outperforms the control group and negative if the opposite is true. Figure 3 shows the difference in differences. The average of the differences in difference scores at 180 days was .20 (SD = .41). This is statistically significantly different compared to zero using a one-sided t-test ($P = .0346$).

4. Discussion

This study demonstrated that an individualized assessment and care planning system, the QOL.SRI, can produce meaningful and lasting improvements in resident QOL. The system was developed to be straightforward to implement and provide a high level of accountability within a traditional nursing home management structure.

The intervention group experienced improvements in all QOL domains at 90 days with the exception of functional competence. This area is closely linked with physical function and can be expected to decline over time in this population. We note that the decrease in QOL scores in this domain was lower in the treatment group than in the control group (the small sample size precludes statistical significance testing of this comparison). At 180 days, the treatment group still experienced higher levels of QOL than the control group. The overall difference was slightly smaller and in two domains (individuality and food enjoyment) was actually negative. This is particularly important considering that the QOL care plan tasks were not updated or changed between 90 and 180 days. Thus, residents in the treatment group were still receiving the benefit of personalized attention to an issue raised approximately six months earlier.

Previous individual-level intervention research in the nursing home setting has focused on modifying specific factors related to the broad concept of QOL, such as autonomy [18, 19], psychological well-being [19], pain [20], physical function [21], or physical comfort (positioning) [22]. Certainly, reducing the use of physical restraints is clearly in service of improving QOL and has been shown to reduce injuries [23, 24]. Other studies have found that personal relationships [25] and quality of communication

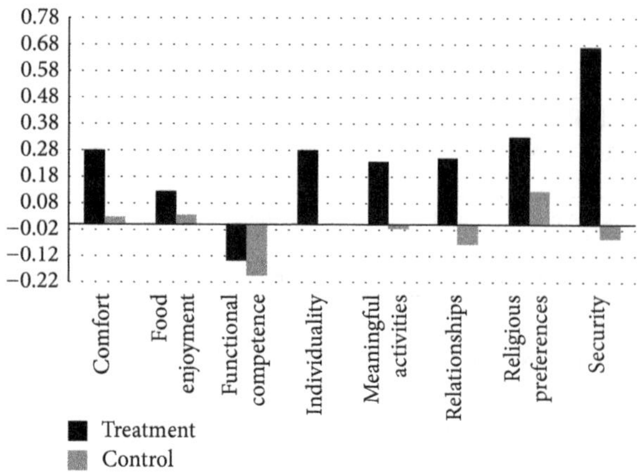

FIGURE 2: Change in quality of life domain scores by QOL care plan target.

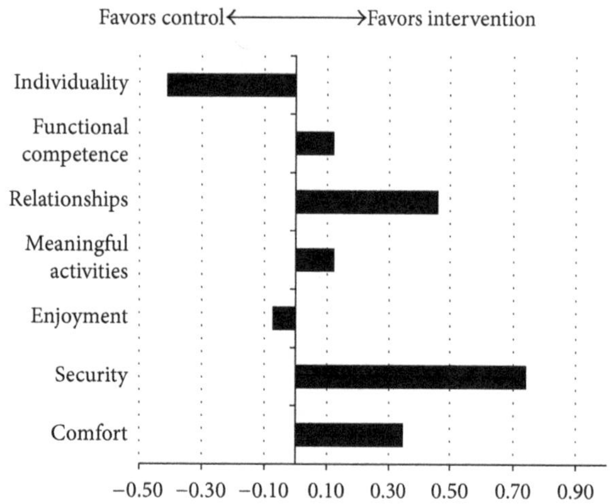

FIGURE 3: Difference between treatment and control at 180 days.

[26] between residents and staff can be enhanced and that simple interventions can improve the mealtime experience [27]. Activities programs such as gardening [28] demonstrate improvement in socialization and physical function. Life reminiscence [29] and programs, such as TimeSlips [30] which use creative storytelling with demented residents, have been shown to improve general QOL and reduce depressive symptoms [31, 32].

There have been several noteworthy facility-wide interventions that place priority on resident-centered care and have the potential to improve QOL. Wellspring [33] is a quality improvement program based on staff empowerment and resident directed. Anecdotal evidence suggests that residents in Wellspring facilities experienced improved QOL; however the evaluation did not include a quantitative measure of QOL. Likewise, the Green House model is a comprehensive alternative to the traditional nursing home, involving completely different architecture, staffing, and operations [34]. Results of the evaluation show that residents in the Green House experience better quality of life than those in traditional nursing homes (an average of .39 points on a 4-point scale) [35].

This study builds on previous research on measuring QOL that found that 91% of the variation in resident self-reported QOL scores can be attributed to differences among individual residents rather than between facilities [36]. Even though it is possible to rank order nursing homes based on resident QOL scores, the variation in ranks cannot be fully explained by organizational factors [37]. Taken together, these findings suggest that effective interventions need to be tailored to the individual resident. Facility-wide improvements are important, however, and should not be forgone. However, the best improvements are ones that enable staff to identify and act on individual residents' preferences.

The QOL.SRI takes about 30 minutes to administer. This is not a trivial commitment for most facilities, given the constant challenges of staffing and competing demands for limited resources. An important benefit of the system, in addition to improving individual resident QOL, is that it generates data about resident QOL that can be aggregated to the unit or facility level in order to track performance and support quality improvement efforts. These data can be compared to the experience of other facilities in order to benchmark improvement over time.

In this study, we repeated the assessment at 90 and 180 days in order to determine whether QOL improvements would persist. We had found that QOL changes reverted; we would be in a position to argue that these issues should be discussed more frequently with residents. However, the results were somewhat mixed on this point. Although residents continued to experience better QOL on average, anecdotally, several of the more cognitively intact residents indicated at the 180-day interview that they were expecting their care plans to be refreshed and asked why further improvements had not been made.

Facilities may elect to use the QOL.SRI on an annual basis. This would reduce the amount of data available to monitor individual and aggregate change. However, staff would be able to return to the answers to the ID component throughout the year and raise new issues at the quarterly care conference. This would likely provide a richer and more systematic source of information about resident preferences than is currently available and, as residents experience decline in their cognitive function, can serve as a historical record of their likes and dislikes.

4.1. Limitations. Resident QOL has been found to be associated with physical function, cognitive function, and various facility factors. Longitudinal research found that decline in resident health is associated with decline in QOL; however, the amount of variation explained by these factors is relatively small. The potential exists that residents in the treatment group experienced greater declines in such factors than the control group. Although the sample sizes were small, there is no evidence of differential decline over time.

The relatively small sample size limits our ability to conduct extensive multivariate or subgroup analyses. The study was constrained by the time required to recruit, randomize, and follow up on residents. The decision to exclude short-stay residents was based on the expectation that many would not be available for the 90-day follow-up. However, that decision eliminated a large number of potential residents from participation and limits the generalizability to the long-stay population. We were limited to three nonprofit nursing homes in the Pittsburgh area. A larger study with more facilities would be able to identify organizational factors associated with fidelity of implementation and outcomes.

The assessments were conducted and care plans were written by a member of the study team (NB). This individual had a similar profile to a nursing home social worker in terms of training and experience. After a short period, facility staff accepted her presence and treated her as a colleague. By the same token, residents came to identify her as the "QOL person." Since her role and function were independent from the facility, it is possible that residents felt more comfortable discussing problems with care staff than they might have been with a nursing home employee.

5. Conclusion

The QOL.SRI provides a system for nursing homes to conduct a tailored and individualized assessment of resident QOL that can be used to inform care planning. The approach has been shown to lead to improvements in resident QOL. The materials are available without charge from a publicly accessible website: http://www.improvingqol.pitt.edu.

Conflict of Interests

The authors declare that there is no conflict of interests regarding the publication of this paper.

Acknowledgments

The authors wish to acknowledge the contributions of their Technical Advisory Panel: Rosalie A. Kane, Ph.D., University of Minnesota; Lois Cutler, Ph.D., University of Minnesota; Barbara A. Bowers, Ph.D., University of Wisconsin; Debra Saliba, M.D., RAND and University of California Los Angeles; and Robert Connolly. The main funding for this research was from a grant from the Commonwealth Fund. Additional funding was received from the University of Pittsburgh Institute on Aging.

References

[1] M. P. Lawton, "Environment and other determinants of well-being in older people.," *Gerontologist*, vol. 23, no. 4, pp. 349–357, 1983.

[2] P. Erickson, E. A. Kendall, J. P. Anderson, and R. M. Kaplan, "Using composite health status measures to assess the nation's health," *Medical Care*, vol. 27, no. 3 supplement, pp. S66–S76, 1989.

[3] S. M. Haley, C. A. McHorney, and J. E. Ware Jr., "Evaluation of the MOS SF-36 physical functioning scale (PF-10): I. Unidimensionality and reproducibility of the Rasch item scale," *Journal of Clinical Epidemiology*, vol. 47, no. 6, pp. 671–684, 1994.

[4] Institute of Medicine (U.S.), "Committee on improving quality in long-term care," in *Improving the Quality of Long-Term Care*, G. S. Wunderlich and P. O. Kohler, Eds., p. 326, National Academy Press, Washington, DC, USA, 2001.

[5] Institute of Medicine, *Improving the Quality of Care in Nursing Homes*, National Academy Press, Washington, D.C., USA, 1986.

[6] J. N. Morris, K. Murphy, and S. Nonemaker, *Long Term Care Facility Resident Assessment Instrument (RAI) User's Manual for Version 2.0.*, Health Care Financing Administration, Baltimore, Md, USA, 1995.

[7] J. N. Morris, S. Nonemaker, K. Murphy et al., "A commitment to change: Revision of HCFA's RAI," *Journal of the American Geriatrics Society*, vol. 45, no. 8, pp. 1011–1016, 1997.

[8] D. R. Zimmerman, S. L. Karon, G. Arling et al., "Development and testing of nursing home quality indicators," *Health Care Financing Review*, vol. 16, no. 4, pp. 107–127, 1995.

[9] Centers for Medicare and Medicaid Services, *Nursing Home Compare*, US Department of Health and Human Services, Washington, DC, USA, 2006, http://www.medicare.gov/NHCompare.

[10] V. Mor, K. Berg, J. Angelelli, D. Gifford, J. Morris, and T. Moore, "The quality of quality measurement in U.S. nursing homes," *Gerontologist*, vol. 43, no. 2, pp. 37–46, 2003.

[11] N. G. Castle and T. J. Lowe, "Report cards and nursing homes," *Gerontologist*, vol. 45, no. 1, pp. 48–67, 2005.

[12] D. B. Mukamel and W. D. Spector, "Quality report cards and nursing home quality," *Gerontologist*, vol. 43, no. 2, pp. 58–66, 2003.

[13] D. Saliba and J. Buchanan, *Development & Validation of a Revised Nursing Home Assessment Tool: Mds 3.0*, RAND Corporation, Washington, DC, USA, 2008.

[14] Centers for Medicare and Medicaid Services, "Long-term care facility resident assessment instrument user's manual," Tech. Rep., 2012.

[15] Centers for Medicare and Medicaid Services, "State operations manual appendix PP: guidance to surveyors for long term care facilities," Report No.: Contract No.: 100-07, Washington, DC, USA, 2004.

[16] R. A. Kane, K. C. Kling, B. Bershadsky et al., "Quality of life measures for nursing home residents," *Journals of Gerontology—Series A Biological Sciences and Medical Sciences*, vol. 58, no. 3, pp. 240–248, 2003.

[17] H. B. Degenholtz, D. Liu, J. Rosen et al., "Psychometric properties of a brief quality of life instrument for nursing home residents," in *Proceedings of the Academy Health Annual Research Meeting*, Boston, Mass, USA, June 2005.

[18] R. Schulz, "Effects of control and predictability on the physical and psychological well-being of the institutionalized aged," *Journal of Personality and Social Psychology*, vol. 33, no. 5, pp. 563–573, 1976.

[19] M. A. Okun, R. W. Olding, and C. M. G. Cohn, "A meta-analysis of subjective well-being interventions among elders," *Psychological Bulletin*, vol. 108, no. 2, pp. 257–266, 1990.

[20] R. R. Baier, D. R. Gifford, G. Patry et al., "Ameliorating pain in nursing homes: a collaborative quality-improvement project," *Journal of the American Geriatrics Society*, vol. 52, no. 12, pp. 1988–1995, 2004.

[21] J. G. Ouslander, P. C. Griffiths, E. McConnell, L. Riolo, M. Kutner, and J. Schnelle, "Functional incidental training: a randomized, controlled, crossover trial in Veterans Affairs nursing homes," *Journal of the American Geriatrics Society*, vol. 53, no. 7, pp. 1091–1100, 2005.

[22] S. R. Herzberg, "Positioning the nursing home resident: an issue of quality of life," *The American Journal of Occupational Therapy*, vol. 47, no. 1, pp. 75–77, 1993.

[23] R. R. Neufeld, L. S. Libow, W. J. Foley, J. M. Dunbar, C. Cohen, and B. Breuer, "Restraint reduction reduces serious injuries among nursing home residents," *Journal of the American Geriatrics Society*, vol. 47, no. 10, pp. 1202–1207, 1999.

[24] N. G. Castle and V. Mor, "Physical restraints in nursing homes: a review of the literature since the Nursing Home Reform Act of 1987," *Medical Care Research and Review*, vol. 55, no. 2, pp. 139–176, 1998.

[25] K. S. McGilton, L. L. O'Brien-Pallas, G. Darlington, M. Evans, F. Wynn, and D. M. Pringle, "Effects of a relationship-enhancing program of care on outcomes," *Journal of Nursing Scholarship*, vol. 35, no. 2, pp. 151–156, 2003.

[26] K. N. Williams, T. B. Ilten, and H. Bower, "Meeting communication needs: topics of talk in the nursing home," *Journal of Psychosocial Nursing and Mental Health Services*, vol. 43, no. 7, pp. 38–45, 2005.

[27] B. A. D. Nolan and R. M. Mathews, "Facilitating resident information seeking regarding meals in a special care unit: an environmental design intervention," *Journal of Gerontological Nursing*, vol. 30, no. 10, pp. 12–56, 2004.

[28] V. M. Brown, A. C. Allen, M. Dwozan, I. Mercer, and K. Warren, "Indoor gardening older adults: effects on socialization, activities of daily living, and loneliness," *Journal of Gerontological Nursing*, vol. 30, no. 10, pp. 34–42, 2004.

[29] E. A. Cook, "Effects of reminiscence on life satisfaction of elderly female nursing home residents," *Health Care for Woman International*, vol. 19, no. 2, pp. 109–118, 1998.

[30] T. Fritsch, J. Kwak, S. Grant, J. Lang, R. R. Montgomery, and A. D. Basting, "Impact of TimeSlips, a creative expression intervention program, on nursing home residents with dementia and their caregivers," *Gerontologist*, vol. 49, no. 1, pp. 117–127, 2009.

[31] E. D. Jones, "Reminiscence therapy for older women with depression. Effects of nursing intervention classification in assisted-living long-term care," *Journal of Gerontological Nursing*, vol. 29, no. 7, pp. 26–33, 56-57, 2003.

[32] C. Rattenbury and M. J. Stones, "A controlled evaluation of reminiscence and current topics discussion groups in a nursing home context," *Gerontologist*, vol. 29, no. 6, pp. 768–771, 1989.

[33] R. I. Stone, S. C. Reinhard, B. Bowers et al., "Evaluation of the wellspring model for improving nursing home quality," Tech. Rep., Institute for the Future of Aging Services, American Association of Homes and Services for the Aging, Washington, DC, USA, 2002.

[34] J. Rabig, W. Thomas, R. A. Kane, L. J. Cutler, and S. McAlilly, "Radical redesign of nursing homes: applying the green house concept in Tupelo, Mississippi," *Gerontologist*, vol. 46, no. 4, pp. 533–539, 2006.

[35] R. A. Kane, T. Y. Lum, L. J. Cutler, H. B. Degenholtz, and T.-C. Yu, "Resident outcomes in small-house nursing homes: a longitudinal evaluation of the Initial Green House Program," *Journal of the American Geriatrics Society*, vol. 55, no. 6, pp. 832–839, 2007.

[36] H. B. Degenholtz, R. A. Kane, R. L. Kane, B. Bershadsky, and K. C. Kling, "Predicting nursing facility residents' quality of life using external indicators," *Health Services Research*, vol. 41, no. 2, pp. 335–356, 2006.

[37] R. L. Kane, B. Bershadsky, R. A. Kane et al., "Using resident reports of quality of life to distinguish among nursing homes," *The Gerontologist*, vol. 44, no. 5, pp. 624–632, 2004.

3

The de Morton Mobility Index: Normative Data for a Clinically useful Mobility Instrument

E. M. Macri,[1] J. A. Lewis,[2] K. M. Khan,[1,3] M. C. Ashe,[1,3] and N. A. de Morton[2]

[1] *Centre for Hip Health and Mobility, University of British Columbia, Vancouver, BC, Canada V5Z 1M9*
[2] *Department of Physiotherapy, Monash University, Melbourne, VIC 3800, Australia*
[3] *Department of Family Practice, University of British Columbia, Vancouver, BC, Canada V6T 1Z4*

Correspondence should be addressed to E. M. Macri, erin.macri@hiphealth.ca

Academic Editor: Richard D. Semba

Determining mobility status is an important component of any health assessment for older adults. In order for a mobility measure to be relevant and meaningful, normative data are required for comparison to a healthy reference population. The DEMMI is the first mobility instrument to measure mobility across the spectrum from bed bound to functional levels of independent mobility. In this cross-sectional observational study, normative data were obtained for the DEMMI from a population of 183 healthy, community-dwelling adults age 60+ who resided in Vancouver, Canada and Melbourne, Australia. Older age categories had significantly lower DEMMI mobility mean scores ($P < 0.05$), as did individuals who walked with a mobility aid or lived in semi-independent living (assisted living or retirement village), whereas DEMMI scores did not differ by sex ($P = 0.49$) or reported falls history ($P = 0.21$). Normative data for the DEMMI mobility instrument provides vital reference scores to facilitate its use across the mobility spectrum in clinical, research, and policymaking settings.

1. Introduction

The International Classification of Functioning (ICF) defines mobility as "moving by changing body position or location or by transferring from one place to another, by carrying, moving or manipulating objects, by walking, running or climbing, and by using various forms of transportation" [1]. Mobility is an important marker and predictor of physical abilities, independence, morbidity, and mortality [2–7]. Loss of mobility can result in a decline in independence, rendering individuals reliant on caregivers to meet their basic needs, or being unable to remain living independently. Such functional decline can also lead to injury and increased hospital admissions [8].

Determining mobility status is an important component of any medical or health assessment for older adults, whether an individual is acutely ill, living with chronic comorbidity, or is a healthy community dweller. Accurately measuring mobility can help a clinician determine an individual's abilities at a single time point to identify potential impairment or to establish a baseline for comparison following a subsequent reassessment. Mobility measures can also (i) help determine whether an individual's mobility has changed, (ii) identify early signs of decline, and (iii) assist with guiding therapeutic intervention, goal setting, and discharge planning in both inpatient and outpatient programs. Given the diverse functional abilities and complex health status of older adults, an ideal measure of mobility is clinimetrically sound, robust, and spans the spectrum of functionally relevant mobility tasks. Recent systematic reviews have revealed a plethora of mobility instruments for both acute medical patients and healthy community dwellers [9, 10]. Most of these instruments have many limitations, including the tendency to be designed for narrowly defined populations, resulting in floor or ceiling effects; lack of external validation or reliability testing; and/or demonstrated lack of responsiveness to change [9, 10].

The de Morton Mobility Index (DEMMI) was rigorously developed in response to clinical needs and has been previously shown to be a valid, reliable, and robust mobility instrument that can be used across the spectrum of mobility and across clinical settings [11–15]. It is easy to use, requires minimal equipment, and can be administered in a very short period of time, making uptake of this instrument into clinical practice both simple and attractive [11]. An important next step for improving usability of this instrument is the development of reference intervals (or "normative data"). Normative data regarding mobility are important for clinicians, researchers, and policy makers. Applied to individuals, they provide a comparison of the expected mobility levels for sex- and age-matched community-dwelling peers. Normative data can also provide richness to interpretation of population data, offering guidelines to help identify at risk populations or shape public health policy; it provides information that critically enhances interpretability.

Just as reference values are critical for the usefulness of measuring blood pressure, having accurate benchmarks for detecting mobility changes is essential for treatment, goal setting, and can serve to motivate both patients and clinicians. Given that normative data have such important, meaningful, and broad applications, the purpose of this study was to assess the mobility of community-dwelling older adults using the DEMMI and to develop reference intervals for healthy men and women over 60 years old.

2. Methods

2.1. Study Design. This was a cross-sectional observational study.

2.2. Participants. The study population comprised community-dwelling adults aged 60 years and older in large cities from two countries: Vancouver, Canada; Melbourne, Australia. We defined community dwelling as living in a house, apartment, or assisted living (AL)/retirement village. This decision was based on current definitions of AL in British Columbia, Canada [16] and retirement village in Victoria, Australia [17]. In both regions, this form of residence provides accommodation and some services that are distinct from the services provided in residential care/nursing home environments, and requires that residents are able to make decisions and otherwise live independently. An alternative definition of "community dwelling" includes those living in a house or apartment, but not AL (because AL is often described as "semi-independent"). We therefore presented our data both as a complete sample (i.e., using our working definition of community dwelling, provided remaining inclusion criteria were met); further separated our data into "independent" (defined as living independently in a house or apartment) and "semi-independent" (defined as living in AL or a retirement village), thus satisfying both definitions of "community dwelling" and achieving broader applicability.

Prior to participation, interested individuals were screened for eligibility to ensure they had no clinical conditions that might affect their mobility, including neuromuscular, orthopaedic, or cardiovascular impairments. All participants were required to speak English and were screened for cognitive limitations that would preclude the provision of informed consent. Where the ability to read was limited, the consent form was read aloud for these participants. All participants provided informed written consent. This study was approved for Canadian data collection by the Clinical Research Ethics Board at the University of British Columbia and by Vancouver Coastal Health Authority. The Australian portion of the study was approved by the Monash University Human Research Ethics Committee.

2.3. Recruitment. In Canada, recruitment strategies for this convenience sample included advertisements in local newspapers and on bulletin boards in seniors' centres, as well as word-of-mouth advertising by local fitness instructors. In Australia, a retirement village and Returned and Services League (RSL) members were invited to participate. Fliers were distributed to residents of the retirement village. Interested individuals contacted researchers by telephone to arrange an appointment for screening and participation or signed up at a specific site on the day of the assessments.

2.4. Data Collection. In Vancouver, Canada, assessments took place at eight different sites, including one AL residence, community centres, seniors' activity centres, and onsite at the Centre for Hip Health and Mobility, University of British Columbia. In Melbourne, Australia, assessments took place at two sites, one retirement village and one RSL centre. Each assessment lasted between 40–60 minutes. For the remainder of the paper we will use the term assisted living (AL) to include "retirement village", since the terminology is simply a matter of dialect, and the two terms are virtually synonymous.

The primary outcome of interest, the DEMMI, is a performance-based instrument that assesses mobility through 15 hierarchical items that begin with bed mobility and progress through chair tasks, static balance, gait, and finally dynamic balance tasks. A raw ordinal score is converted (through Rasch analysis) to an interval score out of 100, with a higher score representing greater mobility. The DEMMI has been described in detail elsewhere [11, 18] and copies of the instrument are available in the original DEMMI publication [11] and at http://www.demmi.org.au/.

Demographic information gathered comprised age, sex, use of mobility aids, living situation, and medical comorbidities/history.

Research assistants or physiotherapists screened interested individuals for eligibility, obtained written informed consent, and conducted interviews, and administered the questionnaires. A physiotherapist conducted the DEMMI in Vancouver; in Melbourne, the DEMMI was administered by either a physiotherapist or a physiotherapy undergraduate honors student. The DEMMI was demonstrated by the test developer (NAD) to all persons who administered the test. A 30-minute instructional DVD (video available through http://www.demmi.org.au/) was also provided prior to data collection in Vancouver. The DEMMI instrument developer (NAD) was present during data collection in Australia and Canada to ensure procedural consistency.

2.5. Statistical Analysis. Exploratory data analysis included graphical exploration of the data, with descriptive statistics

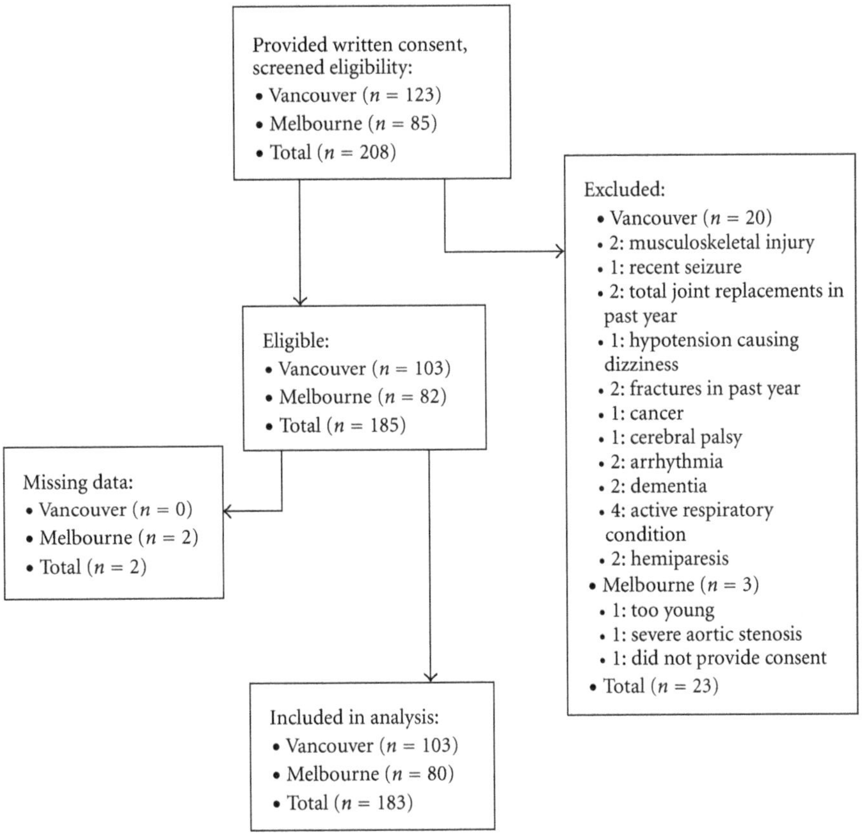

FIGURE 1: Flow diagram.

presented in tables. The DEMMI scores were explored by age category (60–69, 70–79, 80–89, and 90+), sex, and other categories such as living situation and use of mobility aid (e.g., cane, walker). The potential for a ceiling effect was investigated by calculating the percentage of participants achieving the maximum possible score of 100.

For normative data, reference intervals were constructed using empirical centiles (5th, 50th, and 95th) for the purposes of individual comparisons [19]; means and 95% confidence intervals were presented for purposes of population comparisons.

Visual inspection of univariate data as well as a scatter plot of the DEMMI by age and sex with overlying LOWESS (locally weighted scatterplot smoothing) was used to guide analysis. Welch's two-sampled t-tests were used to compare groups to account for heteroscedasticity. All statistical analysis was done using Stata Intercooled 12.0 (StataCorp, Texas, USA).

3. Results

Initially, 208 individuals were screened for eligibility, and 23 were excluded, leaving 185 participants who completed the assessment (see Figure 1 for flow chart). Two participants had missing data for age and were therefore excluded from the analysis (see Figure 1).

A description of the 183 participants included in the analysis, including scores on questionnaires, is presented in Table 1. The majority of the participants lived in Vancouver, Canada ($n = 103$, 56%) with the remainder in Melbourne, Australia ($n = 80$, 44%). Over half the participants were in their 70s and approximately one-quarter were men. Twenty-one percent of participants reported at least 1 fall during the past year; not surprisingly, this is less than the anticipated rate of 35% of all adults > 65 years old [20] (our sample was limited to healthy community dwellers, and included younger participants age 60–64).

DEMMI scores are presented visually by age categories in 10-year increments (Figures 2 and 3). Normative data are provided for comparing group means (Table 2) as well as for comparing scores for individuals (Table 3). The second column of each table provides overall group scores. The next column labeled "independent" provides scores for those living fully independently in the community. Scores for men and women living independently are provided separately in the adjacent columns (though sex was not a statistically significant variable in this analysis, $P = 0.49$). Finally, a column labeled "semi-independent" includes men and women living in AL.

The mean DEMMI scores (Table 2) demonstrate a significant difference between age categories, with a lower score for each older age category (P values presented in Table 4). Reference intervals were presented in centiles (Table 3).

Table 1: Description of study participants ($N = 183$).

	n	%
Vancouver, Canada	103	56
Melbourne, Australia	80	44
Age mean (SD)	74.6 (6.7)	
60–69	43	23
70–79	96	52
80–89	43	23
90+	1	1
Women	136	74
≥1 fall in past year	8	21
Used mobility aid	28 (4/24)*	15
Lived in house or apartment#	120 (95/25)*	66
Assisted living/retirement village#	62 (8/54)*	34
Lived alone	92	50

*n separated by location (Vancouver/Melbourne) to illustrate that participant living arrangements varied by country due to site selection during study design.
#Data incomplete for 1 participant, therefore $n = 182$.

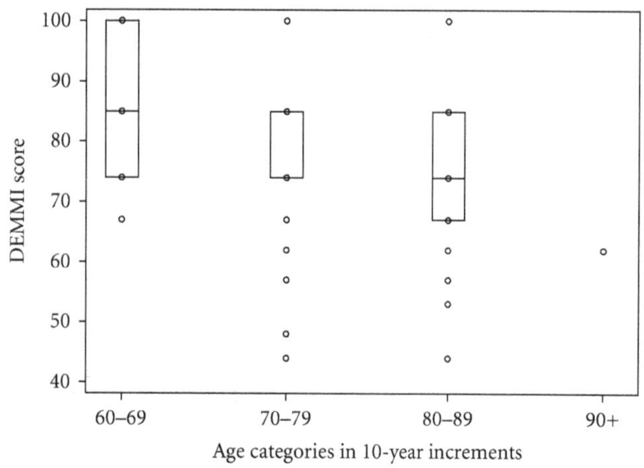

Figure 2: Box plot of DEMMI scores by age category with interquartile ranges (nb in age 70–79, median is the same as the 75th percentile; also, the oldest age category has only one observation).

The median score was maintained across each column with the exception of a lower median score for semi-independent in the 70–79 age category as well as semi-independent overall. Our finding that the 95th percentile was consistently high, with the exception of the semi-independent dwellers (and the overall sample which includes semi-independent dwellers), reflects the fact that 17.5% of the study sample scored the maximum of 100.

A priori, we were interested in comparing the DEMMI scores as a function of key variables including age category, sex, living situation, use of a mobility aid, country of origin, and falls history. For these categorical variables, we used Welch's two sampled t-tests to account for unequal variance between groups. Unadjusted P values (Table 4) showed statistical significance for age category, country, living situation, and mobility aid. Further exploration revealed that only 3 participants using mobility aids did not live in AL and only 4 participants using mobility aids lived in Vancouver (1 of whom also lived in AL). In addition, we noted the difference in DEMMI score by country (mean score in Canada 85.1 versus Australia 75.8, $P = 0.00$) was explained in part by the significant age difference by country (Australia 76.8 versus Canada 72.8, $P = 0.00$), and also by the proportion of individuals who resided in AL (Australia, 68.4% versus Canada, 7.8%, $P = 0.00$). The living situation could also be partly explained by age difference (AL 77.2 versus independent 73.1, $P = 0.00$). DEMMI scores did not differ by sex ($P = 0.49$) or reported falls history ($P = 0.21$).

4. Discussion

This study generates normative data for the DEMMI mobility instrument for adults over 60 years old who live independently or semi-independently in the community. We found that DEMMI mean scores generally decreased across increasing age categories, with the exception of independent-living men, whose average scores were highest in the 70–79 age category. Median scores on the other hand were generally maintained in the 60–69 and 70–79 age categories, with the exception of semi-independent 70–79-year olds, whose median score dropped to 74. Ninety-five percent of older adults living independently in the community demonstrated DEMMI scores ≥67, and 95% of those living semi-independently scored ≥48. Scores were as low as 44, though it was more likely that these individuals were using supports such as a mobility aid or living in AL. Overall, 17.5% of this sample scored the maximum possible of 100.

These normative data can be used either for comparing aggregate data or for comparisons of an individual. For example, in public health, one may wish to compare populations within a specific region (e.g., by neighbourhood or socioeconomic class) to inform policy makers regarding community accessibility, program evaluation, or city planning. In this case, the sample mean for a hypothetical population of fully independent community dwellers is 81.6. Looking at the bottom row of column 3 ("Independent") in Table 2, this DEMMI mean score is below the lower limit of the 95% confidence interval of 82.5, important evidence that this region's older adult population overall demonstrates lower mobility compared to a healthy peer reference group.

More commonly, normative data is referred to when a clinician wishes to know how their patient compares to age- and sex-matched peers. For example, a family member may bring a 78-year-old female relative for evaluation as a result of concerns about increasing difficulties with activities of daily living such as managing her grocery shopping or maintaining her home. The clinician would obtain a DEMMI score during the initial assessment, then compare the patient's score of 62 to the reference intervals in row 3 ("Age 70–79"), column 4 ("Independent Women") in Table 3 to see that a comparable healthy independent community-dwelling woman would score a median of 85, with 95 percent of the population scoring above 67. The clinician would then be able to use the results of this assessment to engage in meaningful education and goal setting with the

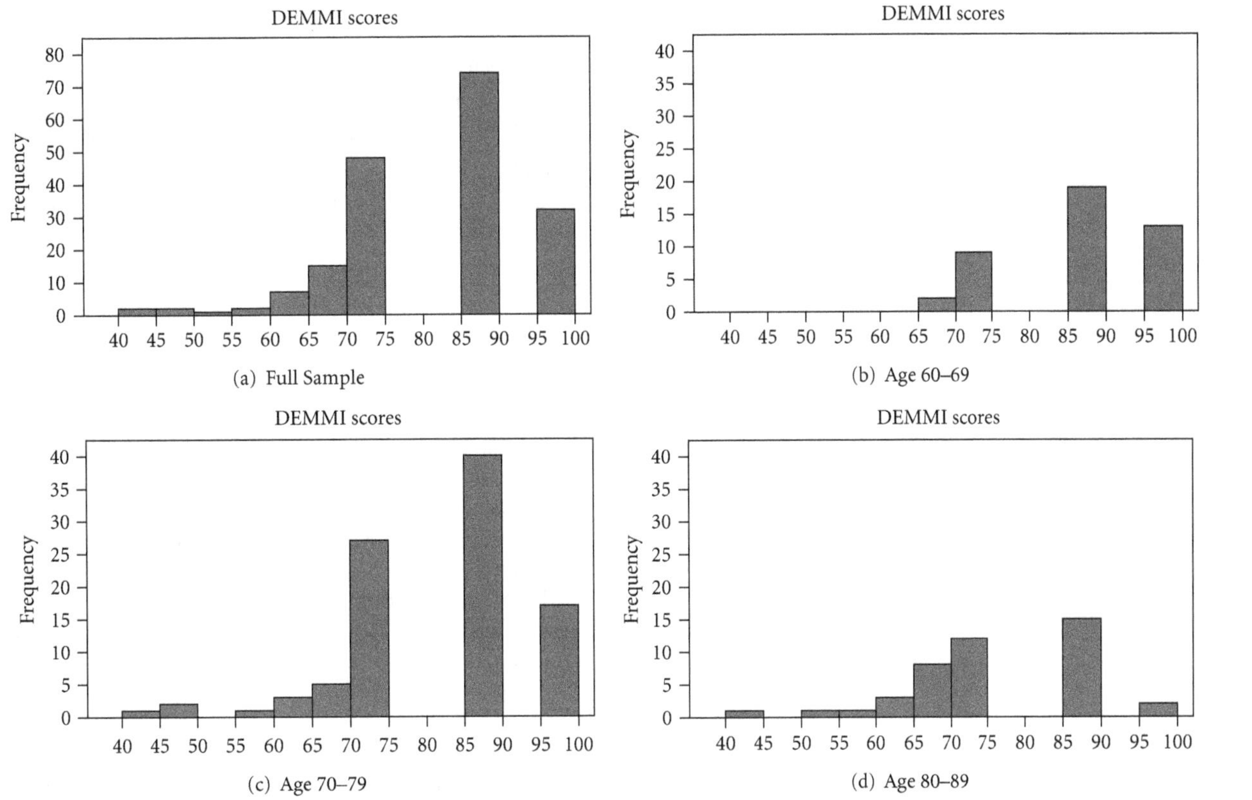

FIGURE 3: Histogram showing DEMMI scores for (a) total sample and (b) through (d) by age category (note category 90+ contained only 1 participant, therefore not represented graphically.

TABLE 2: DEMMI normative Scores for group comparisons: mean, 95% confidence interval, and number in each subsample.

Age category	Overall	Independent	Independent women	Independent men	Semi-independent
			Mean (95% CI) Number		
	86.4	**86.2**	**87.2**	**82.8**	**87.4**
60–69	(83.2, 89.6)	(82.9, 89.6)	(83.3, 91.1)	(75.4, 90.1)	(70.4, 100)
	$n = 43$	$n = 38$	$n = 30$	$n = 8$	$n = 5$
	81.4	**84.3**	**83.4**	**88.4**	**77.2**
70–79	(78.9, 83.9)	(81.5, 87.1)	(80.2, 86.6)	(82.1, 94.6)	(72.9, 81.6)
	$n = 96$	$n = 57$	$n = 47$	$n = 10$	$n = 39$
	75.3	**77.9**	**78.6**	**76.0**	**71.9**
80–89	(71.8, 78.9)	(73.3, 82.5)	(73.3, 83.8)	(63.10, 88.9)	(65.9, 77.9)
	$n = 43$	$n = 24$	$n = 18$	$n = 6$	$n = 18$
90+	**62**	**62**	—	**62**	—
	$n = 1$	$n = 1$		$n = 1$	
	81.0	83.5	83.7	82.6	76.5
Total	(79.3, 82.8)	(82.5, 85.4)	(81.4, 85.9)	(77.9, 87.2)	(73.1, 79.9)
	$n = 183$	$n = 120$	$n = 95$	$n = 25$	$n = 62$

patient and her family. Over the course of treatment, the DEMMI would be periodically re-administered to evaluate the patient's response to treatment and to guide ongoing treatment planning. An end goal for treatment could be set in consultation with the patient that either targeted a certain score (e.g., 74) or identified an item the patient would like to achieve (e.g., pick a pen up off the floor).

In a previous study, De Morton et al. [13] revealed that older adults with acute medical hospital admissions were discharged home with mean DEMMI scores of 60. The current

Table 3: DEMMI reference intervals for individual comparisons, median (5th, 95th percentiles). Please refer to Table 2 for subsample sizes.

Age category	Overall	Independent	Independent women	Independent men	Semi-independent
			Median (p5, p95)		
60–69	**85** (74,100)	**85** (74, 100)	**85** (74,100)	**85** (74,100)	**85** (67, 100)
70–79	**85** (62,100)	**85** (67, 100)	**85** (67,100)	**85** (74,100)	**74** (48, 100)
80–89	**74** (57,85)	**74** (62, 100)	**85**(57,100)	**74** (67,100)	**74** (44, 85)
90+	**62***	**62***	—	**62***	—
Total	85 (62,100)	85 (67, 100)	85 (67,100)	85 (67,100)	74 (48, 100)

* Only 1 observation.

Table 4: Unadjusted P-values from Welch's two sample t-tests comparing DEMMI scores amongst variables of interest.

Variable	P-value
Age 70–79 (versus 60–69)	0.02
Age 80–89 (versus 60–69)	0.00
Age 80–89 (versus 70–79)	0.01
Sex	0.49
Falls history	0.21
Independent versus semi-independent living	0.00
Country	0.00
Mobility aid use	0.00

study reveals higher mean scores than this, for community dwellers aged 60+ (Table 2). However, it would be expected that those recovering from acute illness and hospitalization would very likely demonstrate lower mobility at the time of discharge; mobility would be expected to improve with ongoing recovery and rehabilitation ("rehab potential" is an important factor in discharge planning). Therefore, the current study supports previous findings and demonstrates that means will likely differ between healthy community dwellers compared to community dwellers recovering from acute illness. The reference data obtained in this study could be used in the hospital setting to facilitate physiotherapy discharge planning and to support decision making for funding expenditure for inpatient and community-based rehabilitation services after acute hospital discharge.

We note limitations with this study. First, this was a relatively small sample ($N = 183$), just 25% of whom were men. Previous studies have developed normative data for health instruments from sample populations as small as 32 [21], though most commonly have over 100 participants [22, 23]. Nonetheless, a larger sample would provide greater representation across all age groups (especially those 80–89 and 90+, given the expected shift in population demographics in the coming years) and therefore better confidence in the reference value estimates reported in this study. Further, our sample was one of convenience, and therefore brings into question how well our sample represents the population of interest. Finally, the current study demonstrated 17.5% of community-dwelling older adults scored the maximum possible score of 100, which raises concerns of a ceiling effect. McHorney and Tarlov suggest that up to 15% of participants scoring at either scale extreme is acceptable [24]; and Barber-Westin et al. report up to one third of participants scoring the highest or lowest-possible scores is acceptable [25]. Recognizing this, the DEMMI was designed to measure across a broad spectrum of abilities (acutely hospitalized to healthy community dwellers) with a targeted use for clinical settings, where documenting improvements among those with excellent health is not a primary goal [26]. During the development of the DEMMI, one of the hardest items (standing on one leg with eyes closed) [11] was removed as there were no participants who could complete this item in an acutely hospitalized older population, and this item hence negatively impacted on some of the clinimetric properties of the DEMMI. The present study does not provide convincing evidence to suggest that the inclusion of this item is warranted.

A strength of this study is its important contribution of reference data to the DEMMI mobility instrument, critical in its broad application to older adults across the mobility spectrum from acutely ill, and hospitalized to healthy community dwellers. Additionally, gathering data from ten different community sites in two different countries provide broader generalizability to the reference intervals provided in this study.

5. Conclusions

This study is the first to report normative data for the DEMMI and provides important reference data on community dwelling older adults for clinicians and researchers. Normative data for this instrument will improve the interpretability of DEMMI scores, giving instrument users the ability to compare individual or group scores with known scores of an age- and sex-matched population. Its applicability is broad and can be used for population health applications; annual screening for early signs of mobility decline; therapeutic goal setting; evaluation of changes in mobility during recovery; discharge planning. As the focus of healthcare continues to shift from acute to community care and preventative health approaches, the DEMMI will assist in enhancing the continuity of patient care across clinical settings.

Acknowledgments

This study was funded by the Canadian Institutes of Health Research (CIHR) Mobility in Aging Team Grant, Vincent

Fairfax Churchill Fellowship, and National Health and Medical Research Council of Australia (NHMRC) Post-doctoral Research Fellowship (ID 519555). The authors are enormously grateful for the generous donation of time and support provided by Fabio Feldman, Debbie Chong, Vanessa Young, Vina Tan, Shane Belvedere, and Sarah Davenport. Thanks are also due to the ten sites and each individual for so eagerly supporting and actively participating in this study.

References

[1] World Health Organisation, *International Classification of Functioning, Disability and Health*, Geneva, Switzerland, 2001.

[2] W. D. Warren and R. Knight, "Mortality in relation to the functional capacities of people with disabilities living at home," *Journal of Epidemiology and Community Health*, vol. 36, no. 3, pp. 220–223, 1982.

[3] M. C. Corti, J. M. Guralnik, M. E. Salive, and J. D. Sorkin, "Serum albumin level and physical disability as predictors of mortality in older persons," *Journal of the American Medical Association*, vol. 272, no. 13, pp. 1036–1042, 1994.

[4] L. J. Donaldson, D. G. Clayton, and M. Clarke, "The elderly in residential care: mortality in relation to functional capacity," *Journal of Epidemiology and Community Health*, vol. 34, no. 2, pp. 96–101, 1980.

[5] J. M. Guralnik, L. P. Fried, and M. E. Salive, "Disability as a public health outcome in the aging population," *Annual Review of Public Health*, vol. 17, pp. 25–46, 1996.

[6] S. Studenski, S. Perera, D. Wallace et al., "Physical performance measures in the clinical setting," *Journal of the American Geriatrics Society*, vol. 51, no. 3, pp. 314–322, 2003.

[7] J. Dumurgier, A. Elbaz, P. Ducimetière, B. Tavernier, A. Alpérovitch, and C. Tzourio, "Slow walking speed and cardiovascular death in well functioning older adults: prospective cohort study," *British Medical Journal*, vol. 339, no. 7731, p. 1187, 2009.

[8] Kellog International Work Group, "The prevention of falls in later life: a report of the Kellogg International Work Group on the Prevention of Falls by the Elderly," *Danish Medical Bulletin*, vol. 34, supplement 4, pp. 1–24, 1987.

[9] S. J. Davenport, S. Paynter, and N. de Morton, "What instruments have been used to assess the mobility of community-dwelling older adults?" *Physical Therapy Reviews*, vol. 13, pp. 345–354, 2008.

[10] N. A. de Morton, D. J. Berlowitz, and J. L. Keating, "A systematic review of mobility instruments and their measurement properties for older acute medical patients," *Health and Quality of Life Outcomes*, vol. 6, article 44, 2008.

[11] N. A. de Morton, M. Davidson, and J. L. Keating, "The de Morton Mobility Index (DEMMI): an essential health index for an ageing world," *Health and Quality of Life Outcomes*, vol. 6, article 63, 2008.

[12] N. A. de Morton, N. K. Brusco, L. Wood, K. Lawler, and N. F. Taylor, "The de Morton Mobility Index (DEMMI) provides a valid method for measuring and monitoring the mobility of patients making the transition from hospital to the community: an observational study," *Journal of Physiotherapy*, vol. 57, no. 2, pp. 109–116, 2011.

[13] N. A. De Morton, M. Davidson, and J. L. Keating, "Validity, responsiveness and the minimal clinically important difference for the de Morton Mobility Index (DEMMI) in an older acute medical population," *BMC Geriatrics*, vol. 10, article 72, 2010.

[14] N. A. De Morton and K. Lane, "Validity and reliability of the de Morton Mobility Index in the subacute hospital setting in a Geriatric Evaluation and Management population," *Journal of Rehabilitation Medicine*, vol. 42, no. 10, pp. 956–961, 2010.

[15] M. P. Jans, V. C. Slootweg, C. R. Boot et al., "Reproducibility and validity of the Dutch translation of the de Morton Mobility Index (DEMMI) used by physiotherapists in older patients with knee or hip osteoarthritis," *Archives of Physical Medicine & Rehabilitation*, vol. 92, pp. 1892–1899, 2011.

[16] Community Care and Assisted Living Act, Part 1, Paragraph 1, Government of British Columbia, Canada, 2002.

[17] Retirement Villages Act, Number 126. Version 064, Section 3, Government of Victoria, Australia, 1986.

[18] S. J. Davenport and N. A. De Morton, "Clinimetric properties of the de morton mobility index in healthy, Community-dwelling older adults," *Archives of Physical Medicine and Rehabilitation*, vol. 92, no. 1, pp. 51–58, 2011.

[19] E. M. Wright and P. Royston, "Calculating reference intervals for laboratory measurements," *Statistical Methods in Medical Research*, vol. 8, no. 2, pp. 93–112, 1999.

[20] A. J. Campbell, J. Reinken, B. C. Allan, and G. S. Martinez, "Falls in old age: a study of frequency and related clinical factors," *Age and Ageing*, vol. 10, no. 4, pp. 264–270, 1981.

[21] H. Cohen, L. G. Heaton, S. L. Congdon, and H. A. Jenkins, "Changes in sensory organization test scores with age," *Age and Ageing*, vol. 25, no. 1, pp. 39–44, 1996.

[22] C. Blake, M. B. Codd, and Y. M. O'Meara, "The short form 36 (SF-36) health survey: normative data for the Irish population," *Irish Journal of Medical Science*, vol. 169, no. 3, pp. 195–200, 2000.

[23] R. W. Bohannon, "Comfortable and maximum walking speed of adults aged 20–79 years: reference values and determinants," *Age and Ageing*, vol. 26, no. 1, pp. 15–19, 1997.

[24] C. A. McHorney and A. R. Tarlov, "Individual-patient monitoring in clinical practice: are available health status surveys adequate?" *Quality of Life Research*, vol. 4, no. 4, pp. 293–307, 1995.

[25] S. D. Barber-Westin, F. R. Noyes, and J. W. McCloskey, "Rigorous statistical reliability, validity, and responsiveness testing of the Cincinnati knee rating system in 350 subjects with uninjured, injured, or anterior cruciate ligament-reconstructed knees," *The American Journal of Sports Medicine*, vol. 27, pp. 402–416, 1999.

[26] A. B. Bindman, D. Keane, and N. Lurie, "Measuring health changes among severely III patients: the floor phenomenon," *Medical Care*, vol. 28, pp. 1142–1152, 1990.

4

Is Self-Reported Physical Activity Participation Associated with Lower Health Services Utilization among Older Adults? Cross-Sectional Evidence from the Canadian Community Health Survey

Koren L. Fisher,[1,2] Elizabeth L. Harrison,[3] Bruce A. Reeder,[4] Nazmi Sari,[5] and Karen E. Chad[2]

[1]*Department of Kinesiology, California State University, Fullerton 800 N. State College Boulevard, Fullerton, CA 92831, USA*
[2]*Department of Kinesiology, University of Saskatchewan, 87 Campus Drive, Saskatoon, SK, Canada S7N 5B2*
[3]*School of Physical Therapy, University of Saskatchewan, 1121 College Drive, Saskatoon, SK, Canada S7N 0W3*
[4]*Department of Community Health and Epidemiology, University of Saskatchewan, Box 7, Health Science Building, 107 Wiggins Road, Saskatoon, SK, Canada S7N 5E5*
[5]*Department of Economics, University of Saskatchewan, Arts 815, 9 Campus Drive, Saskatoon, SK, Canada S7N 5A5*

Correspondence should be addressed to Koren L. Fisher; kofisher@fullerton.edu

Academic Editor: Enrica Menditto

Purpose. To examine relationships between leisure time physical activity (LTPA) and health services utilization (H) in a nationally representative sample of community-dwelling older adults. *Methods.* Cross-sectional data from 56,652 Canadian Community Health Survey respondents aged ≥ 50 years (48% M; 52% F; mean age 63.5 ± 10.2 years) were stratified into three age groups and analysed using multivariate generalized linear modeling techniques. Participants were classified according to PA level based on self-reported daily energy expenditure. Nonleisure PA (NLPA) was categorized into four levels ranging from mostly sitting to mostly lifting objects. *Results.* Active 50–65-year-old individuals were 27% less likely to report any GP consultations (OR_{adj} = 0.73; $P < 0.001$) and had 8% fewer GP consultations annually (IRR_{adj} = 0.92; $P < 0.01$) than their inactive peers. Active persons aged 65–79 years were 18% less likely than inactive respondents to have been hospitalized overnight in the previous year (OR_{adj} = 0.82, $P < 0.05$). Higher levels of NLPA were significantly associated with lower levels of HSU, across all age groups. *Conclusion.* Nonleisure PA appeared to be a stronger predictor of all types of HSU, particularly in the two oldest age groups. Considering strategies that focus on reducing time spent in sedentary activities may have a positive impact on reducing the demand for health services.

1. Introduction

The importance of physical activity (PA) in reducing chronic disease and maintaining good health and functional independence has been well documented [1–5]. The health benefits of exercise, including enhanced cardiovascular functioning, improved glucose tolerance, and obesity reduction, are well known [1–3, 6]. Improvements in conditions such as osteoporosis, sarcopenia, and certain forms of cancer [1, 2, 4, 5, 7], positive changes in mental health, particularly related to depression and stress management, and improvements in cognitive ability, quality of life, and well-being [4, 5] have also been linked to increased PA levels. Although the importance of being physically active is widely acknowledged among the Canadian population, levels of physical activity remain low, particularly among older adults, with fewer than 15% attaining the recommended 150 minutes per week of moderate-vigorous PA [8, 9].

Physical inactivity among older adults is of particular concern in many industrialized countries, including Canada, because of the important societal implications associated with population aging [10]. By 2036 it is expected that 1 in 4 Canadians will be 65 years of age or older, the majority of whom will have at least one chronic condition [11–13]. Given that the average life expectancy at 65 years of age is now 21.5 years for women and 18.3 years for men, a significant proportion of the population will require ongoing, long-term medical care to manage their conditions [14]. There is great concern that the increasing chronic care needs of older adults will place considerable strain on the health care system, in terms of both its capacity to meet an increasing demand for services and its ability to sustain the current level of service provision in the face of increasing costs [15, 16]. Among policymakers and health providers alike, there is growing interest in the potential role of PA as a strategy to mitigate these challenges [10, 17, 18].

Physical inactivity has been shown to be positively associated with health service utilization and costs; however, the literature in this area is quite limited, particularly as it pertains to older adults [19, 20]. Recently published estimates of the economic burden of physical inactivity indicate that between 3.6% and 3.8% of total health care costs, or $6.8 billion, can be attributed to physical inactivity in Canada [21–23]. Studies examining the relationship between PA and health services utilization among older adults have shown mixed results. Woolcott et al. [24] compared “general health visits” (including general practitioner and specialist physicians as well as other health care providers) between active and inactive respondents in a nationally representative sample of 24,281 older adults aged 65 years and older. In this study, physically active seniors reported significantly fewer “general health visits” than their inactive counterparts (8.15 versus 11.76 visits/yr). In contrast, Plotnikoff et al. [25] found that PA was not significantly associated with either general practitioner (GP) or specialist visits in a sample of 2300 individuals with type 1 diabetes (T1D) or type 2 diabetes (T2D).

The results of studies of PA and hospital services utilization are also somewhat inconsistent. Sari [26] recently examined the association between PA and the demand for hospital services in adults who are 65 years of age and older and found leisure time PA (LTPA) to be inversely associated with hospital stays, concluding that even small increases in LTPA could translate into a decrease in hospital stays of 16% to 19% in inactive older adults. In a similar study, Woolcott et al. [24] reported that physically inactive older adults were 84% more likely to be hospitalized in the previous 12 months and spent, on average, more than three times the number of days in hospital compared to their active counterparts. In contrast to these studies, Plotnikoff et al. [25] failed to find a significant association between LTPA and the number of hospital visits in their sample of adults with T1D and T2D, after adjusting for other factors associated with health services utilization.

Although these studies are encouraging, there remain considerable gaps in our understanding of the relationship between physical activity and health services utilization, particularly among older adults [20, 27]. Along with the general lack of Canadian data, wide variations in study methodologies limit the extent to which we can draw conclusions from the literature [20]. The purpose of this study was to examine the relationship between PA and health services utilization, while controlling for a comprehensive set of observed covariates, in a nationally representative sample of community-dwelling adults aged 50 years and older in order to gain better insight into the relationship between physical activity and health services utilization.

2. Methods

This study involved a secondary analysis of data from Cycle 3.1 of the Canadian Community Health Survey (CCHS). The CCHS is a nationally representative cross-sectional health survey designed to provide information related to health determinants, health status, and health services utilization for the Canadian population aged 12 or older [28, 29]. Access to the confidential microdata files for Cycle 3.1 of the Canadian Community Health Survey (CCHS) was carried out through the Saskatchewan Research Data Centre at the University of Saskatchewan following an evaluation of the proposed research by the RDC-Access Granting Committee.

Data collection for CCHS Cycle 3.1 took place from January to December 2005 by means of computer-assisted personal and telephone interviews. In total 168,464 households were selected to participate. A response was obtained for 143,076 of the selected households, resulting in a household-level response rate of 84.9%. Of the 143,076 individuals selected (one person per household) to participate, valid interviews were conducted with 132,947 individuals yielding an individual-level response rate of 92.9%. When sample weights are applied, CCHS data represents approximately 98% of the Canadian population living in private and occupied dwellings in all provinces and territories [29, 30]. The present analysis was restricted to those respondents aged 50 years and older with nonmissing PA and health services utilization data, resulting in an unweighted sample of 56,652 adults.

2.1. Dependent Variables. Health services utilization was characterized as the use of general physician (GP) services, specialist physician (SP) services, and hospital services in the 12-month period prior to the survey. Both service contacts (services used versus services not used) and volume of service use were of interest because of the probable differences in the determinants of each type of utilization [31].

2.1.1. Physician Services. Respondents were asked to report the number of consultations, including telephone consultations, with GP and specialist physicians in the 12-month period preceding the survey [32]. In addition to two continuous variables indicating volume of service use (one for each type of physician), two dichotomous variables (use versus nonuse) were constructed to indicate the incidence of contact with both types of physicians.

2.1.2. Hospital Services. Two variables were used to describe the use of hospital services based on questions asking if the respondent had stayed overnight as a patient in a hospital and the total number of nights spent in hospital in the preceding 12 months: a dichotomous variable indicating if the respondent had been hospitalized in the previous year and, for those respondents reporting a hospitalization, a continuous variable indicating the total number of nights spent in hospital.

2.2. Independent Variables. The main independent variable of interest was self-reported LTPA over the 3 months prior to the survey interview. Respondents were asked about their participation in 21 specified physical activities, participation frequency, and average activity duration, using an adaptation of the Minnesota Leisure Time Physical Activity Questionnaire (MLTPAQ) [32]. An index variable was used to categorize respondents as active (>3.0 kilocalories per kilogram per day; KKD), moderately active (1.5 to 3.0 KKD), and inactive (<1.5 KKD), according to the average daily energy expenditure as determined by the reported frequency, duration, and metabolic cost associated with all the leisure time physical activity [32].

2.3. Control Variables. The control variables included in the analysis were chosen *a priori* based upon the Andersen-Newman model of health services utilization [33, 34]. Within this framework, individual determinants of health services utilization are categorized as "predisposing," "enabling," and "need" factors, all of which are thought to influence the decision to seek medical care. Table 1 summarizes the predisposing, enabling, and need factors associated with health services utilization that were available in the CCHS Cycle 3.1 [29] and included as control variables in all statistical models. Selected environmental factors, including those related to the health system, the external environment, and the community, were also included, given their influence on health services utilization [35].

Table 1: Predisposing, enabling, health need, personal health practices, environmental, and community control variables included in the multivariate analyses.

Control variables	Factors
Predisposing factors	Age; gender; marital status; education; ethnicity; immigration
Enabling factors	Annual household income; employment status; speaks English and/or French; has regular doctor; household size; dwelling size
Need factors	Self-rated general health; self-rated mental health; injury in the previous 12 months; limitations in ADLs; number of chronic conditions; chronic conditions[†]; BMI classification
Personal lifestyle factors	Smoking status; exposure to second hand smoke; alcohol consumption; walking/cycling for transportation; typical daily physical activity outside of leisure time
Environmental factors	Province; urban-rural residence

[†]Specified chronic conditions include hypertension, cardio-/cerebrovascular disease (heart disease, stroke); COPD (emphysema, chronic bronchitis); asthma; diabetes; cancer (currently have/ever had); neurological conditions (chronic fatigue, syndrome, migraines, Alzheimer's, other dementia, epilepsy); rheumatological conditions (fibromyalgia, arthritis/rheumatism); back problems; gastrointestinal conditions (intestinal/stomach ulcers; Crohn's disease/ulcerative colitis/irritable bowel syndrome/bowel incontinence); mood/anxiety disorders; other mental health conditions (schizophrenia, autism/other developmental disorder, eating disorder); conditions not otherwise listed.

2.4. Statistical Analyses. All analyses were carried out at the Saskatchewan Research Data Centre using SPSS 19.0 (SPSS Inc., Chicago, IL) and STATA 10 (Statacorp LP, College Station, TX). To account for unequal probability of selection in the CCHS Cycle 3.1 due to the complex sampling design, sample weights were applied in all analyses in order to obtain population-based estimates [29]. Unless otherwise indicated, a significance level of $P < 0.05$ was applied.

In order to describe the characteristics of the study population, frequencies or means ± SD were determined as appropriate for all independent variables of interest. The sample was stratified on the basis of age and PA level into three age groups (50–64 years, 65–79 years, and 80 years and older) and three activity levels (active, moderately active, and inactive). The decision to stratify by age was made *a priori*, in recognition of the considerable heterogeneity within the demographic subgroups of the older adult population relative to PA, health, and health services utilization [15, 16, 26, 36].

Dependent variables were assessed separately for each age group. The distributions of all dependent variables were compared between PA groups using chi square and ANOVA for categorical and continuous variables, respectively. When the assumptions for these tests were not met, Fisher's exact test, Mann-Whitney *U* test, or the Kruskal Wallis test were used, as appropriate.

General linear modeling procedures were employed in order to assess the association between LTPA and each dependent variable. Multiple logistic regression models were used to obtain odds ratios (OR) describing the association between LTPA and the dichotomous variables indicating use or nonuse of physician services. Negative binomial (NB) regression modeling was used to obtain incident rate ratios (IRR) in order to assess the relationship between LTPA and the annual number of GP and specialist physician consultations [26, 37]. The association between LTPA and overnight hospitalizations and the total number of nights spent in hospital was assessed using ORs and IRRs obtained through multiple logistic regression and NB regression techniques, respectively. In all analyses, the reference group was the inactive category.

Bootstrap resampling procedures were used to produce corrected standard errors to calculate confidence intervals and to test for statistical significance. This technique is recommended for estimating sample variances in surveys with a large number of strata and multiple primary sampling units per stratum where exact design effects are not known

[38]. A bootstrap macro specific to the CCHS Cycle 3.1 was provided by Statistics Canada.

3. Results

Key sociodemographic, health, and lifestyle characteristics of respondents are presented by age group and PA level in Table 2. In the 50 to 64 and 65 to 79 years age groups, the majority of the population was married and had completed high school. Most respondents in the oldest age group were not married and although the majority had completed high school, this age group was more evenly split across education levels. Across all age groups, less than 5% of the population self-identified as Aboriginal. The vast majority were born in Canada and lived in urban areas (>66% and ≥79%, resp.).

With regard to income, more than half of older adults under the age of 65 reported annual household incomes greater than $30,000; however fewer than 30% of respondents over the age of 65 reported annual incomes exceeding $30,000 per year. Approximately two-thirds of the population aged 50 to 64 years and 10% of those aged 65 to 79 years were employed. The majority of respondents under the age of 80 years reported living in a household with two or more people while close to half of those 80 years and older lived alone.

The vast majority (>90%) of respondents reported having a regular family doctor and this increased with increasing age. With the exception of inactive respondents in the two oldest age groups, more than 80% of respondents reported their general health to be excellent, very good, or good; more than 90% of respondents, regardless of age group, reported their mental health to be at the same level. At the same time, close to 80% of respondents under the age of 65 and 90% of those over the age 65 reported having at least one chronic condition. In each age group, the proportion of active older adults reporting no chronic conditions was higher than in the inactive and moderately active groups. The most prevalent chronic conditions were arthritis/rheumatologic conditions (24.5%–56%), hypertension (21%–49%), back problems (17%–26%), and cardio-/cerebrovascular conditions (6%–31%). The prevalence of most conditions was higher in older age groups and lower with increasing PA. One notable exception was in the case of mood/anxiety disorders, where the prevalence was lower in the older age groups compared to the youngest age group.

With regard to personal health practices, the vast majority of respondents (>75%) were nonsmokers or former smokers and most (>65%) reported that they did not consume alcohol. Except for inactive respondents in the oldest age group, at least 50% of respondents reported spending, on average, more than 1 hour daily walking to work and/or to complete errands while fewer than 5% reported cycling daily to do the same. The majority of respondents (40%–59%) reported standing or walking as their usual or typical daily activity. In each age group, the proportion of respondents reporting their usual activity as sitting was lower as the activity level increased.

Descriptive data for all health service utilization variables, stratified by age group and LTPA level, are presented in Table 3. In all age groups, the number of GP and specialist consultations differed significantly ($P < 0.001$) between each LTPA level. With the exception of specialist consultations in the oldest age groups, the moderately active group reported fewer GP and specialist consultations than the inactive group and the active group reported fewer GP and specialist consultations than either the moderately active or the inactive group. The majority of respondents reported having between 1 and 4 GP consultations and no specialist consultations in the previous year. In the youngest age group, between 16.5% and 22% of respondents had no visits to their GP in the previous year while, in the oldest age group, fewer than 13% had no visits. Across all age groups, between 29% and 36% of respondents reported at least one contact with a specialist physician in the previous 12 months.

Across all age groups, fewer than 20% of individuals had been hospitalized in the previous 12-month period. The proportion of respondents who had been hospitalized was highest in the inactive group and lowest in the active group regardless of age group. The number of nights spent in hospital differed significantly ($P < 0.001$) according to LTPA level, with the number of nights in hospital decreasing with increasing LTPA, across all age groups.

3.1. Regression Analyses. The results of regression analyses are presented separately for each age group.

3.1.1. 50 to 64 Years Age Group. The results of the regression analyses pertaining to the 50 to 64 years age group are presented in Table 4. After adjusting for other factors related to health services utilization, active individuals in this youngest age group were 27% less likely than their inactive counterparts to have had contact with a GP in the 12-month study period ($OR_{adj} = 0.73$; $P < 0.001$). Being physically active was also associated with 8% fewer GP consultations over the 12-month study period (IRR = 0.92; $P < 0.01$). In contrast, moderately active and active 50- to 64-year-olds were as likely as their inactive counterparts to have at least one contact with a specialist physician ($OR_{adj} = 0.85$–0.94; $P > 0.05$) and were no more or less likely to be a high user of specialist services. Lastly, after adjusting for other determinants of hospital services ($OR_{adj} = 0.77$–0.93; $P > 0.05$) utilization, moderately active and active 50- to 64-year-olds were 8% and 3% less likely, respectively, to have had an overnight hospitalization in the previous 12 months; however, this was not statistically significant. Furthermore, LTPA was not significantly associated with the number of nights spent in hospital across activity level in this age group.

3.1.2. 65 to 79 Years Age Group. The results of the regression analyses pertaining to the 65 to 79 years age group are presented in Table 5. In this age group, no significant associations were found between LTPA and the use of either GP or specialist physician services. While the adjusted analyses showed that moderately active or active individuals did have 4% fewer GP consultations than their inactive counterparts (IRR = 0.96), these groups were 3% ($P < 0.05$) and 13%

Table 2: Population characteristics, stratified by age group and activity level ($N = 56{,}652$).

Predisposing factors	50–64 yrs. ($n = 29{,}914$)			65–79 yrs. ($n = 20{,}183$)			80 yrs. and older ($n = 6{,}555$)		
	Inactive ($n = 15{,}393$)	Mod. active ($n = 7{,}882$)	Active ($n = 6{,}639$)	Inactive ($n = 11{,}109$)	Mod. active ($n = 5{,}027$)	Active ($n = 4{,}047$)	Inactive ($n = 4{,}772$)	Mod. active ($n = 1{,}101$)	Active ($n = 682$)
Age (mean ± SD)	56.2 ± 4.2	56.4 ± 4.3	56.5 ± 4.2	71.5 ± 4.3	70. 9 ± 4.2	70.6 ± 3.9	84.2 ± 3.6	83.2 ± 3.2	83.0 ± 2.9
Gender (%)									
Male	49.3	47.9	52.6	41.0	47.4	57.8	31.0	41.4	52.9
Female	50.7	52.1	47.4	59.0	52.6	42.2	69.0	58.6	47.1
Marital status (%)									
Married	76.0	78.9	79.5	64.8	69.6	72.5	37.0	41.1	53.5
Not married/missing	24.0	21.1	20.5	35.2	30.4	27.5	63.0	58.9	46.5
Education (%)									
Completed secondary	76.4	84.4	85.6	52.3	63.4	67.1	44.6	55.1	59.1
<Secondary	20.7	13.2	12.2	43.3	33.9	29.7	49.0	40.4	36.5
Missing	2.9	2.3	2.2	4.4	2.7	3.2	6.4	4.5	4.4
Household income (%)									
<\$15,000	5.8	3.8	4.1	9.1	7.2	5.7	14.4	9.4	9.9
\$15,000–\$29,999	29.4	24.0	23.4	49.4	47.5	47.5	45.4	44.4	44.2
≥\$30,000	50.0	59.4	59.7	19.8	27.5	27.1	12.0	20.4	23.0
Missing	14.7	12.7	12.8	21.7	17.8	19.7	28.3	25.8	22.9
Employment status (%)									
Not employed	30.4	32.7	37.3	85.6	89.2	87.7	100	100	100
Employed	67.2	65.0	60.7	11.7	9.1	10.1			
Missing	2.4	2.3	2.0	2.6	1.7	2.2			
Has regular family doctor (%)									
Yes	90.3	91.8	90.9	94.6	96.1	93.9	96.2	96.6	95.4
No/missing	9.7	8.2	9.1	5.4	3.9	6.1	3.8	3.4	4.6
Self-rated general health (%)									
Excellent/very good/good	80.8	88.8	91.9	69.8	83.6	88.0	63.5	81.2	82.5
Fair/poor/missing	19.2	11.2	8.1	30.2	16.4	12.0	36.5	18.8	17.5
Self-rated mental health (%)									
Excellent/very good/good	93.1	95.2	96.7	93.7	96.6	97.0	91.0	95.9	95.3
Fair/poor/missing	6.9	4.8	3.3	6.3	3.4	3.0	9.0	4.1	4.7
Number of chronic conditions (%)									
None/missing	20.3	20.0	23.3	10.1	10.7	14.1	7.7	10.9	13.1
1 condition	25.1	28.9	30.3	17.4	21.3	23.9	13.7	19.3	20.1
2 conditions	21.7	22.0	22.3	21.8	24.9	24.8	20.1	23.8	26.7
3 conditions	23.8	21.9	17.7	37.1	30.7	26.6	41.4	34.3	26.5
≥4 conditions	9.0	7.2	6.3	13.6	12.5	10.6	17.1	11.7	13.7
Typical daily PA (%)									
Usually sitting	27.5	21.6	17.0	30.4	12.3	7.4	48.1	21.5	11.0
Standing or walking	43.2	46.1	48.0	48.2	58.1	53.8	40.9	56.9	58.9
Lifting light/heavy loads	28.5	31.7	34.6	20.1	28.7	38.0	9.0	20.5	29.3
Missing	0.8	0.6	0.4	1.3	0.9	0.9	2.1	1.1	0.8

Table 3: Health services utilization, stratified by age group and PA level.

	50–64 yrs. (n = 29,914)			65–79 yrs. (n = 20,183)			80 yrs. and older (n = 6,555)		
	Inactive (n = 15,393)	Mod. active (n = 7,882)	Active (n = 6,639)	Inactive (n = 11,109)	Mod. active (n = 5,027)	Active (n = 4,047)	Inactive (n = 4,772)	Mod. active (n = 1,101)	Active (n = 682)
GP consultations*									
Mean (SD)	3.5 (5.3)	3.1 (4.7)	2.7 (4.2)	4.2 (5.2)	3.6 (3.9)	3.3 (4.4)	5.4 (7.6)	4.4 (4.7)	3.9 (3.8)
None (%)	17.9	16.3	21.8	12.7	11.4	14.8	9.7	12.6	11.3
1 consultation (%)	20.2	23.4	23.8	14.4	16.9	20.8	11.0	14.4	16.4
2 to 4 consultations (%)	41.0	42.4	40.0	43.9	49.1	45.7	41.5	40.8	45.8
5 to 8 consultations (%)	11.8	11.3	9.2	16.1	13.5	11.7	19.0	17.3	16.0
9 or more consultations (%)	9.1	6.6	5.1	12.9	9.0	7.0	18.9	14.9	10.5
†Specialist consultations*									
Mean (SD)	1.1 (3.8)	1.0 (4.3)	0.8 (2.5)	1.0 (3.2)	0.8 (2.1)	0.8 (1.9)	0.9 (2.7)	0.8 (2.4)	0.8 (2.2)
None (%)	67.7	69.1	71.0	64.5	65.4	66.1	68.4	65.9	69.6
1 consultation (%)	13.9	13.8	14.5	14.9	16.4	15.8	12.3	15.8	16.8
2 consultations (%)	6.9	7.4	5.8	8.6	9.2	9.0	7.8	9.6	3.5
3 or more consultations (%)	11.5	9.7	8.7	12.0	9.0	9.1	11.4	8.6	10.1
Hospital admission in past year* (%)									
Yes	7.8	6.1	5.7	14.1	9.9	8.5	19.7	14.4	10.5
No	92.2	93.9	94.3	85.9	90.1	91.5	80.3	85.6	89.5
††Total number of hospital nights*									
Mean (SD)	9.2 (21.2)	9.3 (23.4)	7.2 (16.8)	11.0 (21.2)	9.4 (20.1)	8.0 (17.6)	13.4 (25.8)	10.3 (16.1)	9.7 (12.6)

†Specialist consultations include all specialist physicians except eye specialists.
††Mean number of hospital nights for individuals reporting a hospital admission in previous 12 months.
*Within each age group, PA groups were significantly different ($P < 0.001$) on all health service utilization variables.

Table 4: The association between LTPA and health services utilization in the 50 to 64 years age group (N = 29,914).

	50 to 64 years age group					
	OR/IRR[a]	Unadjusted (95% C.I.)	Sig	OR/IRR	Adjusted (95% C.I.)	Sig
GP services						
At least 1 GP contact						
Moderately active	1.12	(0.99–1.26)	0.061	1.01	(0.88–1.17)	0.854
Active	0.78	(0.70–0.88)	<0.001	0.73	(0.63–0.84)	<0.001
Number of GP consultations[a]						
Moderately active	0.88	(0.83–0.94)	<0.001	0.97	(0.92–1.03)	0.308
Active	0.78	(0.74–0.84)	<0.001	0.92	(0.87–0.97)	0.002
Specialist physician services*						
At least 1 specialist contact						
Moderately active	0.94	(0.86–1.02)	0.138	0.99	(0.89–1.09)	0.792
Active	0.85	(0.77–0.95)	0.002	0.99	(0.87–1.12)	0.882
Number of specialist consultations[a]						
Moderately active	0.93	(0.80–1.08)	0.339	1.01	(0.90–1.13)	0.858
Active	0.77	(0.65–0.90)	0.002	1.04	(0.90–1.21)	0.557
Hospital services†						
Overnight hospitalization						
Moderately active	0.77	(0.65–0.90)	0.001	0.92	(0.76–1.12)	0.416
Active	0.71	(0.58–0.86)	0.001	0.97	(0.77–1.23)	0.822
Number of nights in hospital[a]						
Moderately active	1.01	(0.69–1.49)	0.940	1.15	(0.94–1.43)	0.181
Active	0.78	(0.49–1.25)	0.303	1.03	(0.80–1.33)	0.816

[a]The estimate is an incidence rate ratio (IRR).

Note: analyses adjusted for the following (reference category in italics): age; sex (*male*/female); marital status (married: *yes*/no); education (graduated secondary: *yes*/no); ethnicity (*non-Aboriginal*/Aboriginal); employment status (employed: *no*/yes); household size (*1*, 2, 3, or more people); dwelling size (*<3 bedrooms*, 3 bedrooms, >3 bedrooms); immigration status (*nonimmigrant*, immigrant); injury in previous 12 months (*no*/yes); limitation in ADLs (*no*/yes); smoking status (*never smoked*/former smoker/nonsmoker); exposed to 2nd hand smoke (*no*/yes); alcohol consumption (*<1 drink daily*/at least 1 drink daily); BMI (*<25.0* $kg{\cdot}m^2$/25.0–29.9 $kg{\cdot}m^2$/≥30 $kg{\cdot}m^2$ or greater); time spent walking to work or to run errands (*none*/<1 hour/≥1 hour); cycling to work or to run errands (*no*/yes); typical daily activity level (*usually sitting*/standing or walking/lifting light and/or heavy loads); annual household income (*<$15,000*; $15,000–$29,999; ≥$30,000; missing); province (*ON*, MB, AB, BC, SK, QC, NB, NS, PE, NL, YT/NT/NU); urban-rural classification (*urban*/rural); language (able to speak English and/or French: *yes*/no); has regular family doctor (*yes*/no); self-rated general health (*excellent/very good/good*; fair/poor); self-rated mental health (*excellent/very good/good*; fair/poor); diagnosed with hypertension, cardiovascular disease (including stroke), COPD, asthma, diabetes, cancer, neurological conditions, rheumatological conditions, back problems, gastrointestinal disorders, mood/anxiety disorders, or other chronic conditions (*no*/yes for each); number of chronic conditions (*none*/1 condition/2 conditions/3 conditions/4 or more conditions).

*Analyses of specialist services also adjusted for number of GP consultations.

†Analyses of hospital services also adjusted for specialist physician consultations (yes/*no*).

(P < 0.05) more likely, respectively, to have had at least one contact with a specialist physician.

Lastly, after adjusting for other determinants of hospital services utilization, active 65- to 79-year-olds were 18% less likely to have had an overnight hospitalization in the previous 12 months (OR = 0.82, P < 0.05). Although PA was associated with between 3% and 7% fewer nights in hospital in this age group, this was not statistically significant.

3.1.3. 80 Years and Older Age Group. The results of the regression analyses pertaining to the oldest age group are presented in Table 6. In this age group, no significant associations were found between LTPA and the use of either GP or specialist physician services. Moderately active or active individuals had 7–10% fewer GP consultations over the 12-month study period (P > 0.05). While LTPA was not significantly associated with the use of specialist physician services, moderately active and active individuals aged 80 years and older were 10% and 26% more likely, respectively, than their inactive counterparts to have had at least one contact with a specialist physician (P = 0.068 and P = 0.570, resp.) and active individuals also reported 6% more specialist visits (P > 0.05) over the 12-month study period.

The use of hospital services was not significantly associated with LTPA in the 80 years and older age group; however, moderately active and active individuals were 11% and 32% less likely, respectively, to report being hospitalized during

TABLE 5: The association between LTPA and health services utilization in the 65 to 79 years age group (N = 20,183).

	65 to 79 years age group					
	OR/IRR[a]	Unadjusted (95% C.I.)	Sig	OR/IRR	Adjusted (95% C.I.)	Sig
GP services						
At least 1 GP contact						
Moderately active	1.13	(0.97–1.32)	0.122	1.13	(0.95–1.34)	0.173
Active	0.84	(0.72–0.97)	0.016	0.99	(0.82–1.21)	0.959
Number of GP consultations[a]						
Moderately active	0.86	(0.81–0.90)	<0.001	0.96	(0.92–1.01)	0.123
Active	0.77	(0.72–0.82)	<0.001	0.96	(0.90–1.01)	0.122
Specialist physician services*						
At least 1 specialist contact						
Moderately active	0.96	(0.87–1.06)	0.427	1.03	(0.90–1.18)	0.658
Active	0.93	(0.83–1.04)	0.217	1.13	(0.98–1.31)	0.098
Number of specialist consultations[a]						
Moderately active	0.81	(0.73–0.91)	<0.001	1.02	(0.90–1.15)	0.780
Active	0.80	(0.71–0.90)	<0.001	1.02	(0.91–1.15)	0.709
Hospital services†						
Overnight hospitalization						
Moderately active	0.67	(0.57–0.78)	<0.001	0.90	(0.76–1.07)	0.229
Active	0.57	(0.49–0.66)	<0.001	0.82	(0.68–0.98)	0.032
Number of nights in hospital[a]						
Moderately active	0.85	(0.62–1.17)	0.328	0.97	(0.77–1.22)	0.795
Active	0.72	(0.52–1.01)	0.058	0.93	(0.71–1.22)	0.589

[a]The estimate is an incidence rate ratio (IRR).
Note: analyses adjusted for (reference category in italics) the following: age; sex (*male*/female); marital status (married: *yes*/no); education (graduated secondary: *yes*/no); ethnicity (*non-Aboriginal*/Aboriginal); employment status (employed: *no*/yes); household size (*1*, 2, 3, or more people); dwelling size (*<3 bedrooms*, 3 bedrooms, >3 bedrooms); immigration status (*nonimmigrant*, immigrant); injury in previous 12 months (*no*/yes); limitation in ADLs (*no*/yes); smoking status (*never smoked*/former smoker/nonsmoker); exposed to 2nd hand smoke (*no*/yes); alcohol consumption (*<1 drink daily*/at least 1 drink daily); BMI (*<25.0* $\text{kg}\cdot\text{m}^2$/25.0–29.9 $\text{kg}\cdot\text{m}^2$/≥30 $\text{kg}\cdot\text{m}^2$ or greater); time spent walking to work or to run errands (*none*/<1 hour/≥1 hour); cycling to work or to run errands (*no*/yes); typical daily activity level (*usually sitting*/standing or walking/lifting light and/or heavy loads); annual household income (*<$15,000*; $15,000–$29,999; ≥$30,000; missing); province (*ON*, MB, AB, BC, SK, QC, NB, NS, PE, NL, YT/NT/NU); urban-rural classification (*urban*/rural); language (able to speak English and/or French: *yes*/no); has regular family doctor (*yes*/no); self-rated general health (*excellent/very good/good*; fair/poor); self-rated mental health (*excellent/very good/good*; fair/poor); diagnosed with hypertension, cardiovascular disease (including stroke), COPD, asthma, diabetes, cancer, neurological conditions, rheumatological conditions, back problems, gastrointestinal disorders, mood/anxiety disorders, or other chronic conditions (*no*/yes for each); number of chronic conditions (*none*/1 condition/2 conditions/3 conditions/4 or more conditions).
*Analyses of specialist services also adjusted for number of GP consultations.
†Analyses of hospital services also adjusted for specialist physician consultations (yes/*no*).

the 12-month study period (P = 0.483 and P = 0.087, resp.). Among those reporting a hospitalization, active individuals spent approximately 20% more nights in hospital, although this was also not statistically significant (P = 0.401).

While not the primary variable of interest in this study, significant associations were found between typical daily activity and several of the dependent variables such that a brief presentation of these findings is warranted (see Table 7). Respondents were asked to choose the best description of their usual daily activities or work habits outside of their LTPA (sitting; mostly standing or walking; mostly lifting light or heavy loads) and, across all age groups, higher levels of usual activity were associated with lower health services utilization. In the 50- to 64-year-old age group, those reporting lifting light or heavy loads had significantly fewer GP consultations (IRR = 0.91; $P < 0.05$) and were 15% less likely to use specialist physician services ($P < 0.05$) compared to those reporting sitting as their typical daily activity. Among 65- to 79-year-olds, respondents reporting the highest level of usual activity were 23% significantly less likely to have contact with a GP physician ($P < 0.05$), had 13% fewer GP ($P < 0.001$) and 14% fewer specialist physician consultations (P = 0.065), were 32% less likely to be hospitalized overnight ($P < 0.001$), and spent 42% fewer nights in hospital than their sitting counterparts ($P < 0.05$). In the oldest age group, standing/walking and lifting light or heavy loads were associated with lower levels of GP and specialist physician service utilization compared to those whose typical activity

TABLE 6: The association between LTPA and health services utilization in the 80 years and older age group ($N = 6,555$).

	80 years and older age group					
	Unadjusted			Adjusted*		
	OR/IRR[a]	(95% C.I.)	Sig	OR/IRR	(95% C.I.)	Sig
GP services						
At least 1 GP contact						
Moderately active	0.74	(0.55–1.01)	0.058	0.77	(0.52–1.15)	0.199
Active	0.84	(0.60–1.19)	0.324	1.26	(0.78–2.03)	0.340
Number of GP consultations[a]						
Moderately active	0.82	(0.74–0.92)	<0.001	0.93	(0.83–1.04)	0.225
Active	0.72	(0.65–0.81)	<0.001	0.90	(0.79–1.02)	0.113
Specialist physician services*						
At least 1 specialist contact						
Moderately active	1.12	(0.92–1.37)	0.263	1.26	(0.98–1.61)	0.068
Active	0.95	(0.74–1.21)	0.660	1.10	(0.80–1.50)	0.570
Number of specialist consultations[a]						
Moderately active	0.91	(0.69–1.20)	0.516	0.98	(0.80–1.21)	0.865
Active	0.91	(0.68–1.21)	0.506	1.06	(0.81–1.40)	0.661
Hospital services†						
Overnight hospitalization						
Moderately active	0.69	(0.53–0.89)	0.004	0.89	(0.65–1.22)	0.483
Active	0.48	(0.34–0.67)	<0.001	0.68	(0.43–1.06)	0.087
Number of nights in hospital[a]						
Moderately active	0.77	(0.55–1.08)	0.132	0.99	(0.69–1.43)	0.966
Active	0.72	(0.48–1.09)	0.119	1.19	(0.79–1.79)	0.401

[a]The estimate is an incidence rate ratio (IRR).

Note: analyses adjusted for the following (reference category in italics): age; sex (*male*/female); marital status (married: *yes*/no); education (graduated secondary: *yes*/no); ethnicity (*non-Aboriginal*/Aboriginal); employment status (employed: *no*/yes); household size (*1*, 2, 3, or more people); dwelling size (*<3 bedrooms*, 3 bedrooms, >3 bedrooms); immigration status (*nonimmigrant*, immigrant); injury in previous 12 months (*no*/yes); limitation in ADLs (*no*/yes); smoking status (*never smoked*/former smoker/nonsmoker); exposed to 2nd hand smoke (*no*/yes); alcohol consumption (*<1 drink daily*/at least 1 drink daily); BMI (*<25.0* $\text{kg}\cdot\text{m}^2$/25.0–29.9 $\text{kg}\cdot\text{m}^2$/≥30 $\text{kg}\cdot\text{m}^2$ or greater); time spent walking to work or to run errands (*none*/<1 hour/≥1 hour); cycling to work or to run errands (*no*/yes); typical daily activity level (*usually sitting*/standing or walking/lifting light and/or heavy loads); annual household income (*<$15,000*; $15,000–$29,999; ≥$30,000; missing); province (*ON*, MB, AB, BC, SK, QC, NB, NS, PE, NL, YT/NT/NU); urban-rural classification (*urban*/rural); language (able to speak English and/or French: *yes*/no); has regular family doctor (*yes*/no); self-rated general health (*excellent/very good/good*; fair/poor); self-rated mental health (*excellent/very good/good*; fair/poor); diagnosed with hypertension, cardiovascular disease (including stroke), COPD, asthma, diabetes, cancer, neurological conditions, rheumatological conditions, back problems, gastrointestinal disorders, mood/anxiety disorders, or other chronic conditions (*no*/yes for each); number of chronic conditions (*none*/1 condition/2 conditions/3 conditions/4 or more conditions).

*Analyses of specialist services also adjusted for number of GP consultations.

†Analyses of hospital services also adjusted for specialist physician consultations (yes/*no*).

was sitting (IRR = 0.66–0.89; $P < 0.05$). Lifting light or heavy loads was also associated with 48% fewer nights in hospital in this age group ($P < 0.001$).

4. Conclusion

The primary purpose of this study was to examine relationships between leisure time PA and health services utilization in a nationally (Canadian) representative sample of community-dwelling older adults. Rather than classifying all respondents as one homogeneous group, these relationships were explored separately for 3 age groups: 50 to 64 years, 65 to 79 years, and 80 years and older in order to add precision to the existing knowledge base [15]. The descriptive analysis showed that the use of health services generally increased with increasing age, with the exception of consultations with specialist physicians. Between 10% and 22% of respondents reported that they did not consult with a GP physician in the 12-month period, somewhat of a concerning finding from a health perspective given that it may mean that older adults are going without preventative health care or are having difficulty accessing necessary care. An alternative explanation may be that these individuals received health services from providers other than general practitioners, such as nurse practitioners, naturopathic physicians, chiropractors, and physiotherapists; however, this was not assessed in the present study.

The multivariate analyses showed that, in general, higher LTPA was associated with lower health services utilization; however, few of the associations were statistically significant.

TABLE 7: The association between differing levels of typical daily activity[a] and health services utilization, stratified by age.

	50 to 64 years n = 29,914			65 to 79 years n = 20,183			80 years and older n = 6,555		
	OR/IRR[b]	95% CI	P	OR/IRR[b]	95% CI	P	OR/IRR[b]	95% CI	P
General physician services									
At least 1 contact with a GP									
Standing or walking	1.13	(0.96–1.32)	0.143	1.19	(0.96–1.47)	0.107	0.73	(0.50–1.07)	0.104
Lifting light/heavy loads	0.90	(0.76–1.06)	0.221	0.77	(0.61–0.98)	0.030	0.77	(0.46–1.28)	0.312
Number of GP consultations[b]									
Standing or walking	0.97	(0.92–1.02)	0.298	0.97	(0.92–1.02)	0.239	0.89	(0.81–0.99)	0.027
Lifting light/heavy loads	0.91	(0.86–0.97)	0.002	0.87	(0.82–0.93)	<0.001	0.84	(0.73–0.95)	0.006
Specialist physician services									
At least 1 contact with a specialist									
Standing or walking	0.95	(0.85–1.06)	0.366	0.88	(0.77–1.00)	0.048	0.85	(0.68–1.07)	0.169
Lifting light/heavy loads	0.85	(0.75–0.97)	0.020	0.86	(0.74–1.01)	0.065	0.72	(0.52–0.99)	0.041
Number of specialist consultations[b]									
Standing or walking	0.80	(0.70–0.93)	0.002	0.86	(0.75–0.98)	0.023	0.76	(0.63–0.92)	0.005
Lifting light/heavy loads	0.74	(0.64–0.86)	<0.001	0.82	(0.71–0.95)	0.006	0.66	(0.50–0.88)	0.005
Hospital services									
Overnight hospitalization									
Standing or walking	0.93	(0.77–1.12)	0.431	0.85	(0.72–1.01)	0.060	0.80	(0.62–1.03)	0.081
Lifting light/heavy loads	0.88	(0.70–1.09)	0.243	0.68	(0.56–0.84)	<0.001	0.92	(0.64–1.34)	0.678
Number of nights in hospital[b]									
Standing or walking	0.78	(0.64–0.94)	0.008	0.84	(0.68–1.03)	0.095	0.78	(0.59–1.02)	0.072
Lifting light/heavy loads	0.85	(0.67–1.09)	0.204	0.58	(0.45–0.76)	<0.001	0.52	(0.36–0.76)	0.001

[a]Typical daily activity is a 3-level categorical variable describing respondents' usual level of daily activity outside of LTPA. The reference group (not shown in table) is "usually sitting."

[b] The estimate is an incidence rate ratio (IRR).

Note: adjusted for (reference category in italics) the following: age; sex (*male*/female); marital status (married: *yes*/no); education (graduated secondary: *yes*/no); ethnicity (*non-Aboriginal*/Aboriginal); employment status (employed: *no*/yes); household size (*1*, 2, 3, or more people); dwelling size (*<3 bedrooms*, 3 bedrooms, >3 bedrooms); immigration status (*nonimmigrant*, immigrant); injury in previous 12 months (*no*/yes); limitation in ADLs (*no*/yes); smoking status (*never smoked*/former smoker/nonsmoker); exposed to 2nd hand smoke (*no*/yes); alcohol consumption (*<1 drink daily*/at least 1 drink daily); BMI (*<25.0* kg·m^2/25.0–29.9 kg·m^2/≥30 kg·m^2 or greater); time spent walking to work or to run errands (*none*/<1 hour/≥1 hour); cycling to work or to run errands (*no*/yes); typical daily activity level (*usually sitting*/standing or walking/lifting light and/or heavy loads); annual household income (*<$15,000*; $15,000–$29,999; ≥$30,000; missing); province (*ON*, MB, AB, BC, SK, QC, Other); urban-rural classification (*urban*/rural); language (able to speak English and/or French: *yes*/no); has regular family doctor (*yes*/no); self-rated general health (*excellent/very good/good*; fair/poor); self-rated mental health (*excellent/very good/good*; fair/poor); diagnosed with hypertension, cardiovascular disease (including stroke), COPD, asthma, diabetes, cancer, neurological conditions, rheumatological conditions, back problems, gastrointestinal disorders, mood/anxiety disorders, or other chronic conditions (*no*/yes for each); number of chronic conditions (*none*/1 condition/2 conditions/3 conditions/4 or more conditions); number of GP consultations.

Leisure time PA was significantly associated with lower use of GP physician services in the 50 to 64 years age group, with active individuals 27% less likely to have contact with a GP and reporting 8% fewer GP consultations than their inactive counterparts in the 12-month study period. These findings are consistent with those of Woolcott et al. [24], as well as Wang et al. [39], who found that regular PA was associated with significantly lower outpatient health care costs in a group of Medicare retirees. Similarly, Mitchell et al. [40] also found physician visits to be inversely associated with physical fitness among 6,679 men aged 20–79 years. It is, however, important to note that the findings in this area are somewhat equivocal, with several studies reporting no significant association between LTPA and physician visits [27, 41, 42].

A significant association was also evident between LTPA and hospital services in the 65 to 79 years age group, where active individuals were 8% less likely to be hospitalized than their inactive counterparts. This partially supports the findings of recent studies by Woolcott et al. [24] and Sari [26] which found that LTPA was associated with a decreased likelihood of hospitalization and fewer nights spent in hospital among Canadians aged 65 years and older. While LTPA was mostly associated with fewer nights spent in hospital in the present study, these associations were not statistically significant. In the oldest age group, active respondents were actually more likely to report more nights in hospital. One explanation for the different findings may be related to the stratification of the sample of the present study. The studies by Woolcott et al. [24] and Sari [26] examined CCHS respondents aged 65 years and older as a single study population. There is considerable heterogeneity within the older adult population relative to PA, health, and health services utilization and it is possible that the stratification of the sample in the present study revealed differences in health services utilization that were obscured in studies which examined the population as a whole [15].

Although not statistically significant, the results pertaining to the use of specialist services revealed an interesting pattern. In the two oldest age groups, moderately active and active individuals were more likely than their inactive counterparts to have consulted a specialist in the previous 12 months. One possible explanation may be that moderately active and active older adults may be more health conscious and/or more health "literate" and therefore may seek referrals to specialists more frequently than inactive older adults [43]. The data related to specialist physician visits in the CCHS preclude an in-depth analysis of the physician specialty or the reasons underlying visits to specialists, both of which would provide important insights into the utilization of specialist physician services. However, despite its importance from a policy perspective, very few studies have examined the relationship of PA and specialist physician visits separate from visits to other physicians.

The lack of agreement between studies of PA and health services utilization may be due, in part, to considerable variation in sample populations, study design, and methods. There is no single "gold standard" measure of health services utilization and differences between studies in its operationalization make it difficult to form generalizations based on the available literature. Likewise, beyond the use of self-reported PA measures, there is very little consistency between studies in how PA is assessed. While most studies examining PA and health services utilization in older adults have used populations aged 65 years and older, the present study used a sample aged 50 years and older. There is significant heterogeneity in health status, PA participation, and health services utilization in the older adult population [15, 16, 36]. Also, there are a number of significant life transitions that typically occur after the age of 50, such as retirement and bereavement, which may have implications for health and health services utilization. Stratifying the data into smaller age groups coinciding with key transition periods and adjusting for age within each age group allows for a more precise analysis and comprehensive examination of the association between LTPA and health services utilization in this diverse population. For example, 50 to 65 years is the age range when many chronic conditions emerge and are diagnosed, hence the increased association with physician visits in this age group. In middle age group (65 to 79 years), chronic conditions may be worsening, resulting in stronger associations with hospitalizations. In both instances, LTPA may play an important role by either delaying the clinical manifestation of certain conditions or slowing progression of the disease process, thereby helping to delay or prevent this type of utilization in younger older adults.

Another notable difference between this analysis and previous studies was the inclusion of a wide-ranging set of control variables. A number of factors influence one's decision to seek medical care and the majority of earlier studies are lacking in their ability to account for other determinants of health services utilization, be they demographic and socioeconomic factors, physical and mental health status and medical comorbidities, or personal health practices such as smoking and drinking [26, 27, 37]. It is likely that physical activity affects health care utilization through its relationship with overall health [27]. By including a comprehensive set of health-related control we were also able to account for variations in health that may affect both the level of physical activity and healthcare utilization [26, 27, 37].

While LTPA was the primary focus of this study, respondents' typical daily activity outside of LTPA was also examined and appeared to be a stronger predictor of all types of health services utilization, particularly in the two oldest age groups. Even in the youngest age group, typical daily activity was significantly associated with the use of specialist services, where LTPA was not. One possible explanation may be that the typical daily activity variable may provide an indication of sedentary behavior, which is also associated with the development and chronic health conditions and poorer health status, independent of LTPA [44]. Among younger older adults still in the workforce, the amount of PA accrued during a typical day may exceed that accrued through LTPA due to the number of hours spent working; therefore this type of PA may be a more salient predictor of health services utilization. Another explanation may have to do with how respondents classified their own PA. Older adults typically participate in activities such as housework, gardening, and caregiving more frequently than other types of LTPA [45, 46]. Given that these types of PA were not specified in the CCHS instrument, respondents may have considered them as part of their usual daily activities. This highlights the importance of implementing measures of PA that are appropriate for older adults, given the types of PA typically reported in this population. It is possible that a more appropriate measure of LTPA may have revealed more significant associations with health services utilization. Lastly, among respondents aged 80 years and older, typical daily PA may be reflective of greater mobility and health status and, thus, be a stronger predictor of health services utilization.

Prior research in the area of PA and health services utilization has predominantly been focused on individuals in the workplace. This study is among a small few to examine the relationship between PA and health services utilization in community-dwelling older Canadians. Furthermore, the focus on both LTPA and typical daily PA is unique and provides new insights into the relationship between PA and health services utilization in the older adult population. Nonetheless, this study has certain limitations that should be considered when interpreting the results. The cross-sectional nature of the survey data precludes the inference of causal relationships and one cannot discount the possibility that reverse causality between the outcome measures and one or more independent variables is present. Furthermore, given the self-reported nature of the data, bias due to inaccurate recall or social desirability remains a possibility, particularly in the PA and health services data. Previous studies have shown that older adults tend to overreport contacts with GP physicians and underreport contacts with medical specialists, while recall of events such as hospitalizations appears to be more accurate, perhaps because these events are more highly salient and easily remembered [47, 48]. Likewise, there are issues with the use of self-reported measures of PA in an older population including vision and hearing impairments or disturbances to cognition and short- or long-term memory [49]. Additional problems may include the ability to accurately report activity intensity, because perceptions of what is "hard" activity or "light" activity depend on the tolerance and fitness level of the individual, both of which decline as a person ages [49].

Limitations owing to the CCHS instrument itself, while beyond our control, should also be pointed out. First, the discrepancy in recall periods between the health services utilization and LTPA variables may have made it more difficult to identify significant relationships; however, it would be considerably more difficult to accurately recall PA behaviors over a 12-month period compared to a lower frequency event such as health services utilization over the same period [27]. Furthermore, the measurement of LTPA in the CCHS may underestimate older adults' LTPA, particularly in the oldest age group, for at least two reasons: (1) the instrument does not specifically include more prevalent leisure time activities of older adults, such as housekeeping or caregiving and (2) the questionnaire may not be sensitive enough to detect the typically light and brief activity of elderly people [20, 49].

The above limitations notwithstanding, this study provides a significant contribution to a growing body of evidence suggesting that PA leads to lower health services utilization in community-dwelling older Canadians. Older adults are a very diverse group and this heterogeneity must be considered when examining health services utilization in this population. Although many of the estimates produced in the analyses were not statistically significant, they may have considerable relevance from a clinical perspective. For example, the results showed that moderately active and active respondents in the two oldest age groups were more likely to have at least 1 contact with a specialist and active individuals in the oldest age group appeared to have higher overall utilization of specialist physicians than their inactive or moderately active counterparts. Given that costs associated with specialist physician services are considerably higher than those associated with GP physician services, this finding warrants further exploration. Further studies of the patterns of health services utilization among sedentary, inactive, and active older adults would better clarify the potential role of PA as a strategy to decrease health services utilization and costs. *In addition, these findings suggest that both general and specialist physicians should be engaged in discussions related to physical activity given that older adults seek care from both groups of health professionals.*

In summary, it is possible that interventions aimed at increasing LTPA in this population may result in tangible reductions in health services utilization. The results also suggest that encouraging sedentary and inactive older adults, particularly those over age 65, to maintain or increase their overall daily activity, perhaps simply by reducing time spent in sedentary behaviors, may have an even greater impact on reducing the demand for health services. Given the wide variation in the literature with regard to study populations and methodologies, additional studies, with common outcome measures, appropriate and robust assessments of PA, and sedentary behavior, and adequate controls for confounders, are needed to obtain credible and accurate estimates of the effects of PA. Moreover, prospective longitudinal studies into the causal relationship between PA and health services utilization would provide important information on the potential impact would provide important insights about the potential impact of population-based strategies to increase PA participation among older adults on the health care system.

Acknowledgments

This research received no specific grant from any funding agency in the public, commercial, or not-for-profit sectors; however, Koren L. Fisher received scholarship support from the Saskatchewan Population Health and Evaluation Research (SPHERU) and the Western Region Training Centre for Health Services Research. The analysis presented in this paper was conducted at the Saskatchewan Research Data Centre (SKY-RDC) which is part of the Canadian Research Data Centre Network (CRDCN). The services and activities provided by the SKY-RDC are made possible by the financial or in-kind support of the SSHRC, the CIHR, the CFI, Statistics Canada, the Saskatchewan Health Research Foundation, the Health Quality Council, and the University of Saskatchewan.

References

[1] US Department of Health and Human Services, *Physical Activity and Health: A Report of the Surgeon General*, US Department of Health and Human Services, Public Health Service, CDC, National Center for Chronic Disease Prevention and Health Promotion, Atlanta, Ga, USA, 1996.

[2] D. E. R. Warburton, C. W. Nicol, and S. S. D. Bredin, "Health benefits of physical activity: the evidence," *Canadian Medical Association Journal*, vol. 174, no. 6, pp. 801–809, 2006.

[3] D. E. R. Warburton, S. Charlesworth, A. Ivey, L. Nettlefold, and S. S. D. Bredin, "A systematic review of the evidence for Canada's Physical Activity Guidelines for Adults," *International Journal of Behavioral Nutrition and Physical Activity*, vol. 7, article 39, 2010.

[4] D. H. Paterson, G. R. Jones, and C. L. Rice, "Ageing and physical activity: evidence to develop exercise recommendations for older adults," *Canadian Journal of Public Health*, vol. 98, supplement 2, pp. S69–108, 2007.

[5] D. H. Paterson and D. E. R. Warburton, "Physical activity and functional limitations in older adults: a systematic review related to Canada's Physical Activity Guidelines," *International Journal of Behavioral Nutrition and Physical Activity*, vol. 7, no. 1, article 38, 2010.

[6] P. T. Katzmarzyk and S. A. Lear, "Physical activity for obese individuals: a systematic review of effects on chronic disease risk factors," *Obesity Reviews*, vol. 13, no. 2, pp. 95–105, 2012.

[7] K. Melzer, B. Kayser, and C. Pichard, "Physical activity: the health benefits outweigh the risks," *Current Opinion in Clinical Nutrition & Metabolic Care*, vol. 7, no. 6, pp. 641–647, 2004.

[8] Canadian Fitness & Lifestyle Research Institute, *Physical Activity Levels of Canadians—2008 Physical Activity Monitor*, 2010, http://cflri.ca/.

[9] R. C. Colley, D. Garriguet, I. Janssen, C. L. Craig, J. Clarke, and M. S. Tremblay, "Physical activity of canadian adults: accelerometer results from the 2007 to 2009 canadian health measures survey," *Health Reports*, vol. 22, no. 1, pp. 15–23, 2011.

[10] H. W. Kohl III, C. L. Craig, E. V. Lambert et al., "The pandemic of physical inactivity: global action for public health," *The Lancet*, vol. 380, no. 9838, pp. 294–305, 2012.

[11] Statistics Canada, *Population Projections for Canada, Provinces and Territories*, edited by Demography Division, Ministry of Industry, Government of Canada, Ottawa, Canada, 2010.

[12] H. Gilmour and J. Park, "Dependency, chronic conditions and pain in seniors," *Health Reports*, vol. 16, pp. 21–31, 2006.

[13] P. L. Ramage-Morin, M. Shields, and L. Martel, "Health-promoting factors and good health among Canadians in mid- to late life," *Health Reports*, vol. 21, no. 3, pp. 45–53, 2010.

[14] Organization for Economic Co-Operation and Development, *Health at a Glance 2011: OECD Indicators*, OECD, 2011.

[15] K. Vegda, J. X. Nie, L. Wang, C. S. Tracy, R. Moineddin, and R. E. Upshur, "Trends in health services utilization, medication use, and health conditions among older adults: a 2-year retrospective chart review in a primary care practice," *BMC Health Services Research*, vol. 9, article 217, 2009.

[16] R. Moineddin, J. X. Nie, L. Wang, C. S. Tracy, and R. E. G. Upshur, "Measuring change in health status of older adults at the population level: the transition probability model," *BMC Health Services Research*, vol. 10, no. 1, article 306, 2010.

[17] C. L. Craig, "Evolution and devolution of national physical activity policy in Canada," *Journal of Physical Activity and Health*, vol. 8, no. 8, pp. 1044–1056, 2011.

[18] B. Lankenau, A. Solari, and M. Pratt, "International physical activity policy development: a commentary," *Public Health Reports*, vol. 119, no. 3, pp. 352–355, 2004.

[19] K. M. Herman, C. I. Ardern, C. Mason, S. E. Brien, and P. T. Katzmarzyk, "Trends in physical activity research in Canada," *Applied Physiology, Nutrition and Metabolism*, vol. 32, no. 3, pp. 400–408, 2007.

[20] N. Sari, "Exercise, physical activity and healthcare utilization: a review of literature for older adults," *Maturitas*, vol. 70, no. 3, pp. 285–289, 2011.

[21] P. T. Katzmarzyk, N. Gledhill, and R. J. Shephard, "The economic burden of physical inactivity in Canada," *Canadian Medical Association Journal*, vol. 163, no. 11, pp. 1435–1440, 2000.

[22] P. T. Katzmarzyk and I. Janssen, "The economic costs associated with physical inactivity and obesity in Canada: an update," *Canadian Journal of Applied Physiology*, vol. 29, no. 1, pp. 90–115, 2004.

[23] I. Janssen, "Health care costs of physical inactivity in Canadian adults," *Applied Physiology, Nutrition and Metabolism*, vol. 37, no. 4, pp. 803–806, 2012.

[24] J. C. Woolcott, M. C. Ashe, W. C. Miller, P. Shi, and C. A. Marra, "Does physical activity reduce seniors' need for healthcare? A study of 24 281 Canadians," *British Journal of Sports Medicine*, vol. 44, no. 12, pp. 902–904, 2010.

[25] R. C. Plotnikoff, N. D. Karunamuni, J. A. Johnson, M. Kotovych, and L. W. Svenson, "Health-related behaviours in adults with diabetes: associations with health care utilization and costs," *Canadian Journal of Public Health*, vol. 99, no. 3, pp. 227–231, 2008.

[26] N. Sari, "A short walk a day shortens the hospital stay: physical activity and the demand for hospital services for older adults," *Canadian Journal of Public Health*, vol. 101, no. 5, pp. 385–389, 2010.

[27] M. Y. Martin, M. P. Powell, C. Peel, S. Zhu, and R. Allman, "Leisure-time physical activity and health-care utilization in older adults," *Journal of Aging & Physical Activity*, vol. 14, no. 4, pp. 392–410, 2006.

[28] Y. Beland, "Canadian community health survey—methodological overview," in *Health Reports*, pp. 9–14, 2002.

[29] Statistics Canada, *Canadian Community Health Survey Cycle 3.1 Master Microdata File User Guide*, Statistics Canada, Ottawa, Canada, 2006.

[30] Statistics Canada, *Response Rates by Province/Territory and Health Region. Area Frame, Phone Frames and Total Sample. CCHS Cycle 3.1. January to December 2005*, Statistics Canada, Ottawa, Canada, 2006.

[31] Y. Asada and G. Kephart, "Equity in health services use and intensity of use in Canada," *BMC Health Services Research*, vol. 7, article 41, 2007.

[32] Statistics Canada, *Canadian Community Health Survey Cycle 3.1 Final Questionnaire*, Statistics Canada, Ottawa, Canada, 2005.

[33] R. Andersen and J. F. Newman, "Societal and individual determinants of medical care utilization in the United States," *The Milbank Memorial Fund Quarterly. Health and Society*, vol. 51, no. 1, pp. 95–124, 1973.

[34] R. M. Andersen, "Revisiting the behavioral model and access to medical care: does it matter?" *Journal of Health and Social Behavior*, vol. 36, no. 1, pp. 1–10, 1995.

[35] K. A. Phillips, K. R. Morrison, R. Andersen, and L. A. Aday, "Understanding the context of healthcare utilization: assessing environmental and provider-related variables in the behavioral model of utilization," *Health Services Research*, vol. 33, no. 3, pp. 571–596, 1998.

[36] K. E. Chad, B. A. Reeder, E. L. Harrison et al., "Profile of physical activity levels in community-dwelling older adults," *Medicine & Science in Sports & Exercise*, vol. 37, no. 10, pp. 1774–1784, 2005.

[37] N. Sari, "Physical inactivity and its impact on healthcare utilization," *Health Economics*, vol. 18, no. 8, pp. 885–901, 2009.

[38] S. L. Lohr, *Sampling: Design and Analysis*, Cengage Learning, Inc., Boston, Mass, USA, 2nd edition, 2010.

[39] F. Wang, T. McDonald, B. Reffitt, and D. W. Edington, "BMI, physical activity, and health care utilization/costs among medicare retirees," *Obesity Research*, vol. 13, no. 8, pp. 1450–1457, 2005.

[40] T. L. Mitchell, L. W. Gibbons, S. M. Devers, and C. P. Earnest, "Effects of cardiorespiratory fitness on healthcare utilization," *Medicine & Science in Sports & Exercise*, vol. 36, no. 12, pp. 2088–2092, 2004.

[41] S. Dunlop, P. C. Coyte, and W. McIsaac, "Socio-economic status and the utilisation of physicians' services: results from the Canadian National Population Health Survey," *Social Science & Medicine*, vol. 51, no. 1, pp. 123–133, 2000.

[42] A. J. Perkins and D. O. Clark, "Assessing the association of walking with health services use and costs among socioeconomically disadvantaged older adults," *Preventive Medicine*, vol. 32, no. 6, pp. 492–501, 2001.

[43] E. Costello, M. Kafchinski, J. Vrazel, and P. Sullivan, "Motivators, barriers, and beliefs regarding physical activity in an older adult population," *Journal of Geriatric Physical Therapy*, vol. 34, no. 3, pp. 138–147, 2011.

[44] M. S. Tremblay, R. C. Colley, T. J. Saunders, G. N. Healy, and N. Owen, "Physiological and health implications of a sedentary lifestyle," *Applied Physiology, Nutrition, and Metabolism*, vol. 35, no. 6, pp. 725–740, 2010.

[45] R. A. Washburn, "Assessment of physical activity in older adults," *Research Quarterly for Exercise and Sport*, vol. 71, no. 2, pp. S79–S88, 2000.

[46] S. L. Murphy, "Review of physical activity measurement using accelerometers in older adults: considerations for research design and conduct," *Preventive Medicine*, vol. 48, no. 2, pp. 108–114, 2009.

[47] P. S. Raina, S. A. Kirkland, C. Wolfson et al., "Accessing health care utilization databases for health research: a canadian longitudinal study on aging feasibility study," *Canadian Journal on Aging*, vol. 28, no. 3, pp. 287–294, 2009.

[48] L. L. Roos, M. Brownell, L. Lix, N. P. Roos, R. Walld, and L. MacWilliam, "From health research to social research: privacy, methods, approaches," *Social Science & Medicine*, vol. 66, no. 1, pp. 117–129, 2008.

[49] R. J. Shephard, "Limits to the measurement of habitual physical activity by questionnaires," *British Journal of Sports Medicine*, vol. 37, no. 3, pp. 197–206, 2003.

5

Leisure Engagement: Medical Conditions, Mobility Difficulties, and Activity Limitations—A Later Life Perspective

Ingeborg Nilsson,[1,2] Fredrica Nyqvist,[3] Yngve Gustafson,[4] and Mikael Nygård[3]

[1]*Department of Community Medicine and Rehabilitation, Occupational Therapy, Umeå University, 901 87 Umeå, Sweden*
[2]*Umeå University, Ageing and Living Conditions Program, 901 87 Umeå, Sweden*
[3]*Faculty of Education and Welfare Studies, Social Policy Unit, Åbo Akademi University, 651 01 Vasa, Finland*
[4]*Department of Community Medicine and Rehabilitation, Geriatric Medicine, Umeå University, 901 87 Umeå, Sweden*

Correspondence should be addressed to Ingeborg Nilsson; ingeborg.nilsson@umu.se

Academic Editor: Enrica Menditto

Objectives. This study aims to investigate the impact of medical conditions, mobility difficulties, and activity limitations on older people's engagement in leisure activities. *Methods.* The analyses are based on a cross regional survey carried out in 2010 in the Bothnia region (Northern Sweden and Western Finland). A posted questionnaire, which included questions on different aspects of leisure engagement, medical history, and health, was sent out to older persons in the region. The final sample consisted of 5435 persons aged 65, 70, 75, and 80 years. The data was analyzed by using ordinary least squares (OLS) multivariate regression. *Results.* The most important predictor of leisure engagement abstention among older people is the prevalence of activity limitations, whereas mobility difficulties and medical conditions play less important roles. The strong negative association between activity limitations and leisure engagement remains significant even after we control for individual, sociodemographic characteristics, and country. *Discussion.* This study provides a window into leisure engagement in later life and factors influencing the magnitude of engagement in leisure activities.

1. Introduction

Older people's participation in leisure activities, such as involvement in cultural, social, and physical activities, is known to be positively associated with health and survival [1]. It is therefore important to improve the understanding of the risk factors that might cause a decline in such participation. Accordingly, this study aims to investigate the impact that health-related risk factors, such as medical conditions, mobility difficulties, and activity limitations, may have on older people's engagement in leisure activities.

European countries are currently facing major demographic changes due to substantial increases in longevity (a large reduction in late life mortality) and declines in fertility [2, 3]. As a consequence, the number and proportion of older people will increase. This fact has led to a growing interest in understanding how to meet the needs of an ageing population. It is also a public health priority that includes, among other things, the identification of components that can promote factors to support active and healthy ageing [4, 5]. In an aging population, the prevalence of health-related risk factors such as medical conditions, mobility related difficulties (limits in functions), and activity limitations (inability to perform activities) increase with age [6]. The relation between the above-mentioned health-related risk factors and health is, however, complex and much discussed [7]. According to the World Health Organization, health is a state of complete physical, mental, and social well-being, and to reach this state we must be able to identify and realize aspirations in life, satisfy our needs, and be able to change or cope with the environment [8]. Therefore, the relationship between engaging in activities and becoming healthy is an important perspective of health [9] with a long history [10].

On a general level, engagement in leisure activities has demonstrated positive health-related outcomes [11] and correlates explicitly with increased survival and life expectancies

[12], lower mortality rates [13–17], and higher levels of happiness [18, 19]. Engagement in leisure activities seems therefore to be an important health promoter in the case of older people [17]. Engagement and participation in leisure activities are reported slowly decline over time in later life [20, 21], but how this decline can be promoted is less known. Participation in leisure activities is often studied from the aspect of performing activities as such, while some studies also highlight the importance of incorporating the purpose or motivational aspects for added understanding [22, 23]. Being motivated is a crucial component for making the leisure activities meaningful [11], and therefore the motivation component is an important factor to take into account when conducting research on leisure engagement and its relation to health-related conditions.

Earlier research has shown that functional decline could be an important indicator of ill-health in later life [24, 25]. However, according to the World Health Organization [26], functional decline and limitations might not be the direct cause of the limited ability to perform activities, as the adaptation to the environment or by the person could reduce the negative effect of such decline. Hence, understanding the cause to activity limitations is complex; Wu et al. [27], for example, did not find any associations between medical diseases and activities of daily living (ADL), whereas Gill et al. [24] found change in physical performance as independently associated with ADL dependency. While maintaining healthy habits is described as preventing the deterioration of functional capacity [28, 29], few studies focus on leisure engagement as a result or indicator of a person enjoying good health. Atchley [30] found that limitations in performance affected leisure patterns in older people, but if and how this is true also for mobility difficulties and other important health-related risk factors in later life needs further investigation.

In this study, we therefore wanted to explore potential health-related risk factors related to leisure engagement decline by studying the impact of medical conditions, mobility difficulties, and activity limitations in relation to leisure engagement. While studying this relation, it is important to consider the influence of personal characteristics upon these relationships. For example, it is known that later life health problems seem to vary between genders [31], to be influenced by socioeconomic aspects, and to vary between countries or geographic regions [32]. Therefore, these potential confounders must be considered as having a possible impact on this relation. Specifically, the research questions for this paper are the following.

(1) Is there a relationship between medical conditions, mobility difficulties, activity limitations, and leisure engagement in older people?

(2) Is the relationship influenced by sociodemographic aspects such as gender, age, economy, and geography?

2. Data and Methods

2.1. Sample. The analyses are based on a cross regional survey carried out in 2010 as a part of an interregional EU-funded research project (Gerontological Regional Database and Resource Centre, GERDA). The overall aim of the multidisciplinary project was to map living and health conditions of older adults (aged 65, 70, 75, and 80 years) in the Bothnia region, that is, on both sides of the *Gulf of Bothnia*, in *Västerbotten* in Sweden and in *Österbotten/Pohjanmaa* in Finland (more information about the project is available at the project website (http://web.novia.fi/gerda/)). Although the two regions *Österbotten* and *Pohjanmaa* belong to the same geographical region, they can in fact be treated as two separate regions due to different linguistic conditions (the (technical) division between *Österbotten* and *Pohjanmaa* relates to a language stratification of citizens in this particular West-Finnish region. Elderly Swedish-speaking inhabitants were coded as belonging to *Österbotten* and those with Finnish as their mother tongue were coded as belonging to *Pohjanmaa*). In this paper, however, we do not separate these two areas from each other, since the linguistic characteristics of the Finnish population are controlled for by the language variable.

In 2010, the Swedish region *Västerbotten* consisted of 15 municipalities, including two more densely populated areas (*Umeå* and *Skellefteå*), with an overall population of approximately 260,000 inhabitants. The overall population in the West-Finnish region *Österbotten/Pohjanmaa* (including the town of Vaasa) consisted of approximately 178,000 inhabitants [33]. Although the above-mentioned regions share several common structural features, such as common cultural characteristics and common historical bonds, there are also noticeable differences between them, such as differing linguistic conditions. Finland is an officially bilingual state with a large Finnish-speaking majority and a small Swedish-speaking minority of approximately 6 percent. However, in *Österbotten/Pohjanmaa,* 51 percent of the population belong to the Swedish-speaking group and form to some extent a majority at the local level. In 2010, three out of 17 municipalities in *Österbotten/Pohjanmaa* were officially monolingual (Finnish) whereas Swedish-speakers formed the local majority in nine municipalities. The two language groups in Finland were sent questionnaires in their own language.

A total sample of 10,696 was selected from the National Tax Board in Sweden and the Population Register Centre in Finland. Questionnaires were sent to all people that in 2010 were 65, 70, 75, and 80 years old in rural municipalities, to every second person in the most populous town in Finland and to every third person residing in the two most populous towns in *Västerbotten.* In total, 6 838 persons (64%) replied. The response rate varied between the regions, with 70% responding in *Västerbotten,* 62% in *Österbotten,* and 53% in *Pohjanmaa.* The response rate decreased marginally with age. The response rate was somewhat higher amongst the two younger age groups (66%) than those aged 75 and 80 years (61.9 and 59.2%, resp.).

In order to be selected as a part of the sample, valid responses on leisure engagement were required. This criterion narrowed the final sample down to a total of 5435 older persons. A description of the sample is found in Table 1.

2.2. Data Collection. A posted questionnaire was sent out during late 2010 and included a broad range of questions

Table 1: Frequencies (%) of basic characteristics in the studied sample.

	Total sample $n = 5435$	Finland $n = 2220$	Sweden $n = 3215$
Age			
65	2185 (40.2)	965 (43.5)	1220 (37.9)
70	1357 (25.0)	508 (22.9)	849 (26.4)
75	1091 (20.1)	449 (20.2)	643 (20.0)
80	800 (14.7)	298 (13.4)	502 (15.6)
Gender			
Women	3018 (55.5)	1259 (56.7)	1759 (54.7)
Men	2416 (45.5)	961 (43.3)	1455 (45.3)
Living condition			
Single living	1401 (26.0)	517 (23.5)	884 (27.8)
Living together	3983 (74.0)	1686 (76.5)	2297 (72.2)
Education level			
Shorter (up to 9 yrs)	2469 (46.4)	925 (42.3)	1544 (49.1)
Longer (10 yrs or more)	2857 (53.6)	1255 (57.6)	1602 (50.9)
Income level			
≤1000€	1384 (27.2)	599 (28.3)	786 (26.5)
>1000€	3700 (72.8)	1515 (71.7)	2185 (73.6)
Leisure engagement			
M (SD)	0.28 (0.99)	0.29 (0.97)	0.27 (1.0)
Range	−4.90–5.10	−4.90–5.0	−4.60–5.10

related to aspects of societal engagement, medical history, health, and sociodemography. The battery of questions was developed by the multidisciplinary team of researchers included in the GERDA, and for this paper we analyzed medical conditions (integrating ≥5 pharmaceutical drugs, stroke, heart disease, cancer, and hospital stays during the last 12 months into an index); mobility difficulties (integrating fear of falling and mobility device into an index); activity limitations (integrating independent bathing and independent cleaning into an index); and leisure engagement. The sociodemographic variables included in the analysis were age (65/70/75/80 yrs), language (Swedish/Finnish and other languages), gender (man/women), civil status (single/together), income (≤1000€/>1000€), education (≤9 yrs/≥10 yrs), and country (Finland/Sweden).

Leisure engagement was measured by asking about two aspects of 20 different leisure activities (task): first if the participant had a habit of performing the task and then if the participant was motivated to perform the said task. These questions were a part of the MNPS leisure checklist that has been used in previous similar samples and that has been evaluated for its validity [23, 34].

2.3. Data Analysis. Firstly, we calculated the extension of medical conditions, mobility difficulties, and activity limitations in every person by adding up each component in the index into a number. More specifically, each person was assigned a number that put their medical condition between 0 and 5 based on if they reported using ≥5 pharmaceutical drugs, personal incidence of stroke, heart disease, cancer, or/and hospital stays during the last 12 months. Similarly, a number between 0 and 2 was assigned for mobility difficulties (adding a fear of falling, dependency on mobility devices) and activity limitations (dependency on help for bathing, dependency on help for cleaning). A higher number was interpreted as showing a more severe medical condition, mobility difficulties, or activity limitations.

Secondly, to generate the measures of leisure engagement, the raw data of leisure performance and the raw data of leisure motivation were combined and subjected to the Rasch rating scale analysis by using the WINSTEPS program [35]. This procedure has been used and found to be a valid measurement for groups of older people [36]. The generated data was treated as valid if it met the common criteria for surveys of MnSq ≤ 1.5 and $z \leq 2.0$ [37]. To be included in the study, a valid response regarding leisure engagement was required. In total, data from 1 403 respondents was excluded due to invalid responses. A major reason for this error was that many participants had not answered the question about leisure motivation ("do you want to perform this activity?").

Lastly, we exported the leisure engagement scale measures to IBM SPSS Statistics, version 20, for continued analysis. The relationship between the engagement in leisure activities of older adults, different health indicators and sociodemographic control variables was assessed by using ordinary least squares (OLS) multivariate regression. We used the above-mentioned measure for leisure engagement as our dependent variable as well as three indexes measuring medical condition, mobility difficulties, and activity limitations as independent variables. We also controlled for sociodemographic aspects. Three regression models were calculated. The first model calculated a bivariate regression coefficient for each separate health indicator index on leisure engagement. The second model consisted of multivariate regressions of the above-mentioned health indicator indexes on leisure engagement. The third model was a full model assessing the association between leisure engagement and health indicators while controlling for sociodemographic characteristics.

3. Results

In this study a total of 5435 participants met the inclusion criteria, 1375 from Österbotten (25.3%), 845 from Pohjanmaa (15.5%), and 3215 from Västerbotten (59.2%). The most dominant type of person found in the sample was a 65-year-old (40.2%) women (55.5%) living in Västerbotten, Sweden (59.2%), together with someone (74%) and earning more than 1000€ a month (72.8%). Details about the sample are described in Table 1. The basic characteristics were similarly distributed in Finland and Sweden. Of the total sample 59.2% were Swedes (from Västerbotten, Sweden), 25.3% were Swedish-speaking Finns (from Österbotten, Finland) and 15.5% were Finnish-speaking Finns (from Pohjanmaa, Finland). Leisure engagement varied in the sample between the most engaged (5.10) and the least engaged (−4.60) with a mean 0.28 (SD 0.99).

TABLE 2: Frequencies (%) of medical conditions, mobility difficulties, and activity limitations in the studied group.

	Total sample $n = 5435$	Finland $n = 2220$	Sweden $n = 3215$
Medical conditions			
≥5 pharmaceutical drugs	1074 (20.4)	370 (17.2)	704 (22.5)
Stroke	352 (6.9%)	100 (4.8)	252 (8.2)
Heart disease	435 (8.7)	147 (7.2)	288 (9.7)
Cancer	749 (14.6)	299 (14.4)	450 (14.7)
Hospital care during the last 12 months	1018 (19.3)	409 (19.0)	609 (19.5)
Mobility difficulties			
Mobility device	645 (12.2)	228 (10.5)	417 (13.3)
Fear of falling	1389 (26.4)	454 (21.1)	935 (30.1)
Activity limitations			
Need help with bathing	326 (6.1)	107 (4.9)	219 (6.9)
Need help with cleaning	774 (14.4)	323 (14.8)	451 (14.2)

TABLE 3: The effects of medical conditions, mobility difficulties, and activity limitations on the leisure engagement of older adults. Results from bivariate and multivariate OLS analyses.

Independent variables	Model 1	Model 2	Model 3
Health-related risk factors			
Medical conditions (index)	-0.134^{***}	-0.052^{***}	-0.036^{*}
Mobility difficulties (index)	-0.273^{***}	-0.115^{***}	-0.079^{***}
Activity limitations (index)	-0.504^{***}	-0.196^{***}	-0.168^{***}
Sociodemographic variables			
Age (cont.)			-0.104^{***}
Language: Swedish (ref. Finnish and others)			0.068^{***}
Gender: female (ref. male)			0.056^{***}
Civil status: partnership (ref. single)			0.052^{***}
Income: high (ref. low)			0.062^{***}
Education: high (ref. low education)			0.083^{***}
Country: Sweden (ref. Finland)			-0.015
n		5435	5435
Adjusted R square		0.071	0.101

Note: the first model shows nonstandardised Beta coefficients from bivariate regressions of each health indicator of leisure engagement, whereas models 2 and 3 show standardised Beta coefficients from multivariate regressions. The variables, medical conditions, mobility difficulties, and activity limitations, are indexes. Age is a continuous variable and the other variables are "dummy" variables. $^{*}P < 0.95$ and $^{***}P < 0.999$.

Every fifth participant (about 20%) used 5 or more pharmaceutical drugs and reported a hospital stay during the last 12 months. The most frequently reported medical diagnosis was (some form of) cancer (15%). One quarter of the participants (about 25%) reported a fear of falling and about 14% needed help with cleaning. More details about medical diagnoses, mobility difficulties, and activity limitations are described in Table 2.

The first two models of the OLS regression (see Table 3) indicate that medical conditions, mobility difficulties, and activity limitations all have hampering effects on the leisure engagement of older adults, both when we consider the bivariate associations between each of the three indicators and leisure engagement (model 1) and when their relative importance for leisure engagement (model 2) is taken into consideration. As is shown in the table, the indicator having the biggest impact on the leisure engagement of older adults is activity limitations, while the two other health status indexes play somewhat lesser roles. Interestingly, the strong negative association between activity limitations and leisure engagement remains significant (which is also the case with mobility difficulties) even after we control for individual, sociodemographic characteristics, and country (model 3). This suggests an independent association between activity limitations, mobility difficulties, and leisure engagement. The table also shows that leisure engagement tends to decline with old age and that leisure engagement is higher among Swedish-speaking older adults than among Finnish-speakers and persons with other mother tongues. It is intriguing to note that one's mother tongue seems to play an important role in this respect, although the country variable does not seem to matter a great deal. As it is revealed in the figure, the Swedish-speakers in Finland also show a high rate of leisure engagement, which may explain why the country variable remains insignificant (see Figure 1). Furthermore, Table 3 shows that leisure engagement is higher among women, persons living together with someone else, persons with high incomes (pensions), and persons with higher levels of education.

4. Discussion

In this paper, we have analyzed the relationship between leisure engagement and medical conditions, mobility difficulties, and activity limitations. This study demonstrates that having a fear of falling, using mobility devices, and needing help with bathing and/or cleaning all have a significant impact on the level of leisure engagement in the case of older people. This impact remains significant even after controlling for variables such as gender, age, civil status, income, education, and language group affiliation.

For the purpose of this study, we operationalized mobility difficulties and activity limitations as an index that assessed whether older persons were experiencing a fear of falling and using mobility devices or if they were in need of help in order to bathe or clean themselves, respectively. Even though this is only one way of operationalizing mobility difficulties and activity limitations, it still gives an insight into how mobility issues as well as ability factors influence the extent to which older persons engage in leisure activities. Mobility issues and particularly a fear of falling have previously been studied and found to influence physical leisure activities negatively [38, 39].

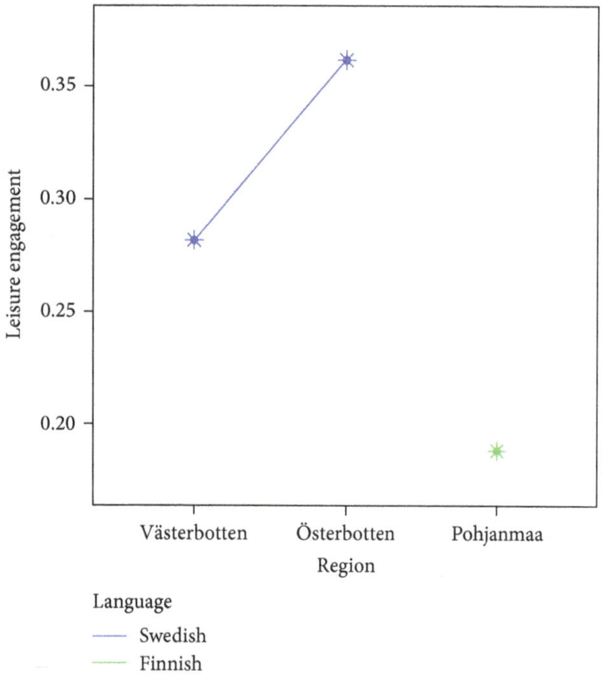

FIGURE 1: Illustration of how leisure engagement varies between Swedish- and Finnish-speakers in the study.

Medical conditions also play a role in predicting the level of leisure engagement. Yet this variable does not seem to play a role as big as that of mobility difficulties and activity limitations. Moreover, the variable of medical conditions loses its strength after controlling for sociodemographic variables. These results are somewhat supported by earlier findings [6, 40], which report that older people may view themselves as healthy despite suffering from chronic illnesses and disabilities. However, the negative link between illnesses or diagnoses and activities is often taken for granted or regarded as obvious (e.g., [41–43]) even though other researchers found that engagement in activities is affected by more than just diseases. Life style factors as well as persons' physical and social environment, for example, have been noted to play a role in the level of engagement in such activities [44–47].

With a regression model explaining about 10% of the variance in leisure engagement, this study demonstrates the need to examine leisure engagement no matter medical conditions, mobility difficulties, or activity limitations. Moreover, this study supports the need to consider age, gender, civil status, and socioeconomic status in terms of income and educational level when examining leisure engagement in the case of older people. In this study, leisure engagement varied between Finnish- and Swedish-speakers, but the country variable as such showed no impact on their engagement in leisure activities. This is an interesting finding that seems to separate the effects of language group affiliation from those of the geographic region where a person is resident (e.g., [32]). The results found in this paper also corroborate the findings from a recent study, which found that good self-rated health was high among Swedish-speakers in Sweden and Finland, respectively, but lower among Finnish-speakers in Finland [48]. Further, being in line with previous research [49], it seems like historical, social, and cultural differences attributed to belonging to a specific language group in Finland are playing an important role in explaining language group differences in leisure engagement. It has been suggested that the Swedish-speaking community in Finland live in tighter social networks as compared to the Finnish-speaking community [49] which might explain the high levels of leisure engagement among the Swedish-speakers in Finland in our study.

To what extent does leisure engagement of older persons depend on their level of activity limitations, their level of mobility difficulties, or their medical diagnoses, and to what may such engagement be related to other factors not examined in the present study? These factors need to be identified and highlighted in future studies. Environmental issues and physical and social factors may also be important here, as suggested in many theories [50–52]. Supports and barriers in the social, physical, or societal environment could, for example, be a part of interventions [53] but are also shown to influence physical activities and suggested to be used as predicting factors [54]. There might also be other, yet unknown, factors of importance to identify and incorporate into future evaluations of leisure engagement.

Earlier research supports a relationship between self-rated health, seen as an overall measure of health, and leisure engagement [55, 56] and this needs to be investigated further. Perhaps self-rated health could go together with medical conditions, mobility difficulties, and activity limitations to create a broader understanding of factors influencing the engagement in leisure activities.

Based on the results, we can question whether medical conditions have a great impact on leisure engagement. Other findings similarly reveal limitations in using medical conditions to predict a decline in the activities of daily living [57]. Hence, it is important to remember that only a few diagnoses and signs of medical conditions were included in this study's medical condition variable. If other diagnoses or signs, such as symptoms of depression and cognitive limitations, were included, the predictive strength of the regression models might be improved in terms of leisure engagement. Another limitation of this study is that self-reports of diseases are prone to be influenced by individual bias, particularly in the case of illnesses perceived as nonthreatening and that do not hamper a person's ability to live normally [58]. These illnesses may nevertheless increase the risks for a decline of a person's ability to function normally and need therefore to be considered. Although we used a population-based cohort, the exclusion from the analyses of participants with invalid responses on leisure engagement measures may have introduced bias and reduced the generalizability of the results. However, as the study is not limited to include only the performance of leisure activities, but also the motivational aspect of these activities, our measure on leisure engagement can arguably be seen as robust.

This study is based on self-reports, that is, on the accounts of older people assessing their engagement in leisure activities as well as their experienced medical diagnoses, mobility difficulties, and activity limitations. Together, this contributes to an understanding about leisure engagement in later life. There is however a great need to study also other variables in the complex field of leisure engagement.

Conflict of Interests

The authors report no conflict of interests.

Acknowledgments

The GERDA Bothnia project and data collection (Gerontological Regional Database 2011, GERDA) are a result of the cooperation between universities in Finland and Sweden: the Novia University of Applied Sciences (Finland), Åbo Akademi University (Finland), and Umeå University (Sweden) during 2004–2012. The GERDA project was financed by the Interreg IV A Botnia-Atlantica programme, the Regional Council of Ostrobothnia, Novia University of Applied Sciences (Finland), Åbo Akademi University (Finland), Umeå University (Sweden), and Umeå Municipality (Sweden). Furthermore, this study was supported financially by the Swedish Research Council's Linnaeus Grant (no. 2006-21576-36119-66), the Swedish Research Council's Strategic Research Programme: Care Science, Umeå University, and the Academy of Finland (Grant no. 250054) as part of the FLARE-2 programme.

References

[1] N. Agahi, "Leisure in late life: pattern of participation and relationship to health," in *Neurobiology, Care Sciences and Society*, Karolinska Institutet, Stockholm, Sweden, 2008.

[2] E. Grundy, "Ageing and vulnerable elderly people: European perspectives," *Ageing and Society*, vol. 26, no. 1, pp. 105–134, 2006.

[3] Eurostat, Europe in figures—Eurostat yearbook, European Commision, 2013, http://epp.eurostat.ec.europa.eu/statistics_explained/index.php/Europe_in_figures_-_Eurostat_yearbook.

[4] A. Walker and T. Maltby, "Active ageing: a strategic policy solution to demographic ageing in the European Union," *International Journal of Social Welfare*, vol. 21, no. 1, pp. S117–S130, 2012.

[5] The Swedish National Institute, "Healthy ageing—a challenge for Europe," Report 29, The Swedish National Institute of Public Health, Stockholm, Sweden, 2007.

[6] P. von Heideken Wågert, J. M. C. Gustavsson, L. Lundin-Olsson et al., "Health status in the oldest old. Age and sex differences in the Umeå 85+ study," *Aging Clinical and Experimental Research*, vol. 18, no. 2, pp. 116–126, 2006.

[7] M. V. Johnston, "Desiderata for clinical trials in medical rehabilitation," *The American Journal of Physical Medicine and Rehabilitation*, vol. 82, no. 10, pp. S3–S7, 2003.

[8] World Health Organization, *The Ottawa Charter for Health Promotion*, Canadian Public Health Association, Ottawa, Canada, 1986.

[9] A. A. Wilcock, "Reflections on doing, being and becoming," *Australian Occupational Therapy Journal*, vol. 46, no. 1, pp. 1–11, 1999.

[10] A. Meyer, "The philosophy of occupational therapy," *Archives of Occupational Therapy*, vol. 1, pp. 1–10, 1922.

[11] K. B. Adams, S. Leibbrandt, and H. Moon, "A critical review of the literature on social and leisure activity and wellbeing in later life," *Ageing and Society*, vol. 31, pp. 683–712, 2010.

[12] T. A. Glass, C. M. de Leon, R. A. Marottoli, and L. F. Berkman, "Population based study of social and productive activities as predictors of survival among elderly Americans," *British Medical Journal*, vol. 319, no. 7208, pp. 478–483, 1999.

[13] N. Agahi and M. G. Parker, "Leisure activities and mortality: does gender matter?" *Journal of Aging and Health*, vol. 20, no. 7, pp. 855–871, 2008.

[14] M. T. Hyyppä, J. Mäki, O. Impivaara, and A. Aromaa, "Leisure participation predicts survival: a population-based study in Finland," *Health Promotion International*, vol. 21, no. 1, pp. 5–12, 2006.

[15] C. Lennartsson and M. Silverstein, "Does engagement with life enhance survival of elderly people in sweden? The role of social and leisure activities," *Journals of Gerontology: Series B Psychological Sciences and Social Sciences*, vol. 56, no. 6, pp. S335–S342, 2001.

[16] F. Nyqvist, B. Pape, T. Pellfolk, A. K. Forsman, and K. Wahlbeck, "Structural and cognitive aspects of social capital and all-cause mortality: a meta-analysis of cohort studies," *Social Indicators Research*, vol. 116, no. 2, pp. 545–566, 2014.

[17] A. Paganini-Hill, C. H. Kawas, and M. M. Corrada, "Activities and mortality in the elderly: the leisure world cohort study," *Journals of Gerontology, Series A, Biological Sciences and Medical Sciences*, vol. 66, no. 5, pp. 559–567, 2011.

[18] M. C. Janke, G. Nimrod, and D. A. Kleiber, "Reduction in leisure activity and well-being during the transition to widowhood," *Journal of Women and Aging*, vol. 20, no. 1-2, pp. 83–98, 2008.

[19] V. H. Menec, "The relation between everyday activities and successful aging: a 6-year longitudinal study," *Journal of Gerontology Series B: Social Sciences*, vol. 58, no. 2, pp. S74–S82, 2003.

[20] M. C. Janke, A. Davey, and D. Kleiber, "Modeling change in older adults' leisure activities," *Leisure Sciences*, vol. 28, no. 3, pp. 285–303, 2006.

[21] M. Silverstein and M. G. Parker, "Leisure activities and quality of life among the oldest old in Sweden," *Research on Aging*, vol. 24, no. 5, pp. 528–547, 2002.

[22] K. M. Everard, H. W. Lach, E. B. Fisher, and M. C. Baum, "Relationship of activity and social support to the functional health of older adults," *Journals of Gerontology—Series B Psychological Sciences and Social Sciences*, vol. 55, pp. S208–S212, 2000.

[23] I. Nilsson, "Occupational engagement among older people: evaluation, repertoire and relation to life satisfaction," in *Community Medicine and Rehabilitation, Occuaptional Therapy*, Umeå University, Umeå, Sweden, 2006.

[24] T. M. Gill, C. S. Williams, C. F. De Mendes Leon, and M. E. Tinetti, "The role of change in physical performance in determining risk for dependence in activities of daily living

among nondisabled community-living elderly persons," *Journal of Clinical Epidemiology*, vol. 50, no. 7, pp. 765–772, 1997.

[25] C. H. Hirsch, P. Bůžková, J. A. Robbins, K. V. Patel, and A. B. Newman, "Predicting late-life disability and death by the rate of decline in physical performance measures," *Age and Ageing*, vol. 41, no. 2, pp. 155–161, 2012.

[26] World Health Organization, *International Classification of Functioning, Disability and Health*, 2006.

[27] H. Wu, J. Flaherty, B. Dong et al., "Impact of geriatric conditions versus medical diagnoses on ADL disability among nonagenarians and centenarians," *Journal of Aging and Health*, vol. 24, no. 8, pp. 1298–1319, 2012.

[28] A. E. Stuck, J. M. Walthert, T. Nikolaus, C. J. Büla, C. Hohmann, and J. C. Beck, "Risk factors for functional status decline in community-living elderly people: a systematic literature review," *Social Science & Medicine*, vol. 48, no. 4, pp. 445–469, 1999.

[29] T. Sulander, H. Heinonen, T. Pajunen, A. Karisto, P. Pohjolainen, and M. Fogelholm, "Longitudinal changes in functional capacity: effects of socio-economic position among ageing adults," *International Journal for Equity in Health*, vol. 11, no. 1, article 78, 2012.

[30] R. C. Atchley, *Continuity and Adaptation in Aging: Creating Positive Experiences*, Johns Hopkins University Press, Baltimore, Md, USA, 1999.

[31] B. Meinow, M. G. Parker, and M. Thorslund, "Complex health problems and mortality among the oldest old in Sweden: decreased risk for men between 1992 and 2002," *European Journal of Ageing*, vol. 7, no. 2, pp. 81–90, 2010.

[32] G. B. Ploubidis, C. Dale, and E. Grundy, "Later life health in Europe: how important are country level influences?" *European Journal of Ageing*, vol. 9, no. 1, pp. 5–13, 2012.

[33] K. Herbets, "Gerda Botnia 2010. Metod och material," Intern Rapport, 2011 (Swedish).

[34] I. Nilsson and A. Fisher, "Evaluating leisure activities in the oldest old," *Scandinavian Journal of Occupational Therapy*, vol. 13, no. 1, pp. 31–37, 2006.

[35] J. M. Linacre, *WINSTEPS Rasch Measurement Computer Software*, 2010.

[36] I. Nilsson, B. Bernspång, A. C. Fisher, Y. Gustafson, and B. Löfgren, "Occupational engagement and life satisfaction in the oldest-old: the Umeå 85+ study," *OTJR Occupation, Participation and Health*, vol. 27, no. 4, pp. 131–139, 2007.

[37] B. D. Wright and J. M. Linacre, "Reasonable mean-square fit values," *Rasch Measurement Transactions*, vol. 8, p. 370, 1994.

[38] I. K. Crombie, L. Irvine, B. Williams et al., "Why older people do not participate in leisure time physical activity: a survey of activity levels, beliefs and deterrents," *Age and Ageing*, vol. 33, no. 3, pp. 287–292, 2004.

[39] C. A. Chase, K. Mann, S. Wasek, and M. Arbesman, "Systematic review of the effect of home modification and fall prevention programs on falls and the performance of community-dwelling older adults," *The American Journal of Occupational Therapy*, vol. 66, no. 3, pp. 284–291, 2012.

[40] L. P. Montross, C. Depp, J. Daly et al., "Correlates of self-rated successful aging among community-dwelling older adults," *The American Journal of Geriatric Psychiatry*, vol. 14, no. 1, pp. 43–51, 2006.

[41] A. F. G. Cicero, S. D'Addato, F. Santi, A. Ferroni, and C. Borghi, "Leisure-time physical activity and cardiovascular disease mortality: the Brisighella Heart study," *Journal of Cardiovascular Medicine*, vol. 13, no. 9, pp. 559–564, 2012.

[42] M. E. Bravell, S. H. Zarit, and B. Johansson, "Self-reported activities of daily living and performance-based functional ability: a study of congruence among the oldest old," *European Journal of Ageing*, vol. 8, no. 3, pp. 199–209, 2011.

[43] E. Orellano, W. I. Colón, and M. Arbesman, "Effect of occupation- and activity-based interventions on instrumental activities of daily living performance among community-dwelling older adults: a systematic review," *The American Journal of Occupational Therapy*, vol. 66, no. 3, pp. 292–300, 2012.

[44] E. E. Femia, S. H. Zarit, and B. Johansson, "Predicting change in activities of daily living: a longitudinal study of the oldest old in Sweden," *Journals of Gerontology Series B: Psychological Sciences*, vol. 52, no. 6, pp. P294–P302, 1997.

[45] E. E. Femia, S. H. Zarit, and B. Johansson, "The disablement process in very late life: a study of the oldest-old in Sweden," *Journal of Gerontology: Psychological Sciences*, vol. 56, no. 1, pp. P12–P23, 2001.

[46] S. Iwarsson, "A long-term perspective on person-environment fit and ADL dependence among older Swedish adults," *The Gerontologist*, vol. 45, no. 3, pp. 327–336, 2005.

[47] A. M. Jette, D. Rooks, M. Lachman et al., "Home-based resistance training: predictors of participation and adherence," *The Gerontologist*, vol. 38, no. 4, pp. 412–421, 1998.

[48] F. Nyqvist and M. Nygård, "Is the association between social capital and health robust across Nordic regions? Evidence from a cross-sectional study of older adults," *International Journal of Social Welfare*, vol. 22, no. 2, pp. 119–129, 2013.

[49] F. Nyqvist, F. Finnäs, G. Jakobsson, and S. Koskinen, "The effect of social capital on health: the case of two language groups in Finland," *Health & Place*, vol. 14, no. 2, pp. 347–360, 2008.

[50] E. A. Townsend and H. J. Polatajko, *Enabling Occupation II: Advancing an Occupational Therapy Vision for Health, Well-Being, & Justice Through Occupation*, CAOT Publications ACE, Ottawa, Canada, 2007.

[51] G. Kielhofner, *Model of Human Occupation: Theory and Application*, Lippincott Williams & Wilkins, Baltimore, Md, USA, 4th edition, 2008.

[52] M. Law, B. Cooper, S. Strong, D. Stewart, P. Rigby, and L. Letts, "The person-environment-occupation model: a transactive approach to occupational performance," *Canadian Journal of Occupational Therapy*, vol. 63, no. 1, pp. 9–23, 1996.

[53] A. C. Pighalls, D. J. Torgerson, T. A. Sheldon, A. E. Drummond, and J. M. Bland, "Environmental assessment and modification to prevent falls in older people," *Journal of American Geriatric Society*, vol. 59, no. 1, pp. 26–33, 2011.

[54] N. Humpel, N. Owen, and E. Leslie, "Environmental factors associated with adults' participation in physical activity: a review," *American Journal of Preventive Medicine*, vol. 22, no. 3, pp. 188–199, 2002.

[55] L. L. Caldwell, "Leisure and health: why is leisure therapeutic?" *British Journal of Guidance & Counselling*, vol. 33, no. 1, pp. 7–26, 2005.

[56] S. Iso Ahola and R. C. Manell, "Leisure and health," in *Work and Leisure*, J. T. Haworth and A. J. Veal, Eds., Routledge, London, UK, 2004.

[57] S. Volpato, G. Onder, M. Cavalieri et al., "Characteristics of nondisabled older patients developing new disability associated with medical illnesses and hospitalization," *Journal of General Internal Medicine*, vol. 22, no. 5, pp. 668–674, 2007.

[58] C. F. Simpson, C. M. Boyd, M. C. Carlson, M. E. Griswold, J. M. Guralnik, and L. P. Fried, "greement between self-report of disease diagnoses and medical record validation in disabled older women: factors that modify agreements," *Journal of the American Geriatrics Society*, vol. 52, no. 1, pp. 123–127, 2004.

6

Transitions among Health States Using 12 Measures of Successful Aging in Men and Women: Results from the Cardiovascular Health Study

Stephen Thielke[1, 2] and Paula Diehr[3]

[1] *Department of Psychiatry, University of Washington, Seattle, WA 98195, USA*
[2] *Geriatrics Research, Education, and Clinical Center, Puget Sound VA Medical Center and Psychiatry and Behavioral Sciences, University of Washington, P.O. Box 356560, Seattle, WA 98195, USA*
[3] *Departments of Biostastitics and Health Services, University of Washington, Seattle, WA 98195, USA*

Correspondence should be addressed to Stephen Thielke, sthielke@u.washington.edu

Academic Editor: Loretta DiPietro

Introduction. Successful aging has many dimensions, which may manifest differently in men and women at different ages. *Methods.* We characterized one-year transitions among health states in 12 measures of successful aging among adults in the Cardiovascular Health Study. The measures included self-rated health, ADLs, IADLs, depression, cognition, timed walk, number of days spent in bed, number of blocks walked, extremity strength, recent hospitalizations, feelings about life as a whole, and life satisfaction. We dichotomized variables into "healthy" or "sick," states, and estimated the prevalence of the healthy state and the probability of transitioning from one state to another, or dying, during yearly intervals. We compared men and women and three age groups (65–74, 75–84, and 85–94). *Findings.* Measures of successful aging showed similar results by gender. Most participants remained healthy even into advanced ages, although health declined for all measures. Recuperation, although less common with age, still occurred frequently. Men had a higher death rate than women regardless of health status, and were also more likely to remain in the healthy state. *Discussion.* The results suggest a qualitatively different experience of successful aging between men and women. Men did not simply "age faster" than women.

1. Introduction

Changes in health status, symptoms, and functioning during aging defy simple description. Despite the inevitability of death, no orchestrated or predictable decrements in health or types of sickness uniformly precede it, and individuals vary widely in how and how successfully they age. Certain groups may experience aging and health differently from others. The most obvious instance is gender: older men and women have been observed to have different lifespans [1, 2], functional trajectories [3], risk factors for disease [4], chronic and acute diseases [5, 6], and use of medical treatments [7]. There is practical and theoretical importance in understanding health changes during aging, especially the maintenance of health and the ability to recuperate from sickness, differ between men and women.

Successful aging is a multidimensional construct, which initially centered on absence of disease and objective physical and social functioning [8]. Recent research has deemphasized medical disease and concentrated more on self-identified successful aging, psychological health, well-being, mobility, and the absence of frailty [9–12]. There is no canonical definition for successful aging, and no single domain or variable captures all of its facets. Most previous analyses of age and gender effects on health status have examined health transitions for single health measures such as disability, depression, self-rated health, body mass index, ADL, or IADLs [13–21]. Because these studies generally focus on a single aspect of successful aging, and they inconsistently examine gender and age as predictors, they offer somewhat limited perspectives and generally cannot be compared.

There is utility in systematically scrutinizing the changes in different aspects of health status that occur with advancing age among men and women. First, evidence from research can help to counter ageist or sexist stereotypes about health during the aging process, which may influence social expectations, clinical care, and patient decision making [22]. Second, interventions to reduce morbidity and mortality can be better targeted by understanding the prevalence, persistence, and resolution of sickness in different populations. Third, observational results can inform both the theory of successful aging and research into the biology of aging. For instance, research has suggested that men "age faster" than women [23], yet this observation has not received much scrutiny in observational studies.

We sought to characterize a variety of measures of successful aging among a group of older adults, with particular attention to the differences between men and women of different ages. To explore changes in health systematically, and to allow age and gender comparisons, we analyzed transition probabilities for 12 different health variables which capture different aspects of psychological, physical, cognitive, and functional status. We hypothesized, for these 12 different domains of successful aging, that (1) the prevalence of health decreases because both the probability of remaining healthy and the probability of returning to a healthy state decline with increasing age, and (2) the prevalence and transition probabilities are different for men and women.

2. Methods

2.1. Data. Data came from the Cardiovascular Health Study (CHS), a population-based longitudinal study of risk factors for heart disease and stroke in 5888 adults aged 65 and older at baseline [24]. Participants were recruited from a random sample of Medicare eligible adults in four US communities, and extensive data were collected during annual clinic visits and telephone calls. The original cohort of 5201 participants, recruited in 1989 and 1990, had up to ten annual clinic examinations. A second cohort of 687 African Americans, enrolled in 1993 and 1994, had up to seven annual examinations.

The 12 variables used in this study were measures of health based on self-report or observation. They were selected in order to capture various aspects of psychological, physical, cognitive, and functional status. All were measured annually. Each value was dichotomized into "Healthy" and "Sick", as shown in Table 1, using either previously published cutoffs or logical thresholds [27]. Some of the domains involved responses inherently suggestive of sickness. For hospitalization (HOSP), bed days (BED), ADL limitations (ADL), IADL limitations (IADL), and poor extremity strength (EXSTR), participants who endorsed the presence of any difficulty or one or more impairments were considered to be sick in that domain. For feelings that life is worthwhile (FLW), answers of "delighted," "pleased," and "mostly satisfied" were considered healthy; those of "mostly dissatisfied," "unhappy," and "terrible" were considered sick. For satisfaction with the purpose of life (SPL), using a 10-point scale between "extremely satisfied" (1) and "not at all satisfied" (10), answers better than "neither satisfied nor unsatisfied" (<4) were used to characterize health. For depression (DEP), a score of less than 10 on the CES-D depression scale was used to characterize health [20, 28]. For self-rated health (SRH), self-reported "excellent," "very good," or "good" general health were defined as healthy, and "fair" or "poor" as sick [29]. Healthy cognitive status (COG) was defined as above 89 points on a 100-point scale, corresponding to 26 or higher on the MMSE, which is suggestive of intact cognition [30]. The sick state for ambulation (TWLK) was defined by a velocity of less than 0.66 feet per second (10 seconds) in a 15-foot walk, which is a marker for low speed [31]. Blocks walked during the last week (BLK) were dichotomized at 28 blocks or more to signify the healthy state [32]. Because the analyses compared age and gender groups within each domain rather than the domains to each other, the variability in the prevalence of healthy and sick states as a result of different cutoffs were unlikely to influence the main results significantly.

In order to simplify comparisons, age was divided into three categories—65–74, 75–84, and 85–94—in accordance with the common definitions of "young old," "old old," and "oldest old". Persons could contribute data to more than one age category, depending on their age at the start of each transition.

Missing data were imputed, after a transformation to recode death as zero health, by interpolating over time between existing data points for each person. Any data that remained missing at the end of a sequence were extrapolated as an average of the last observed value and of transformed self-rated health (which was measured every 6 months and is thus well characterized) [33, 34]. No imputation across participants was performed. All available observations were used, including those that were imputed.

2.2. Statistical Approach. In order to represent and compare prevalence and incidence of healthy and sick states in various domains, and to account for death, we used a transition probability approach. This technique has been used to examine other changes in health among older adults, including self-rated health [13], obesity [14], depression [20], and pain [35]. Transition probability models make the simple assumption that health status measures can be categorized into discrete states, among which individuals can move. The ovals in Figure 1 represent discrete health states, and the arrows show the likelihood of transitioning from one state to another during a single time interval, one year. The number of individuals in each of the states (shown by the ovals) is the relative prevalence of health or sickness in the total population.

When evaluated at two time points, there are thus six possible transitions among these states: remaining healthy (P(HtoH)), becoming sick (P(HtoS)), remaining sick (P(StoS)), becoming healthy (P(StoH)), dying from a state of health (P(HtoD)), and dying from a state of sickness (P(StoD)). Persons move among those states with certain

Table 1: 12 Measures of successful aging.

Category	Abbreviation	Question	Definition of healthy
Not hospitalized	HOSP	"Did you stay overnight in the hospital in the last 6 months?"	No report of being hospitalized
No bed days	BED	"During the past two weeks, how many days have you stayed in bed all or most of the day because of illness or injury?"	No days in bed reported
Life satisfaction	SPL	"How satisfied are you with the meaning and purpose of your life? on a scale of 1–10, with 1 being extremely and 10 being not at all"	Score of 1 to 4
Life as a whole	FLW	"How do you feel about life as a whole?" (1: delighted; 3: mostly satisfied; 6: terrible)	Score of 1–3
Not depressed	DEP	10 questions of the center for epidemiologic studies short depression scale [25], each ranked 0–3	Score < 10, out of a possible 30 points
No limitations in activities of daily living	ADL	"Do you have any difficulty performing this activity?" from a list of walking, transferring, eating, dressing, bathing, or toileting	No difficulties reported
No limitations in independent activities of daily living	IADL	"Do you have any difficulty performing this activity?" from a list of heavy or light housework, shopping, meal preparation, money management, or telephoning	No difficulties reported
Intact extremity strength	EXSTR	"Do you have any difficulty with this activity" from a list of lifting, reaching, or gripping	No difficulty reported
Self-rated health	SRH	"How would you rate your health in general: excellent, very good, good, fair, or poor?"	Excellent, very good, or good self-reported health
Intact cognition	COG	Modified minimental state examination [26], scored from 0 to 100	Score above 89
Ability to ambulate	TWLK	Timed 15 foot walk	Less than 10 seconds
Frequent ambulation	BLK	"During the last week, how many city blocks did you walk?"	>4 blocks per day, on average

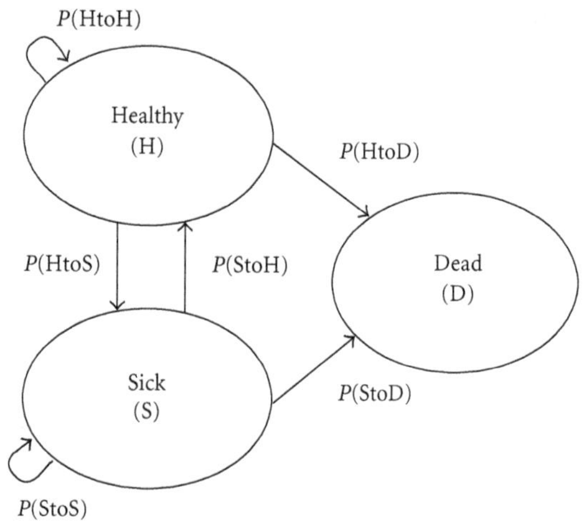

Figure 1: Transition probability model, showing the probability of remaining in a state or moving to another state during specific time intervals (such as one year).

probabilities, which may vary by age, gender, or other characteristics. The equilibrium—or steady state—prevalence of a system can be calculated directly from the transition probabilities [36].

2.3. Analysis. The prevalence of the healthy state of each variable in each wave was calculated as the percentage of living persons who were healthy. The one-year probabilities of transitioning from state to state were estimated from crosstabulation of data collected one-year apart. All cases where a beginning state and a starting state were available were used, for all 5888 participants. General patterns by age and gender groups were described. We estimated one-year transition probabilities for participants starting in each health state (sick or healthy). These transition probabilities, shown in Figure 1, were constructed as a simple fraction: number of moving to other state or remaining in state/ number in the state at the starting time point. Calculations were performed separately for each age and gender grouping. The associations of the estimated transition probabilities with age and gender were tested using cross-sectional time series logistic regression (the xtlogit command in Stata). This form of generalized estimating equation accounts for participants contributing multiple observations. We carried out separate analyses for men and women of the same age group and estimated the statistical significance of the difference using generalized estimating equations.

The level of significance for individual comparisons was set at $P < 0.05$, two tailed, and differences between men and women in the same age group at this degree are shown in bold in the tables. The differences by age are described in the text. We summarize the significant findings across variables, with the reminder that 5% of all significant differences could be due to chance. There was no explicit adjustment for multiple comparisons, because all of the results were shown (i.e., we did not select only the significant results after running multiple models and because of the large number of potential combined hypotheses.)

Analyses were conducted in Stata (StataCorp, College Station, Texas, version 11.2).

3. Findings

45,297 transition pairs (starting and ending state, separated by one year) from the 5888 participants were analyzed. During the study, 1684 participants died. For the whole sample, 13.5% of observations were missing and imputed, with some variability across the 12 domains of health. In the year prior to death, 7% of all observations were missing, which were part of the imputed fraction. The median number of imputed observations per participant was one.

As an illustration of the analytic approach, the prevalences and selected transition probabilities for ADL are shown in Figure 2. "Healthy" was defined as having no difficulties with activities of daily living, and "sick" as having one or more difficulties. The third and fourth lines from the top represent the healthy prevalence (proportion of the living who had no ADL difficulties), with a solid line for males and a dotted line for females. The prevalence is quite high for the youngest group (about 90%) and declines over time. The healthy prevalence is higher for men than for women, and the difference becomes larger with age. The lowermost two lines represent the probability of recovering from the sick state (having ADL difficulties) by transitioning into the healthy state (no ADL difficulties) one year later, labeled as P(StoH). The probability is initially near 0.4 and is higher for women than for men. The two topmost lines in the graph represent the probability of staying in the healthy state, P(HtoH). This probability is initially about 0.9 and is higher for men than for women. This figure shows how transitions and prevalence both change over time and differ between men and women, and also how relatively small differences in transitions accumulate into more pronounced differences in prevalence.

3.1. Prevalence of the Healthy State. The first two lines of Table 2 show the number of observations (transition pairs) in each group, and the mean age, by age category and gender. Mean age did not differ significantly in each category for men and women. The next 12 lines show the prevalence of a healthy state for each variable. For example, for HOSP, 91.3% of the women aged 65–74 were "healthy," defined as "having no hospital days." For men in the same age range, the prevalence of a healthy state was 88.0%. Over the three age groups, women's prevalence for HOSP declined from 91.3% to 87.8% to 84.9%.

Prevalence by Age and Gender. All of the prevalence values in Table 2 declined with age; the prevalence values were significantly lower at each subsequent age group compared with the younger one. The bolded entries in Table 2 show the situations where women or men had a significantly higher prevalence of a healthy state. Women were significantly healthier than men only for HOSP and COG. Men had a significantly higher prevalence of a healthy state than women for all the 33 other domains and age groups, except for three where there was no significant difference.

3.2. Transitions Probabilities for Healthy Persons. Table 3 shows the transition probabilities for persons who were initially in the healthy state. For instance, for HOSP, age 65–74, women who were healthy (without a hospital stay in the first year) had a 0.92 probability of remaining healthy (not having a hospital stay in the next year), a 0.08 probability of becoming sick (having a hospital stay), and a 0.01 probability of dying. The bold entries in the upper and lower tables represent probabilities where women or men became or remained significantly healthier. More than half of the comparisons were found to be statistically significant.

In all three comparisons (remaining healthy, becoming sick, and dying from a healthy state), there was a significant decline with advancing age for almost all the domains of health. Men were more likely than women to remain healthy and less likely to become sick in the majority of comparisons, and men were more likely to die.

3.3. Transition Probabilities for Sick Persons. Table 4 shows the transition probabilities for persons who were initially in the sick state. The bolded entries indicate probabilities of remaining in or recovery from sickness, or probability of death, that were significantly healthier in women (in the top of the table) or in men (in the bottom). For convenience we considered P(StoS), remaining sick, as an unfavorable transition, because the person did not recover, but it could also be considered as favorable because the person did not die.

In almost all domains of health, the probability of recovery from a sick state declined significantly with age, while the probability of dying from a sick state increased with age. Women were significantly more likely than men to recover from a sick state in six of 36 total groups; men were more likely to recover in 12. Men were less likely to remain in a sick state than women in 23 of the 36 groups; in no cases were women significantly less likely than men to remain sick. For every health variable, men were significantly more likely to die from a state of sickness than women were.

4. Discussion

4.1. Overview. This analysis, unlike previous approaches that have focused on one or a few domains of health, examined the prevalence of and transitions in 12 measures of successful aging among a cohort of older adults. The 12 health-related variables, while related, were diverse and included measures of physical and mental health, quality of life, and health behaviors. Some were self-reported and some were measured through objective tests. Some were subjective single item questions while others were based on structured

Table 2: Prevalence of a healthy state among men and women, with health defined separately for each domain. Bolded entries represent significantly higher prevalence of health in women (left columns) or men (right columns). The differences between groups based on age are described in the text.

	Female			Male		
	65–74	75–84	85–94	65–74	75–84	85–94
Number of observations	12261	12433	2183	7801	8867	1752
Mean age	71.0	78.6	87.5	71.1	78.6	87.7
HOSP: no hospital days	**91.3**	**87.8**	**84.9**	88.0	85.6	81.7
BED: no bed days	94.3	92.3	89.3	**95.9**	**94.6**	**91.3**
SPL: Satisfied with purpose of life	75.7	69.8	59.6	**80.7**	**75.2**	**67.4**
DEP: not depressed	80.2	73.8	64.3	**87.6**	**81.4**	**70.9**
ADL: no ADL difficulties	86.3	76.1	56.7	**90.2**	**82.7**	**67.6**
FLW: feel life is worthwhile	94.4	91.0	83.6	**95.3**	91.7	85.6
EXSTR: good extremity strength	67.6	57.6	42.1	**84.6**	**78.8**	**65.4**
SRH: high self-rated health	79.0	70.8	60.7	80.0	**73.6**	**64.7**
TWLK: walk 10 feet < 10 seconds	64.3	44.5	16.9	**73.8**	**58.6**	**30.0**
IADL: no IADL difficulties	71.8	58.7	39.5	**80.9**	**70.5**	**50.7**
COG: 3 MSE > 90	**70.9**	**54.6**	**27.6**	67.2	53.1	25.7
BLK: walked 4+ blocks per day	33.3	20.9	8.5	**47.7**	**37.8**	**22.3**

Table 3: One-year transition probabilities for those starting in a healthy state for 12 different variables. Bolded entries indicate a significantly healthier transition (more likely remaining healthy, less likely remaining sick, or less likely dying) among women compared to men (top half) or men compared to women (bottom half). The differences between groups based on age are described in the text.

	Age 65–74			Age 75–84			Age 85–94		
	P(HtoH)	P(HtoS)	P(HtoD)	P(HtoH)	P(HtoS)	P(HtoD)	P(HtoH)	P(HtoS)	P(HtoD)
Female									
HOSP	**0.92**	**0.08**	**0.01**	**0.88**	**0.10**	**0.02**	**0.80**	**0.13**	**0.07**
BED	0.95	0.05	**0.01**	0.92	0.06	**0.02**	0.86	0.08	**0.06**
SPL	0.85	0.15	**0.01**	0.80	0.18	**0.02**	0.70	0.27	**0.04**
DEP	0.88	0.11	**0.01**	0.84	0.14	**0.02**	0.77	0.19	**0.04**
ADL	0.90	0.09	**0.01**	0.85	0.14	**0.02**	0.72	0.24	**0.04**
FLW	**0.96**	0.04	**0.01**	0.92	0.06	**0.02**	**0.85**	0.11	**0.05**
EXSTR	0.83	0.17	**0.01**	0.77	0.21	**0.02**	0.66	0.30	**0.03**
SRH	**0.90**	**0.30**	**0.01**	0.85	0.37	**0.01**	0.73	**0.40**	**0.04**
TWLK	0.83	0.17	**0.00**	0.72	0.27	**0.01**	0.54	0.45	**0.01**
IADL	0.85	0.15	**0.01**	0.77	0.21	**0.02**	0.61	0.35	0.05
COG	**0.86**	**0.13**	**0.01**	**0.81**	**0.18**	**0.01**	0.67	0.30	0.04
BLK	0.65	0.01	**0.00**	0.55	**0.01**	**0.01**	0.49	0.03	0.03
Male									
HOSP	0.88	0.10	0.02	0.85	0.12	0.03	0.76	0.15	0.09
BED	0.95	**0.03**	0.02	0.92	**0.04**	0.04	0.84	0.07	0.10
SPL	**0.86**	**0.12**	0.02	**0.82**	**0.16**	0.03	0.71	**0.21**	0.08
DEP	**0.91**	**0.08**	0.02	**0.86**	**0.11**	0.03	0.76	**0.16**	0.07
ADL	**0.92**	**0.06**	0.02	**0.87**	**0.11**	0.03	0.75	**0.18**	0.07
FLW	0.95	**0.03**	0.02	0.92	0.05	0.03	0.82	0.10	0.08
EXSTR	**0.90**	**0.08**	0.02	**0.85**	**0.12**	0.03	0.74	**0.20**	0.06
SRH	0.89	0.35	0.01	0.84	**0.34**	0.03	0.75	0.45	0.06
TWLK	**0.85**	**0.13**	0.02	**0.76**	**0.22**	0.02	0.61	**0.34**	0.05
IADL	**0.88**	**0.11**	0.01	**0.81**	**0.17**	0.02	0.64	**0.30**	0.06
COG	0.83	0.15	0.02	0.78	0.20	0.03	0.62	0.33	0.05
BLK	**0.72**	0.02	0.01	**0.63**	0.02	0.02	0.54	0.04	0.03

TABLE 4: One-year transition probabilities for those starting in a sick state for 12 different variables. Bolded entries indicate a significantly healthier transition (more likely becoming healthy, less likely remaining sick, or less likely dying) among women compared to men (top half) or men compared to women (bottom half). The differences between groups based on age are described in the text.

	Age 65–74			Age 75–84			Age 85–94		
	P(StoH)	P(StoS)	P(StoD)	P(StoH)	P(StoS)	P(StoD)	P(StoH)	P(StoS)	P(StoD)
Female									
HOSP	0.68	0.26	0.06	**0.61**	0.29	**0.11**	0.54	0.27	**0.20**
BED	0.55	0.37	**0.08**	**0.44**	0.41	**0.15**	0.34	0.37	**0.30**
SPL	0.37	0.60	**0.03**	0.30	0.64	**0.06**	0.24	0.61	**0.16**
DEP	0.35	0.62	**0.03**	0.29	0.64	**0.07**	0.20	0.63	**0.17**
ADL	**0.36**	0.59	**0.05**	0.25	0.67	**0.08**	0.15	0.70	**0.15**
FLW	**0.37**	0.54	**0.09**	**0.29**	0.56	**0.15**	0.18	0.53	**0.29**
EXSTR	0.31	0.66	**0.03**	0.23	0.72	**0.05**	0.14	0.74	**0.12**
SRH	0.31	0.64	**0.04**	0.25	0.67	**0.07**	**0.24**	0.61	**0.15**
TWLK	0.29	0.68	**0.03**	0.16	0.80	**0.05**	0.06	0.84	**0.10**
IADL	0.30	0.67	**0.03**	0.22	0.73	**0.05**	0.16	0.73	**0.11**
COG	0.27	0.70	**0.03**	0.17	0.78	**0.05**	0.07	0.83	**0.11**
BLK	0.14	0.84	**0.02**	0.08	0.88	**0.04**	0.03	0.88	**0.09**
Male									
HOSP	0.63	0.29	0.08	0.56	0.28	0.16	0.49	0.23	0.28
BED	0.49	0.35	0.15	0.33	0.36	0.32	0.26	0.33	0.41
SPL	**0.41**	**0.53**	0.06	0.32	**0.56**	0.12	0.24	**0.54**	0.22
DEP	0.37	**0.54**	0.08	0.27	**0.57**	0.16	0.18	0.58	0.25
ADL	0.31	0.59	0.10	0.23	**0.60**	0.17	0.13	**0.63**	0.24
FLW	0.29	0.55	0.16	0.20	0.52	0.28	0.15	0.46	0.39
EXSTR	**0.37**	**0.57**	0.07	**0.31**	**0.56**	0.14	**0.20**	**0.56**	0.24
SRH	0.32	**0.60**	0.08	0.25	**0.62**	0.13	0.18	0.59	0.24
TWLK	**0.34**	**0.61**	0.05	**0.21**	**0.70**	0.09	**0.08**	**0.76**	0.16
IADL	**0.34**	**0.59**	0.08	**0.24**	**0.64**	0.12	0.17	**0.64**	0.19
COG	0.27	0.69	0.04	0.18	**0.74**	0.08	0.07	**0.78**	0.15
BLK	**0.21**	**0.76**	0.04	**0.14**	**0.79**	0.07	**0.08**	**0.77**	0.15

responses. Despite these differences, most of the measures of successful aging performed in very similar ways with regard to their associations with age and gender.

4.2. Age Trends. Overall, the trends in prevalence suggest both high initial rates of health and consistent incremental declines in health with advancing age. First, the prevalence of emotional and functional health shown in Table 2 remained quite high, even at advanced ages. For instance, about 85% of 85–94-year-old individuals expressed the belief that life is worthwhile. Second, health declined with advancing age across all the domains: there were no areas that were spared the effects of aging. Some aspects declined more dramatically, especially the functional measures of cognition, timed walk, and blocks walked. In these domains, the proportion of participants who were healthy in the oldest group was less than half the proportion of who were healthy in the youngest group. Nevertheless, the majority of men and women aged 85–94 in this community cohort had no hospital days, no bed days, no ADL difficulties, were not depressed, had high self-rated health, and felt that life was worthwhile. These findings are a testament to overall successful aging among the old old and oldest old, and challenge stereotypes about the high prevalence of sickness and disability in these groups.

4.3. Prevalence and Incidence by Gender and Age. Men were observed to have a higher prevalence of a healthy state except for hospitalization and cognitive status. In Table 4, P(HtoS) is consistently higher for men than for women only for these domains of health; Table 3 shows smaller and less consistent differences in P(StoH). Most of the gender difference is thus driven by difference in incidence of sickness rather than difference in recovery from it. In other words, men seem to be healthier because they are less likely to transition *into* sick states, while men and women show roughly the same return to health. This implies an aging process for men in which the sickest persons are consistently removed by recovery or death, while for women the sickest persons are less likely to be removed. A different trend is seen for the age effects: with increasing age, the probability of staying healthy becomes lower than the probability of staying sick, which decreases the prevalence of health. Older adults are thus less healthy than younger adults mainly as a result of less likely recovery from sickness combined with higher probability of death. These findings may have some implications for disease prevention and treatment programs [37].

4.4. Patterns of Aging in Men and Women. We found several key differences in aging based on gender. Men died more often than women from a state of either sickness or health, remained more healthy than women while alive, and were more likely to recover from being sick. These differences were not characterized by similar transitions offset by a period of years, as might happen if men's health trajectories were simply premature or accelerated versions of women'strajectories. Comparing the adjacent age categories for men and women (for instance, 65–7-year-old men compared to 75–84-year-old women) shows that younger men's transitions were more similar to older women'stransitions than younger women's transitions to older men's transitions for 58 (60%) of the 96 possible comparisons. This is seen graphically for ADL status in Figure 2, where the transition probabilities for men are consistently higher for P(HtoH) but lower for P(StoH), and there is no transformation of the women's transitions (as by moving the lines for women to the left, or by compressing the curves) that would make them match those for men.

These results demonstrate qualitative differences in health transitions between men and women during aging, not just that men "age faster", as has been suggested [23]. If this had been the case, men would have developed sickness sooner than women, remained sick as much as women, and had equal likelihood of dying from a state of sickness as women. Not only was this effect not seen but also in many cases opposite effects were observed. The findings suggest that men may show more compression or squaring of mortality than women [38]. Put another way, the occurrence of sickness—regardless of the operational definition—does not seem to be the key intermediary which makes men die sooner than women, and no other factor associated with gender well accounts for this effect.

The observed differences in incidence and prevalence of health between men and women encourage speculation about their etiology in human gender dimorphism and argue for fundamental differences between how men and women age. Historical analyses suggest that the environmental pressures of infectious disease and resource availability have caused women to live longer [39]. Some research suggests that lower mortality among women could be attributable to a low-risk, healthy lifestyle [40, 41], or to lack of male hormones such as testosterone [42]. Other factors include the unequal distribution of chronic conditions, health behaviors like smoking, and differential effects of diseases on mortality [40]. Women may assess their health differently, for instance by applying different anchoring points to define sick and healthy states, or by being more willing to assume the sick role. [43, 44]. This latter possibility is supported by the fact that hospitalization and cognitive status, the only variables where women were healthier than men, are relatively objective measures. Nonetheless, timed walk, another objective measure of health, favored men. In order to understand the underlying factors behind these gender differences better, it might be useful to repeat these analyses using other variables, datasets, and age groups, with

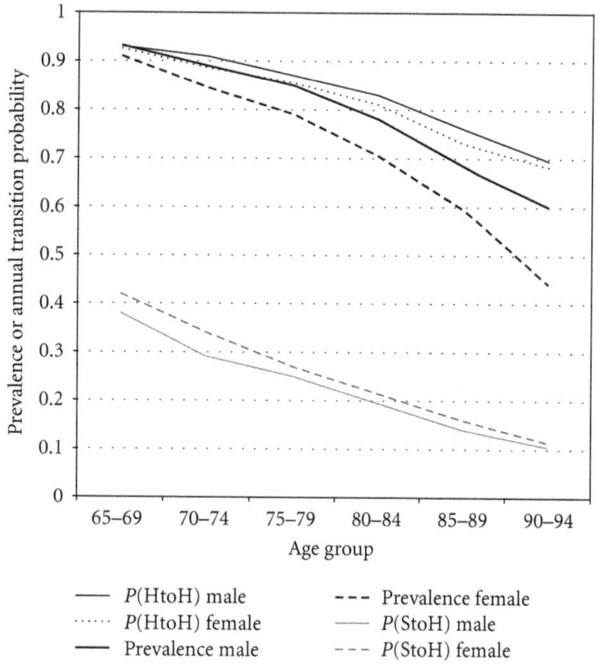

FIGURE 2: Prevalence, maintenance, and recovery for ADL Health by age and sex. The prevalence estimates are the proportion with no ADL difficulties. The transition probability estimates are the likelihoods of remaining healthy (P(HtoH)) and of returning to health (P(HtoS)) over one-year intervals.

attention to differences in self-reported and performance measures.

4.5. Limitations. First, about one-tenth of the data were missing and had to be imputed. The ascertainment of death, however, was essentially complete. The approach we used for imputation, using interpolation and extrapolation, may have minimized changes by assuming that the missing health status was mainly consistent with the data before and after the missing measurement and declined close to death. There was no difference in missingness between men and women, and it is unlikely that this imputation method would intensify group differences. Second, the individual significance tests that are reported here should be considered as descriptive rather than definitive, due to the large number of comparisons that were made in this analysis. Third, the category of "healthy" in the various outcome measures should not be interpreted literally, since the cutoffs for healthy and sick states were assigned by categorizing each variable individually, and not by cross-validating them with other metrics for subjective or objective health. Most of the cutoffs have face validity as markers of health. Fourth, in the interests of generating straightforward descriptive results, we did not adjust for other patient-level health or sociodemographic characteristics which might confound the associations between age, gender, and health. Investigating these could help understand how men and women differ in the aging process.

5. Summary and Conclusion

Transition probabilities among various states of health during aging, and separately for men and women, are rarely reported in ways that can be compared. We calculated the gender-specific transition probabilities for 12 health-related variables across different domains of health and believe that these have utility for organizing future research and for characterizing the changes that happen during aging. In general, the 12 variables all behaved similarly. Recuperation from sickness declined with age, but still occurred frequently. Men and women experienced different types of change in health over time, with men showing more health and less sickness, but greater likelihood of dying. Men did not simply age faster compared to women. They exhibited a more "square" pattern of health status over time, with dropoff at younger ages than women. There is no simple explanation for the differences observed between men and women; they may partly relate to women's health-related behaviors or perceptions of health, or to more biologically fundamental gender dimorphisms. Future study can help to clarify how health is constructed and changes in different groups during aging.

Acknowledgments

The research reported in this paper was supported by contracts N01-HC-85239 and N01-HC-85079 through N01-HC-85086, N01-HC-35129, N01 HC-15103, N01 HC-55222, N01-HC-75150, and N01-HC-45133 and Grant HL080295 from the National Heart, Lung, and Blood Institute (NHLBI), with additional contribution from the National Institute of Neurological Disorders and Stroke (NINDS). Additional support was provided through AG-023629, AG-15928, AG-20098, and AG-027058 from the National Institute on Aging (NIA). A full list of principal CHS investigators and institutions can be found at http://www.chs-nhlbi.org/pi.htm. Additional support was provided by K23 MH093591 Career Development Award (Thielke).

References

[1] A. C. Carlsson, H. Theobald, and P. E. Wändell, "Health factors and longevity in men and women: a 26-year follow-up study," *European Journal of Epidemiology*, vol. 25, no. 8, pp. 547–551, 2010.

[2] M. O. Baerlocher, "Differences in healthy life expectancy among men and women," *Canadian Medical Association Journal*, vol. 177, no. 10, p. 1174, 2007.

[3] K. Schultz-Larsen, N. Rahmanfard, and C. Holst, "Physical activity (PA) and the disablement process: a 14-year follow-up study of older non-disabled women and men," *Archives of Gerontology and Geriatrics*, vol. 55, no. 1, pp. 25–30, 2012.

[4] N. Goldman, M. Weinstein, J. Cornman, B. Singer, T. Seeman, and M. C. Chang, "Sex differentials in biological risk factors for chronic disease: estimates from population-based surveys," *Journal of Women's Health*, vol. 13, no. 4, pp. 393–403, 2004.

[5] L. M. Verbrugge, "Females and illness: recent trends in sex differences in the United States," *Journal of Health and Social Behavior*, vol. 17, no. 4, pp. 387–403, 1976.

[6] C. Rius, G. Pérez, M. Rodríguez-Sanz, and E. Fernàndez, "Comorbidity index was successfully validated among men but not in women," *Journal of Clinical Epidemiology*, vol. 61, no. 8, pp. 796–802, 2008.

[7] S. A. K. Stock, B. Stollenwerk, M. Redaelli, D. Civello, and K. W. Lauterbach, "Sex differences in treatment patterns of six chronic diseases: an analysis from the German Statutory Health Insurance," *Journal of Women's Health*, vol. 17, no. 3, pp. 343–354, 2008.

[8] J. W. Rowe and R. L. Kahn, "Successful aging," *Gerontologist*, vol. 37, no. 4, pp. 433–440, 1997.

[9] E. A. Phelan, L. A. Anderson, A. Z. LaCroix, and E. B. Larson, "Older adults' views of "successful aging"—how do they compare with researchers' definitions?" *Journal of the American Geriatrics Society*, vol. 52, no. 2, pp. 211–216, 2004.

[10] R. A. Parslow, V. J. Lewis, and R. Nay, "Successful aging: development and testing of a multidimensional model using data from a large sample of older Australians," *Journal of the American Geriatrics Society*, vol. 59, no. 11, pp. 2077–2083, 2011.

[11] K. A. Lowry, A. N. Vallejo, and S. A. Studenski, "Successful aging as a continuum of functional independence: lessons from physical disability models of aging," *Aging and Disease*, vol. 3, no. 1, pp. 5–15, 2012.

[12] I. V. Vahia, T. W. Meeks, W. K. Thompson et al., "Subthreshold depression and successful aging in older women," *American Journal of Geriatric Psychiatry*, vol. 18, no. 3, pp. 212–220, 2010.

[13] P. Diehr and D. L. Patrick, "Probabilities of transition among health states for older adults," *Quality of Life Research*, vol. 10, no. 5, pp. 431–442, 2001.

[14] P. Diehr, E. S. O'Meara, A. Fitzpatrick, A. B. Newman, L. Kuller, and G. Burke, "Weight, mortality, years of healthy life, and active life expectancy in older adults," *Journal of the American Geriatrics Society*, vol. 56, no. 1, pp. 76–83, 2008.

[15] P. Diehr, A. Derleth, A. B. Newman, and Liming Cai, "The number of sick persons in a cohort," *Research on Aging*, vol. 29, no. 6, pp. 555–575, 2007.

[16] S. E. Hardy, J. A. Dubin, T. R. Holford, and T. M. Gill, "Transitions between states of disability and independence among older persons," *American Journal of Epidemiology*, vol. 161, no. 6, pp. 575–584, 2005.

[17] M. H. Chin, J. X. Zhang, and P. J. Rathouz, "Transitions in health status in older patients with heart failure," *Southern Medical Journal*, vol. 96, no. 11, pp. 1096–1106, 2003.

[18] S. E. Hardy, H. G. Allore, Z. Guo, and T. M. Gill, "Explaining the effect of gender on functional transitions in older persons," *Gerontology*, vol. 54, no. 2, pp. 79–86, 2008.

[19] D. A. Wolf and T. M. Gill, "Modeling transition rates using panel current-status data: hsow serious is the bias?" *Demography*, vol. 46, no. 2, pp. 371–386, 2009.

[20] S. M. Thielke, P. Diehr, and J. Unutzer, "Prevalence, incidence, and persistence of major depressive symptoms in the Cardiovascular Health Study," *Aging and Mental Health*, vol. 14, no. 2, pp. 168–176, 2010.

[21] S. G. Leveille, B. W. J. H. Penninx, D. Melzer, G. Izmirlian, and J. M. Guralnik, "Sex differences in the prevalence of mobility disability in old age: the dynamics of incidence, recovery, and mortality," *Journals of Gerontology B*, vol. 55, no. 1, pp. S41–S50, 2000.

[22] B. Levy, "Stereotype embodiment: a psychosocial approach to aging," *Current Directions in Psychological Science*, vol. 18, no. 6, pp. 332–336, 2009.

[23] M. V. Blagosklonny, "Why men age faster but reproduce longer than women: mTOR and evolutionary perspectives," *Aging*, vol. 2, no. 5, pp. 265–273, 2010.

[24] L. P. Fried, N. O. Borhani, P. Enright et al., "The cardiovascular Health Study: design and rationale," *Annals of Epidemiology*, vol. 1, no. 3, pp. 263–276, 1991.

[25] L. L. Radoff, "The CESD Scale: a self-report depression scale for research in the general population," *Applied Psychological Measurement*, vol. 1, pp. 385–401, 1977.

[26] E. L. Teng and H. C. Chui, "The Modified Mini-Mental State (MMS) examination," *Journal of Clinical Psychiatry*, vol. 48, no. 8, pp. 314–318, 1987.

[27] P. Diehr, S. Thielke, E. O'Meara, A. L. Fitzpatrick, and A. Newman, "Comparing years of healthy life, measured in 16 ways, for normal weight and overweight older adults," *Journal of Obesity*, vol. 2012, Article ID 894894, 13 pages, 2012.

[28] E. M. Andresen, J. A. Malmgren, W. B. Carter, and D. L. Patrick, "Screening for depression in well older adults: evaluation of a short form of the CES-D," *American Journal of Preventive Medicine*, vol. 10, no. 2, pp. 77–84, 1994.

[29] P. Diehr, J. Williamson, D. L. Patrick, D. E. Bild, and G. L. Burke, "Patterns of self-rated health in older adults before and after sentinel health events," *Journal of the American Geriatrics Society*, vol. 49, no. 1, pp. 36–44, 2001.

[30] J. T. Tschanz, K. A. Welsh-Bohmer, B. L. Plassman et al., "An adaptation of the modified mini-mental state examination: analysis of demographic influences and normative data. The Cache County Study," *Neuropsychiatry, Neuropsychology and Behavioral Neurology*, vol. 15, no. 1, pp. 28–38, 2002.

[31] J. E. Graham, G. V. Ostir, Y. F. Kuo, S. R. Fisher, and K. J. Ottenbacher, "Relationship between test methodology and mean velocity in timed walk tests: a review," *Archives of Physical Medicine and Rehabilitation*, vol. 89, no. 5, pp. 865–872, 2008.

[32] D. Mozaffarian, C. D. Furberg, B. M. Psaty, and D. Siscovick, "Physical activity and incidence of atrial fibrillation in older adults the cardiovascular health study," *Circulation*, vol. 118, no. 8, pp. 800–807, 2008.

[33] P. Diehr, D. L. Patrick, J. Spertus, C. I. Kiefe, M. McDonell, and S. D. Fihn, "Transforming self-rated health and the SF-36 scales to include death and improve interpretability," *Medical Care*, vol. 39, no. 7, pp. 670–679, 2001.

[34] P. Diehr, W. E. Lafferty, D. L. Patrick, L. Downey, S. M. Devlin, and L. J. Standish, "Quality of life at the end of life," *Health and Quality of Life Outcomes*, vol. 5, article 51, 2007.

[35] S. M. Thielke, H. Whitson, P. Diehr et al., "Persistence and remission of musculoskeletal pain in community-dwelling older adults: results from the Cardiovascular Health Study," *Journal of the American Geriatrics Society*, vol. 60, no. 8, pp. 1393–1400, 2012.

[36] P. Diehr, D. Yanez, A. Derleth, and A. B. Newman, "Age-specific prevalence and years of healthy life in a system with three health states," *Statistics in Medicine*, vol. 27, no. 9, pp. 1371–1386, 2008.

[37] P. Diehr, A. Derleth, L. Cai, and A. B. Newman, "The effect of different public health interventions on longevity, morbidity, and years of healthy life," *BMC Public Health*, vol. 7, article 52, 2007.

[38] J. F. Fries, "The compression of morbidity," *Milbank Quarterly*, vol. 83, no. 4, pp. 801–823, 2005.

[39] A. P. Møller, C. L. Fincher, and R. Thornhill, "Why men have shorter lives than women: effects of resource availability, infectious disease, and senescence," *American Journal of Human Biology*, vol. 21, no. 3, pp. 357–364, 2009.

[40] A. Case and C. Paxson, "Sex differences in morbidity and mortality," *Demography*, vol. 42, no. 2, pp. 189–214, 2005.

[41] S. E. Chiuve, T. T. Fung, K. M. Rexrode et al., "Adherence to a low-risk, healthy lifestyle and risk of sudden cardiac death among women," *Journal of the American Medical Association*, vol. 306, no. 1, pp. 62–69, 2011.

[42] E. Nieschlag, U. Kramer, and S. Nieschlag, "Androgens shorten the longevity of women: sopranos last longer," *Experimental and Clinical Endocrinology and Diabetes*, vol. 111, no. 4, pp. 230–231, 2003.

[43] J. A. Salomon, A. Tandon, and C. J. L. Murray, "Comparability of self rated health: cross sectional multi-country survey using anchoring vignettes," *British Medical Journal*, vol. 328, no. 7434, pp. 258–261, 2004.

[44] J. B. Dowd and M. Todd, "Does self-reported health bias the measurement of health inequalities in u.s. adults? evidence using anchoring vignettes from the health and retirement study," *Journals of Gerontology B*, vol. 66, no. 4, pp. 478–489, 2011.

7

Employing a Participatory Research Approach to Explore Physical Activity among Older African American Women

Emerson Sebastião, Kelechi Ibe-Lamberts, Julie Bobitt, Andiara Schwingel, and Wojtek Chodzko-Zajko

Aging and Diversity Lab, Department of Kinesiology and Community Health, University of Illinois, 209 Louise Freer Hall, 906 S Goodwin Avenue, Urbana, IL 61801, USA

Correspondence should be addressed to Emerson Sebastião; esebast2@illinois.edu

Academic Editor: F. R. Ferraro

Introduction. Older African American women are particularly vulnerable to unhealthy lifestyle behaviors such as physical inactivity and the resultant chronic diseases and conditions. This study explored older African American women's perception of physical activity as well as facilitators of and barriers to being physically active in their local environment. *Methods.* Using a participatory research approach, a total of 7 women aged 65 years and over had their PA level assessed objectively through accelerometry. In addition, physical activity was discussed through the photo-elicitation procedure, which was supplemented by semistructured interviews. Qualitative thematic analysis was used to identify patterns and themes emerging from participants' interview. *Results.* Participants exhibited low levels of physical activity and viewed "physical activity" to be a broadly defined, nonspecific construct. Interviews revealed that many participants lack important knowledge about physical activity. A variety of personal, social, and environmental facilitators and barriers were reported by the participants. *Conclusion.* Efforts should be made towards clarifying information on physical activity in this population in order to help them incorporate physical activity into their routines, overcome barriers, and make use of opportunities to be active.

1. Introduction

The exponential growth in numbers of older adults is unprecedented in the history of the United States. Longer life spans and aging baby boomers will double the population of Americans aged 65 years or older during the next couple of decades to about 72 million. Thus, it is expected that, by 2030, older adults will account for nearly 20% of the United States population. Currently, there are approximately 40 million persons aged 65 years and over in the United States. This represents 13% of the United States population, meaning that 1 in every 8 Americans is in this age group [1].

Along with the general aging trends for America's population, a significant increase in racial and ethnic diversity will be also observed. Although young individuals in the United States current reflect diversity more strikingly than their older counterparts, the racial and ethnic makeup of older adults is also changing [1]. African American population is living longer with African American women living longer than men. The African American older population was about 3.3 million in 2010 and is projected to grow over 9.9 million by 2050. Currently, African Americans aged 65 years and over account for approximately 8% of the older population; however, this number is expected to increase to 11% by the year of 2050 [2, 3]. Population aging comes with wide-ranging challenges, not only for the individual, but also for society, especially for the health sector. Expenditures for health care are expected to increase at considerable levels as chronic diseases increasingly affect the growing numbers of older adults in most developed countries [1, 4]. High rates of chronic diseases and disabilities are observed in the older population as recently demonstrated by a Centers for Disease Control and Prevention report [1]. African Americans bear a disproportionate burden of disease morbidity, disabilities, and injuries compared to other racial groups [5]. Health disparities among underserved groups are well documented in the United States. For instance, information shows that in the United States nearly 30% of the population aged 65 years and over has diabetes. Among them, African Americans (18.7%) present the highest prevalence compared to Whites (10.2%) [6]. In addition, other health issues also appear to be disproportionately prevalent in the African American population. For example, African Americans exhibit higher level of disabilities compared to Whites [7, 8]. Different factors, including physical inactivity, have been suggested to explain health disparities, such as higher rates of diseases in African Americans [9–12]. African American women are a particular vulnerable group to unhealthy lifestyles, such as physical inactivity, and the resultant chronic diseases and conditions.

Physical activity has the potential to promote health and well-being, delay the onset of chronic diseases and disabilities, and reduce the risk of premature death [13, 14]. However, for health benefits, it is recommended that adults accumulate at least 150 minutes per week of moderate to vigorous intensity physical activity [15]. Evidence-based interventions focused on lifestyle behavior changing, such as physical activity promotion, have been recommended to enhance health in different age groups including the older adult population [16]. Despite solid evidence of the benefits of physical activity, participation rates are low worldwide with the older population reporting higher levels of inactivity compared to young age groups [17]. However, data from the Behavioral Risk Factor Surveillance System shows that in the United States African American present with very low rates of physical activity participation at recommended levels [18]. Additionally, older African American women appear to be a vulnerable group to physical inactivity [19]. Factors such as health issues, family demands, lack of money, reduced public resources available, and neighborhood safety have been suggested as factors preventing individuals from engaging in physical activity among African Americans and other at risk population groups [20, 21].

However, it is also possible that the lack of physical activity among older African Americans could be related to public health messages. Public health messages used to educate the general public towards physical activity may not be clearly interpreted by, or are not adequately reaching this population [22]. As interventions should be culturally tailored, so should the messages used to promote positive behaviors such as physical activity. Thus, it is essential to first understand how a certain group of interest views a given topic. In this sense, a study aiming to explore how older African American women conceptualize physical activity is of great importance and is a step towards the development of culturally sensitive messages that may have a better impact on this population. Furthermore, cultural values and the legacy of racism, segregation, and discrimination carried by this population may shape their views of opportunities for and barriers to physical activity.

By employing objective assessment of physical activity in conjunction with a participatory research approach, this study explored the understanding of physical activity among inactive older African American women. Moreover, facilitators of and barriers to being physically active in their local environment were also examined. Physical activity is a complex and dynamic behavior that clearly depends on multiple factors as previously mentioned. In this sense, theoretical frameworks are important tools to help investigators better understand and interpret their findings. Ecological models are adequate and effective for better understanding of complex health behaviors that are involved in daily living, such as physical activity. This study was driven by the Social Ecological Model of Health Behavior [23] which suggests that individual behavior does not occur in isolation but emerges from a complex multi-level interaction between the individual, the environment, and the social cultural context where they live. This model provides a useful and important framework for understanding the numerous factors enabling or detracting from participation in this complex and dynamic behavior.

2. Methods

2.1. Study Design. A cross-sectional mixed-methods research design approach employing a participatory research technique was adopted. The Institutional Review Board of the University of Illinois approved the research protocol and signed inform consent was obtained from participants before data collection.

2.2. Sample and Setting. A total of 7 older African American women aged 65 to 75 years living in Urbana-Champaign, IL, were interviewed. The recruitment process involved flyers posted in health centers, senior centers, and local food stores. This procedure was conducted alongside the engagement of community leaders. To be included, participants had to be female and self-identify as African American. Additionally, participants were aged 60 years and older and lived in the community. Participants had to be able to walk independently and to be able to answer questions coherently by themselves. This study did not include older adults living in institutionalized settings (i.e., nursing homes, etc.), as well as individuals with significant cognitive and physical functioning decline. Participants selected to take part in this study were cash compensated throughout each step of the study.

2.3. Data Collection. Participants in this study followed three different steps during the data collection process that occurred during October and November of 2013.

2.3.1. Sociodemographic and Health Data. Participants completed a questionnaire to collect information on age, height, weight, years of education, income level, marital status, self-reported health, number of diagnosed diseases, medications taken, and health insurance coverage. At this phase, participants could select whether to meet at the investigators laboratory/office or at their own home.

2.3.2. Accelerometry and Camera. Participants wore an accelerometer at the hip (Actigraph GT3x plus) for 7 consecutive days for physical activity assessment. Participants were asked to wear the device for at least 10 hours each day.

Additionally, participants were instructed to maintain their normal routine.

Along with the week wearing the accelerometer, participants were given a disposable camera to take pictures of meaningful places (indoor and outdoor) that they go and things they do in their daily lives, as well as people they interact with, which for them were related of being active or physical activity. Participants were instructed to represent both week and weekend days in their pictures. This participatory research approach is known as photo *elicitation* [24]. Photo elicitation is a participatory research technique that invites participants to take photographs of salient features in their lives that are personally meaningful and possess significant explanatory power. After completion, accelerometers and cameras were retrieved for physical activity data analysis and photo development. Participants in this study received previous training on how to handle the devices.

2.3.3. Photo Elicitation Plus Semistructured Interview. After photo development, participants were invited to take part in the individual interview, which was conducted in a quiet room (investigator's office). Among approximately 25 photos, 6 were selected to be part of the interview process. Four meaningful photos were selected by the participants and 2 additional ones were selected by the investigator. The 2 photos selected by the investigator were selected with the goals of providing different insights from the ones selected by the participant, thereby assisting with the physical activity discussion. Interviews were conducted in English and lasted about 60 minutes. During the interview, participants were asked questions about the photos and their representation. Additionally, follow-up questions were used to discuss physical activity (interview guide available upon request with the investigator). At the end of each interview the entire set of photos provided by the participant were displayed in the table. Follow, participants were asked to take one more look on the entire set of photos to talk about anything that was not previously covered in the interview, if any. The interviews were recorded using a digital recorder and transcribed to a word document by native English speakers.

2.4. Data Analysis. The data collected from the questionnaires were analyzed using descriptive data. Accelerometer data were analyzed using ActiLife 6.0 software employing the Freedson et al. adult cut-score equations [25]. The 150 minutes per week of moderate to vigorous physical activity intensity was adopted as the cut point to classify the participants as active or inactive for health benefits [15].

Qualitative data were analyzed using a descriptive thematic approach. The 6 phases described by Braun and Clarke [26] were adopted during the analysis. Thematic analysis consists of the identification of themes that naturally emerge from the data as being important to the description of the phenomenon. Therefore, after transcription, the interviews were coded and analyzed for common themes and key patterns that emerged from the conversations. Credibility and reliability of the data were examined employing investigators' triangulation with 2 other researcher colleagues. A hundred percent agreement was found between the investigators involved in this process.

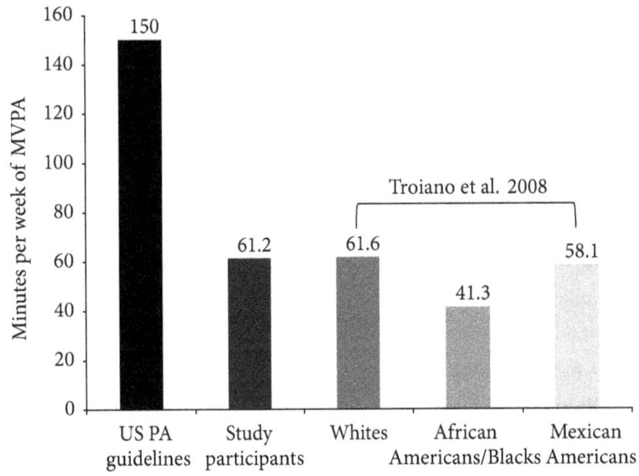

FIGURE 1: Level of moderate to vigorous physical activity (MVPA) recommended by the current United States physical activity guidelines, mean level of MVPA observed in the older African American women participating in this study ($n = 7$) living in Urbana-Campaign, IL, and mean level of MVPA observed in the national sample of older women (60 and plus) reported in the Troiano et al. study [19].

3. Results

Seven older African American women took part in this study (68.43 ± 3.20). All participants were classified as inactive for health benefits according to the criteria adopted above (Figure 1). Table 1 displays, in detail, the sociodemographic and health information of the participants.

Regarding habitual physical activity, accelerometer data showed that none of the 7 participants achieved the recommended level of physical activity for health benefits. Figure 1 displays the current recommendations for physical activity to achieve health benefits, the mean level of physical activity observed in the participants of this study, and the findings observed by Troiano and colleagues [19] study conducted in a national sample in the United States.

After completion of the interviews, the following themes emerged.

3.1. "Physical Activity" Defined as Broad Concept. The women in this study viewed physical activity as a broad concept, which extends beyond traditional exercise routines. Although they did not provide a clear definition of what physical activity is, some of the participants were able to suggest examples of what physical activity means to them. The way the older inactive African American women conceptualized physical activity was generally consistent with a public health definition of physical activity, that is, covering a variety of lifestyle-related activities. The following is an example:

> *"...it is like getting out there and mowing the grass; getting out there and cleaning the gutters,*

Table 1: Sociodemographic and health information of older African American women (n = 7) living in Urbana-Campaign, IL.

Variables	Participants (n = 7)
Age, mean (SD)	68.43 (3.20)
Education	
High school or less	1
Incomplete college	4
College	2
Marital Status	
Divorced/separated	5
Widowed	2
Annual income	
\$10,000–\$14,999	2
\$15,000–\$19,999	1
\$20,000–\$29,999	3
\$50,000 and over	1
Chronic diseases	
0-1	5
2 or more	2
Medication	
0-1	5
2 or more	2
BMI, kg/m^2, and mean (SD)	28.64 (5.74)
Self-reported health, (very good)	7
Health insurance, (yes)	7
Do you think that a person at your age can improve your health through regular exercise or balanced diet or by stopping smoking? (yes)	7

> *painting like I paint. And that is what I think, and apart from that is exercising too." (Female 71)*

3.2. How Much? As Much as You Can. When asked about how much physical activity women in their age should do, and if they ever heard about any government recommendation regarding physical activity, the answers were diverse. The United States guidelines recommend that every adult should accumulate at least 150 minutes per week of moderate to vigorous physical activity for health benefits. However, none of the interviewed women appeared to be aware of the current recommendations. Although they all agreed that being physically active was important, there was a misconception regarding the amount needed. In addition, none of the women talked about intensity, which is an important element within the recommendation along with frequency and duration to achieve health benefits. The following is an example:

> *"...As much as they can... you do what you can! But be consistent you know?... Even if you have a walker, you do that. This is just my opinion." (The same woman said) "... Twenty, ten minutes every morning of physical exercise and that is all the government requires. But that is like selling a product or something so I do not know the validity of those type [sic] of things." (Female 71)*

The interviews revealed that despite agreeing that some physical activity is better than nothing, women in this study understood little about the specific details of physical activity recommendations in terms of frequency, duration, and intensity.

3.3. Facilitators of and Barriers to Physical Activity

3.3.1. Social Facilitators. The older African American women described different factors related to social support, that is, friends; senior centers and churches as facilitators for physical activity. Women talked how having a companion for physical activity could be an encouragement to be active. The following is an example: "*...a buddy system is one of the most effective ways of getting people involved... It takes a different type of courage and strength for people to go and do something...*" *(Female 65)*. Community-based institutions were also viewed as facilitators of physical activity. Women described how they use the community center as a place to be active. For example: "*...most of the time I try to go down to Douglas Center at least for 45 minutes a day maybe not often [sic] Fridays but most of the time for about 45 minutes... The senior building (Douglas Center Annex) in the mornings I would walk over there for, [sic] maybe a half-hour to 45 minutes...*" *(Female 66)*. Moreover, the interviews revealed that church initiatives towards physical activity may be a promising way to promote physical activity among African American women. The following is an example: *"From time to time, we have people. We have students that come through...we have people who come through and we try to do some programming...one young man that comes through and he was teaching us tai chi. He taught tai chi to us and it was kind of fun. So we do have things there..." (Female 68).*

3.3.2. Environmental Facilitators. Participants recognized the importance of green areas and parks nearby as facilitators for physical activity. The following is an example: "*...and this is like in the back of my house... you know there is a big field and there is like a walkway through the park district... they put walkways and bikeways. I just like the nature, it just lifts you up, it is just beauty. It is a beauty of nature and it makes you...eyes get in tune with nature. I love to hear the birds, I love to hear the crickets, I love all of that; the creatures that are on the earth, now does that make sense?" (Female 67).*

3.3.3. Personal Barriers. African American women participating in this study talked about how health problems related to having a chronic physical condition prevent them from being more active. One woman describes her experience when inviting a friend to walk together: "*...Oh need a new knee. I need a new knee replacement* (female talking about reason on *[sic]* why older African Americans are not so active). *I am trying to get my friends to walk more, like I tell my friend [She] now she had a knee replacement and she will say ("You know I cannot walk")" (Female 66).*

Table 2: Summary of the facilitators of and barriers to physical activity that emerged from the interviews with older African American women ($n = 7$) living in Urbana-Campaign, IL.

Category	Factors influencing physical activity
Facilitators	(i) Friends (ii) Senior center (iii) Church; (iv) Green area and parks
Barriers	(i) Health issues (ii) Bad weather (iii) Unsafe environment

3.3.4. Environmental Barriers. Environmental barriers emerged in terms of bad weather and lack of safety in the environment, that is, cracked sidewalks, and neighborhood in the context of fear of crime. Women expressed how the cold weather hinders them from being more active. The following is an example: "*...So it is a lot of walking area; and then sometime I come back down Kirby. So I just... Like I said I like walking; but I do not like walking in the cold...*" *(Female 66).*

In addition, problems in the neighborhood related to lack of infrastructure such as poor sidewalks and fear-related violence were expressed as factors detracting participants from being more active. The following is an example: "*You see this here (... talking about a cracked sidewalk). I almost tripped and fell on my face. My friend ... actually did that and she had to go to the doctor and they had to do a MRI. She fell flat on her head. That is like about 2 inches up and if you are walking and you are not looking, anybody not even an old person but even a child could fall and hurt themselves*" *(female 67)*; and "*When it was nice weather, they have their hoods on their heads. So I got that feeling that something was not quite right if you cover it up, you know. I just feel like it was not really safe anymore. Cause I used to walk around [sic].*" *(Female 68).*

Table 2 summarizes the facilitators and barriers influencing physical activity that emerged from participants' photos and interviews.

4. Discussion

Factors influencing physical activity in different age groups have received increased attention due to concerns regarding physical inactivity and its negative impact on individual health and cost to the society. Few studies have examined perceptions of physical activity among older African American women. This study adopted a mixed-methods approach employing a participatory research technique to explore perceptions of and factors influencing physical activity among older African American women.

It was observed that, on average, women participating in this study perform nearly 61 minutes per week of moderate to vigorous physical activity. This value is less than half of the current recommended level of physical activity to achieve health benefits [15]. However, this value is higher than those reported by Troiano and colleagues [19]. These authors observed in a national sample of older adults in the United States that African Americans/Blacks aged 60 years and over perform on average nearly 41 minutes per week of the recommended level of physical activity. However, the values observed for the women in this study are similar to the values observed by Troiano and colleagues when examining physical activity in older White and Mexican American women of similar age. The averages observed were, respectively, 61.6 and 58.1 minutes per week. Taken together, these findings suggest that physical inactivity continues to be a concern in the older adult population in the United States. In this sense, urged public health actions are needed to mitigate such problem.

Furthermore, it was observed that many participants lack basic knowledge regarding recommended levels of physical activity, especially in terms of frequency, duration, and intensity. Moreover, it was observed that women in this study believe that the amount of physical activity needed for people in their age should be determined by the individual. These findings are similar to those observed by Wilcox et al. [27] in a study of underactive rural women living in South Carolina. Similar to our findings, the authors also observed that their participants held the opinion that frequency, duration, and intensity should be determined by the individual. Taken together, these findings suggest that the promotion of the Physical Activity Guidelines for Americans should be stressed in order to make individuals more aware of the scientific evidence regarding the quantity and intensity of physical activity needed to achieve health benefits. Even though attempts to disseminate information about the Physical Activity Guidelines for Americans [15] exist (e.g., websites), none of the participants in this study heard about any government recommendations for physical activity. Although all women in this study agreed that some physical activity is better than none, the findings suggest that none of them appear to be fully aware of some of the basic recommendations for physical activity to achieve health benefits.

Facilitators of and barriers to physical activity were also explored. Our in-depth interviews suggest that social and environmental factors often serve as facilitators of physical activity in this population. Regarding barriers, a number of personal and environmental factors were found to be barriers to physical activity. These findings are similar to those observed by Mathews et al. [20] in a multicultural study conducted among older adults as well as several other studies in the literature [20, 28–31]. For instance, Mathews and colleagues [20] examined physical activity enablers and barriers in a sample of older Americans composed of 6 racial/ethnic groups (i.e., African Americans, American Indians, Latinos, Chinese, Vietnamese, and Whites). The authors observed that no barriers to physical activity were mentioned in common across all groups; however, barriers discussed frequently by at least 3 racial/ethnic groups included physical health problems, built environment/community design, financial costs, weather, and lack of time. Common facilitators across 5 or more groups were observed by the authors who found that social support, conducive built environment, health benefits, and physical activity programs were reported as physical activity enablers by the participants. Belza and colleagues [21] also found similar findings for both enablers of and barriers to physical activity studying the most prevalent racial/ethnic groups of older adults living in United States. Taken together, the findings from these studies allied to the findings of the present study suggest that most of the barriers and facilitators for physical activity are not exclusive for African Americans. Similar factors positively and negatively affecting physical activity participation have been reported by other racial groups. These findings reinforce current knowledge of factors associated with physical inactivity in older African Americans and older adults in general and constitute important implications for public health initiatives and community-based interventions aiming to promote active living among African Americans.

Both facilitators and barriers related to physical activity expressed by the women participating in this study are in line with proximal and distal factors influencing physical activity proposed by the Social Ecological Model of Health Behavior. Based on the information gathered from the participants, it is noteworthy to highlight the role of the organizational level in both promoting and preventing physical activity. It reinforces the necessity of developing community-based interventions to physical activity to target specific groups.

The present study employed a participatory approach known as photo elicitation along with an objective assessment of physical activity to enhance our knowledge of how physical activity is understood among older inactive African American women. The combination of objective (accelerometry) and subjective (photo elicitation) approaches provides an opportunity to add to the extant literature. Previous studies addressing similar purposes as the present study adopted only focus group or individual interviews along with self-reported or subjective assessments of participant physical activity levels. Since individuals often overestimate their physical activity levels when assessed by self-report methods [32], it is difficult to be confident about their actual activity status. The combination of both qualitative and quantitative approaches has the potential to generate more meaningful and useful information. It is important to highlight that photo elicitation is not a substitute for other methods such as individual interviews or focus group. Instead, the technique serves as a useful supplement to these approaches that have the potential to enhance the quality of the findings. As stated by Hagedorn [33], "*...the images captured in photography invite people to take the lead in inquiry, facilitating their discussion of an experience. Photographic interviews elicit a unique return of insights that might otherwise be impossible to obtain with other techniques. Photographs sharpen memory and give the interview an immediate character of realistic construction and function.*" Moreover, investigators state that the act of sharing and talking about pictures evokes the power of visual images to communicate not only life experience but individuals' expertise and knowledge. Thus, although photo elicitation has the purpose of having people recording and reflecting positive and negative things in their community, it also promotes a critical dialogue about important community issues by the lens of large and small group discussion of photographs; and also can be used as a tool to reach policymakers [34, 35].

Our findings must be interpreted with care due to some limitations. Our study was based on participatory-approach along with in-depth interview of a nonrandomized sample of 7 inactive older African American women. We do not know if the patterns that emerged would have differed if a different cohort of African American women had been selected. Caution is warranted when generalizing the outcomes to the broader population of older African American women and African Americans in general. However, despite the small sample size, it is important to highlight that qualitative studies drastically differ from quantitative studies regarding "ideal" sample size. Moreover, studies adopting partial or full qualitative designs are less concerned with the generalizability of the findings. Instead, the goal is to better understand how particular groups view/perceive a particular phenomenon and extract rich data that can be add to the literature.

Although no amount of physical activity can stop the aging process, there is now compelling evidence that a moderate amount of regular physical activity can minimize the physiological effects of aging and increase active life expectancy by limiting the development and progression of chronic disease and disabling conditions [36]. Culturally, sensitive approaches to physical activity promotion are essential to help reduce heath disparity among older adults. Thomas et al. [37] suggest that it is important to match the cultural characteristics of minority populations with public health interventions to enhance receptivity to, acceptance of, and salience of health information and programs. The authors recognize the importance of factors like belief systems, religious and cultural values, life experiences, and group identity as powerful filters through which information is received. Therefore, such factors should be considered in the development of both interventions aiming to improve chronic diseases through physical activity as well as health communication campaigns. In fact, health communication is believed to be an important aspect for educating and promoting positive behaviors such as physical activity at the population level. As noted by Balbale et al. [22] tailoring and improving the message design for underserved groups is essential if we are to mitigate or eliminate the burden of health disparities.

Conflict of Interests

The authors declare that there is no conflict of interests regarding the publication of this paper.

Acknowledgment

The authors thank Coordenação de Aperfeiçoamento de Pessoal de Nível Superior (CAPES) for the scholarship provided to Emerson Sebastião (Process number BEX 5718/10-4).

References

[1] CDC, "The state of aging and health in America 2013," Report, Center for Disease Control and Prevention Health, Atlanta, Ga, USA, 2013.

[2] U.S. Census Bureau, *The Older Population: 2010. Brief Report*, U.S. Department of Commerce, Economics and Statistics Administration, U.S. Census Bureau Administration, 2010.

[3] AOA, "Aging statistics," Washington, DC, USA, Department of Health & Human Services, 2011, http://www.aoa.gov/AoARoot/Aging_Statistics/index.aspx.

[4] S. Woolhandler, T. Campbell, and D. U. Himmelstein, "Costs of health care administration in the United States and Canada," *New England Journal of Medicine*, vol. 349, no. 8, pp. 768–775, 2003.

[5] OMHD, *About Minority Health Atlanta*, Center for Disease Control and Prevention, Atlanta, Ga, USA, 2007, http://www.cdc.gov/omhd/AMH/AMH.htm.

[6] CDC, Chronic Disease Prevention and Health Promotion: Healthy Aging Atlanta 2011, Center for Disease Control and Prevention, http://www.cdc.gov/chronicdisease/resources/publications/AAG/aging.htm.

[7] J. A. Kelley-Moore and K. F. Ferraro, "The black/white disability gap: persistent inequality in later life?" *Journals of Gerontology B*, vol. 59, no. 1, pp. S34–S43, 2004.

[8] H. E. Whitson, S. N. Hastings, L. R. Landerman, G. G. Fillenbaum, H. J. Cohen, and K. S. Johnson, "Black-white disparity in disability: the role of medical conditions," *Journal of the American Geriatrics Society*, vol. 59, no. 5, pp. 844–850, 2011.

[9] S. B. Wyatt, D. R. Williams, R. Calvin, F. C. Henderson, E. R. Walker, and K. Winters, "Racism and cardiovascular disease in African Americans," *American Journal of the Medical Sciences*, vol. 325, no. 6, pp. 315–331, 2003.

[10] R. J. Thorpe Jr., D. T. Brandon, and T. A. LaVeist, "Social context as an explanation for race disparities in hypertension: findings from the Exploring Health Disparities in Integrated Communities (EHDIC) study," *Social Science and Medicine*, vol. 67, no. 10, pp. 1604–1611, 2008.

[11] G. C. Gee and D. C. Payne-Sturges, "Environmental health disparities: a framework integrating psychosocial and environmental concepts," *Environmental Health Perspectives*, vol. 112, no. 17, pp. 1645–1653, 2004.

[12] W. W. Dressler, K. S. Oths, and C. C. Gravlee, "Race and ethnicity in public health research: Models to explain health disparities," *Annual Review of Anthropology*, vol. 34, pp. 231–252, 2005.

[13] DHHS, *Physical Activity Guidelines for Americans: Chapter 2—Physical Activity Has Many Health Benefits*, DHHS, Washington, DC, USA, 2008, http://www.health.gov/paguidelines/guidelines/chapter2.aspx.

[14] W. J. Chodzko-Zajko, D. N. Proctor, M. A. Fiatarone Singh et al., "Exercise and physical activity for older adults," *Medicine and Science in Sports and Exercise*, vol. 41, no. 7, pp. 1510–1530, 2009.

[15] DHHS, "Physical activity guidelines advisory committee report," Tech. Rep., Department of Health and Human Services, Services DoHaH, Washington, DC, USA, 2008.

[16] G. W. Heath, D. C. Parra, O. L. Sarmiento et al., "Evidence-based intervention in physical activity: lessons from around the world," *The Lancet*, vol. 380, no. 9838, pp. 272–281, 2012.

[17] H. W. Kohl III, C. L. Craig, E. V. Lambert et al., "The pandemic of physical inactivity: global action for public health," *The Lancet*, vol. 380, no. 9838, pp. 294–305, 2012.

[18] BRFSS, "Participated in 150 minutes or more of Aerobic Physical Activity per week," Prevalence and Trends Data, CDC, Atlanta, Ga, USA, 2011, http://apps.nccd.cdc.gov/brfss/page.asp.

[19] R. P. Troiano, D. Berrigan, K. W. Dodd, L. C. Mâsse, T. Tilert, and M. Mcdowell, "Physical activity in the United States measured by accelerometer," *Medicine and Science in Sports and Exercise*, vol. 40, no. 1, pp. 181–188, 2008.

[20] A. E. Mathews, S. B. Laditka, J. N. Laditka et al., "Older adults' perceived physical activity enablers and barriers: a multicultural perspective," *Journal of Aging and Physical Activity*, vol. 18, no. 2, pp. 119–140, 2010.

[21] B. Belza, J. Walwick, S. Shiu-Thornton, S. Schwartz, M. Taylor, and J. LoGerfo, "Older adult perspectives on physical activity and exercise: voices from multiple cultures," *Preventing Chronic Disease*, vol. 1, no. 4, article A09, 2004.

[22] S. N. Balbale, A. Schwingel, W. Chodzko-Zajko, and M. Huhman, "Visual and participatory research methods for the development of health messages for underserved populations," *Health Communication*, vol. 29, no. 7, pp. 728–740, 2014.

[23] D. Stokols, J. Allen, and R. L. Bellingham, "The social ecology of health promotion: implications for research and practice," *American Journal of Health Promotion*, vol. 10, no. 4, pp. 247–251, 1996.

[24] D. Harper, "Talking about pictures: a case fro photo elicitation," *Visual Studies*, vol. 17, no. 1, p. 14, 2002.

[25] P. S. Freedson, E. Melanson, and J. Sirard, "Calibration of the computer science and applications, inc. accelerometer," *Medicine and Science in Sports and Exercise*, vol. 30, no. 5, pp. 777–781, 1998.

[26] V. Braun and V. Clarke, "Using thematic analysis in psychology," *Qualitative Research in Psychology*, vol. 3, no. 2, pp. 77–101, 2006.

[27] S. Wilcox, L. Oberrecht, M. Bopp, S. K. Kammermann, and C. T. McElmurray, "A qualitative study of exercise in older African American and white women in Rural South Carolina: perceptions, barriers, and motivations," *Journal of Women and Aging*, vol. 17, no. 1-2, pp. 37–53, 2005.

[28] S. Gobbi, E. Sebastião, C. B. Papini et al., "Physical inactivity and related barriers: a study in a community dwelling of older brazilians," *Journal of Aging Research*, vol. 2012, Article ID 685190, 8 pages, 2012.

[29] S. G. Trost, N. Owen, A. E. Bauman, J. F. Sallis, and W. Brown, "Correlates of adults' participation in physical activity: review and update," *Medicine and Science in Sports and Exercise*, vol. 34, no. 12, pp. 1996–2001, 2002.

[30] A. A. Eyler, D. Matson-Koffman, D. Rohm Young et al., "Quantitative study of correlates of physical activity in women from diverse racial/ethnic groups. Women's Cardiovascular Health Network Project—introduction and methodology," *American Journal of Preventive Medicine*, vol. 25, no. 3, supplement 1, pp. 5–14, 2003.

[31] Z. Siddiqi, J. A. Tiro, and K. Shuval, "Understanding impediments and enablers to physical activity among African American adults: a systematic review of qualitative studies," *Health Education Research*, vol. 26, no. 6, pp. 1010–1024, 2011.

[32] E. Sebastião, S. Gobbi, W. Chodzko-Zajko et al., "The International Physical Activity Questionnaire-long form overestimates self-reported physical activity of Brazilian adults," *Public Health*, vol. 126, no. 11, pp. 967–975, 2012.

[33] M. Hagedorn, "Hermeneutic photography: an innovative esthetic technique for generating data in nursing research," *Advances in Nursing Science*, vol. 17, no. 1, pp. 44–50, 1994.

[34] C. Wang and M. A. Burris, "Empowerment through photo novella: portraits of participation," *Health Education Quarterly*, vol. 21, no. 2, pp. 171–186, 1994.

[35] C. C. Wang, W. K. Yi, Z. W. Tao, and K. Carovano, "Photovoice as a participatory health promotion strategy," *Health Promotion International*, vol. 13, no. 1, pp. 75–86, 1998.

[36] A. C. Schwingel, "Understanding human aging," in *ACSM's Guide to Exercise for Older Adults*, W. J. Chodzko-Zajko, Ed., p. 15, LLW Press, Philadelphia, Pa, USA, 2013.

[37] S. B. Thomas, M. J. Fine, and S. A. Ibrahim, "Health disparities: the importance of culture and health communication," *American Journal of Public Health*, vol. 94, no. 12, Article ID 2050, 2004.

8

Single Stance Stability and Proprioceptive Control in Older Adults Living at Home: Gender and Age Differences

Dario Riva,[1,2] Carlo Mamo,[3] Mara Fanì,[4] Patrizia Saccavino,[5] Flavio Rocca,[2] Manuel Momenté,[2] and Marianna Fratta[5]

[1] *International Society of Proprioception and Posture, Turin, Italy*
[2] *Proprioception Center, Via Valgioie 85-87, 10146 Turin, Italy*
[3] *Epidemiology Unit, Local Health Unit TO3, Piemonte Region, Grugliasco, Italy*
[4] *Sanitary District 2, Local Health Unit TO1, Piemonte Region, Turin, Italy*
[5] *Department of Functional Rehabilitation, Local Health Unit TO1, Piemonte Region, Turin, Italy*

Correspondence should be addressed to Dario Riva; dario.riva@ispp.eu

Academic Editor: Karl Rosengren

In developed countries, falls in older people represent a rising problem. As effective prevention should start before the risk becomes evident, an early predictor is needed. Single stance instability would appear as a major risk factor. Aims of the study were to describe single stance stability, its sensory components, and their correlation with age and gender. A random sample of 597 older adults (319 men, 278 women) living at home, aged 65–84, was studied. Stability tests were performed with an electronic postural station. The single stance test showed the impairment of single stance stability in older individuals (75–84 yrs). The significant decline of stability in the older subjects may be explained by the impairment of proprioceptive control together with the decrease in compensatory visual stabilization and emergency responses. Younger subjects (65–74 yrs) exhibited better, but still inadequate, proprioceptive control with compensatory visual stabilization. Gender differences appeared in older subjects: women were significantly less stable than men. The measurement of the sensory components of single stance stability could aid in the early detection of a decay in antigravity movements many years before the risk of falling becomes evident. Adequate proprioceptive control could mitigate the effects of all other risks of falling.

1. Introduction

Unstable balance, falls, and loss of independence in the older population are a growing problem in the developed countries [1, 2]. The safety of walking and balance are indispensable requirements to prevent falls and loss of independence [3–6].

Safe mobility is primarily based on the integration of the proprioceptive, visual, and vestibular inputs [7–11].

Afferent proprioceptive inputs are conveyed to different levels of the central nervous system [10, 12, 13], but most remain unconscious and only a very few (approximately one signal out of a million) are able to reach the conscious level [14]. The joint position sense and the joint movement sense (kinesthesia) are the expression of the conscious component, while postural control is mainly based on the unconscious component [13]. In the case of the antigravity movements, proprioceptive control is the expression of the effectiveness of the stabilizing reflexes in controlling vertical stability [12]. By antigravity movements, we mean activities which require the individual to counteract gravity and postural instability with at least a phase of single-limb stance (walking, running, jumping, going up and down stairs, and so forth). Proprioceptive inputs are the most important sensory system in the maintenance of static postural stability at all ages [8, 15].

Several studies have shown that impaired vision reduces postural stability and increases the risk of falling in older people [16–19]. Consequently, maximizing vision is an effective strategy for preventing falls [20]. Other studies have shown that visual field dependence as postural stabilizer is a risk factor [21, 22]. This visual dependence may develop in response to impaired proprioceptive and vestibular systems as a result of age and chronic health problems [21, 22]. Beyond age 65, the contribution made by vision to balance control declines [8].

The role of the vestibular inputs in maintaining postural stability has been investigated mainly in double stance [7], and most studies have shown age-related differences [8, 15]. In order to isolate the function of the vestibular signals, the stability tests were performed excluding the visual information and diminishing the proprioceptive inputs in different ways, for example, by changing the inclination of the base of support [7, 15] or using different compliant surfaces [8]. In both cases the proprioceptive inputs cannot be abolished, and the decrease in the proprioceptive involvement cannot be quantified. Moreover the proprioceptive mitigation could limit the expression of the vestibular responses [8]. While the visual inputs can be excluded without affecting the motor responses based on proprioceptive and vestibular inputs, on the contrary proprioceptive and vestibular inputs cannot be isolated without compromising the responses based on the remaining signals. For these reasons in the measurement of proprioceptive control it could be more useful to include the possible intervention of the vestibular responses in order not to compromise the expression of the proprioceptive potential. Similarly, it might be preferable to assess the full potential of the emergency responses without diminishing the proprioceptive inputs and considering instead how the joint action of the proprioceptive and vestibular systems is able to face an increase in instability.

The fact that the single-limb support period accounts for 80% of the gait cycle at normal walking speed, while the double-support period accounts for 20% [23–25] suggests an important role for single stance stability in the safety of walking. Studies have reported that increasing age is associated with decreased stride length, speed, single support time, and increased stride width [26–29]. However, other studies have reported that aging is not the primary factor for decline in gait parameters [29–31]. Decreased stride length, speed, and single stance phase may in fact be stabilizing adaptations related to fear of falling [9, 26, 29, 30, 32].

For the above reasons, single stance stability could be the key element of the effectiveness and safety of antigravity movements, and the very refined single stance stability of world and Olympic champions [33] enforces this hypothesis. Postural stability has been measured in different sensory conditions (with eyes open and closed, on firm and compliant surfaces) and in different stances (double or single). Age-associated worsening in postural stability and sensori-motor functions has been shown in older people in double stance [8, 15, 34–37]. In single stance, age-related impairment of postural stability has also been shown, but sensori-motor functions were not investigated [35, 38–40]. Gender-related differences are more controversial: some studies in double stance have shown no differences in postural sway [36, 37] while other authors have found that postural sway is higher in women at all ages [34] or under stressing balance conditions [41]. In single stance, gender differences have been investigated only with timed tests and in a few studies: one author has found that men are more stable than women at all ages [38] while a more recent study has shown no differences between genders [40].

The heterogeneity of the study methods and the limited sample size entail that the reported data in literature do not clarify the measure of the decay of single stance stability and of its sensory components associated to aging and gender.

The aims of the present study were to describe, by means of an instrumented test, the characteristics of single stance stability and its proprioceptive and visual components in a representative sample of older adults and their correlation with age and gender. Additionally, single stance stability was compared to double stance stability.

2. Methods

2.1. Study Subjects. A random sample of older men and women resident in Turin (an industrial town in North-western Italy) was recruited by means of a sex-stratified random sampling from the general population. The database of the Turin Longitudinal Study (which includes the whole resident population of Turin) was used as the data source for the sampling [42]. A letter of invitation, presenting the objectives of the study, was sent to 750 men and 750 women in the age class 65–84, resident in the Second Administrative District of the Local Health Unit TO1. It was possible to contact 688 men and 703 women by phone to establish a date for performing the tests. 16 men and 39 women did not meet the inclusion criteria during the phone call. 374 men and 324 women accepted to participate (298 men and 340 women were not interested). 41 men and 37 women did not attend the appointment; 333 men and 287 women were tested, with a response rate of 89%. All subjects signed an informed consent form that summarized the purpose of the study, explained risks and discomforts, and indicated that all information gathered would remain confidential. Prior to the tests, a medical history questionnaire was administered to collect data about the subject's health status. In order to be included in the study, subjects had to be able to walk for at least six meters without an assistive device and to perform the tests. Subjects with cognitive deficits or medical problems were excluded only if the condition prevented them from meeting these inclusion criteria. 14 men and 9 women were excluded from the study because they did not meet the inclusion criteria at the moment of the questionnaire/tests or because their data were not complete. In total, 597 adults (319 men, 278 women), living at home, were included in the study and analysis. Tests and interviews were performed between April and September, 2010. Prior to the study, a pilot study was conducted on 20 subjects in order to check the feasibility and to improve the design of the research. The subjects in the pilot study were not included in the analysis.

2.2. Postural Stability Assessment

2.2.1. Instruments. The stability tests were performed by means of an electronic postural proprioceptive station (DPPS, Delos, Turin, Italy) [43] connected to a personal computer with a specific software (DPPS 5.0). In Figure 1, the

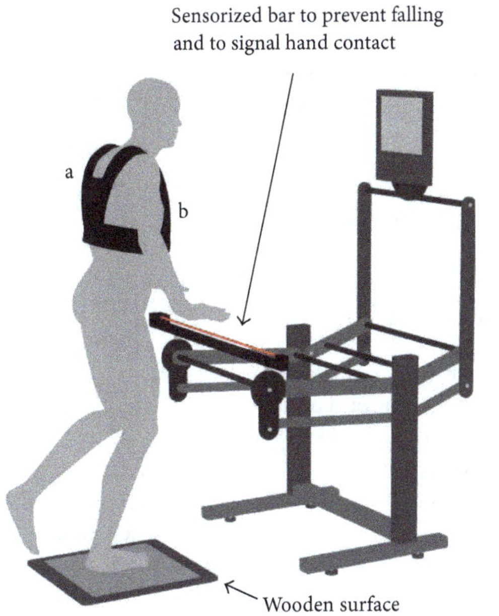

FIGURE 1: The postural proprioceptive station. The red line represents the infrared ray of the sensorized bar. Vest (a) to support the "postural reader", (b) a two-dimensional accelerometer unit, in sternal position.

station included an electronic postural reader (DVC, Delos Vertical Controller), a sensorized bar, and a display. The DVC, applied to the sternum, measured the trunk inclination in the frontal (x) and sagittal (y) plane by means of a two-dimensional accelerometer unit. The rotational radius of the DVC, when applied to the sternum, in most cases lays between 0 and 15 centimeters, never exceeding 30 centimeters. In fact, the trunk of a subject in single stance moves as a segment of a broken line with multiple joints. To minimize the fall risk, subjects could lean on the horizontal bar placed in front of them, at an adjustable height, to regain vertical control rapidly. The bar was equipped with an infrared sensor able to indicate when subjects leant on it.

2.2.2. Algorithms. The data from the postural reader are a stream of acceleration samples taken by converting into digital domain the sensor outputs, at a rate of 100 Hz. These raw data were initially averaged with a 4-tap sliding window, so the 3 dB bandwidth was narrowed to about 11 Hz. A scaling with the calibration data of the DVC was then performed, and an arcsin function was applied to convert the raw data into angles:

$$\alpha(i) = \arcsin\left[2\left(\frac{dx(i) - dx_{-90}}{dx_{+90} - dx_{-90}} - 0.5\right)\right], \quad (1)$$

$$\beta(i) = \arcsin\left[2\left(\frac{dy(i) - dy_{-90}}{dy_{+90} - dy_{-90}} - 0.5\right)\right], \quad (2)$$

where $dx(i)$ and $dy(i)$ are the generic elements of the raw data stream while those with the numerical indexes are calibration data taken at the mechanical limits of the instrument. Due to the nature of the sensor, the raw data are affected by linear accelerations superimposed on the inclination information. The measurement error is mainly proportional to the rotational speed and radius, momentarily counteracting the real movement; in static conditions it disappears. As the disturbance is mainly located at high frequencies, a pole at about 1.1 Hz was digitally applied to the data stream in order to get a good approximation of the position; the validity of this assumption was confirmed by numerical simulation and video recording compared to the system output. In the following parts of this paper, the filter outputs will be taken as angle samples. Each of them had a contact attribute according to the presence or absence of hand contact with the sensorized bar. The postural assessment was based on two components: autonomy (Au) and the average postural instability ($PIxy$). Au is the percentage of the trial without hand contact and was calculated as

$$Au = 100\frac{n - n_c - n_m}{n}, \quad (3)$$

where n is the total number of samples, n_c the number of samples with contact attribute, and n_m a correction amount that will be defined hereafter.

As each hand contact with the sensorized bar has a stabilizing posteffect, consequently multiple very short hand contacts could significantly overestimate the actual value of Au. In order to consider this effect, an additional time (malus time) was applied to each contact period with duration between 0.06 and about 2 seconds. This operation was performed by forcing the contact attribute of a certain number of samples, starting from the end of the considered contact. In case of a further contact, this action was stopped, and the contact time measurement was also restarted in order to eventually apply a correction after this new contact. Au was calculated on the basis of the corrected contact data set. The method of calculating the correction amount (m) was defined empirically, with an inverse relation to the length of the contact period. This correction ranged from a maximum of 0.674 s (for the shortest considered contact period of 0.060 s) to zero (for hand contact periods greater than 2.02 s). If the jth contact has a duration $t_c(j)$, the correction should last (only positive corrections are applied):

$$m(j) = \frac{\log(\mathrm{MM}/t_c(j) - 1) + \mathrm{SF}}{\mathrm{TF}}, \quad (4)$$

where MM = 3.3 s is the malus maximum factor, $t_c(j)$ is the duration of a contact event in seconds, SF = 0.2 is the shift factor, and TF= 2.8 Hz is the twist factor.

Being $Fs = 100$ Hz the sampling rate, the number of samples with forced contact attribute following the end of the jth contact event will be $n_e(j) = Fs \cdot m(j)$ or $n_e(j) < Fs \cdot m(j)$ in case of a new contact interrupting the forced action.

The total number of samples with forced contact attribute will then be

$$n_m = \sum_{j=1}^{C} n_e(j), \quad (5)$$

where C is the total number of contact events.

The second component of the postural assessment is $PIxy$, which derives from the average instability in the frontal and sagittal planes (PIx, PIy). $PIxy$ is an indicator of the average radius of the postural cone of instability. PIx, PIy, and $PIxy$ are expressed in degrees. PIx was calculated as the average of the absolute shifting around the average position α_a:

$$PIx = \frac{1}{n}\sum_{i=1}^{n} \left|\alpha(i) - \alpha_a\right|. \quad (6)$$

The n elements of data vector $\alpha(i)$ were averaged in order to calculate α_a:

$$\alpha_a = \frac{1}{n}\sum_{i=1}^{n} \alpha(i). \quad (7)$$

β_a and PIy were calculated in the same way as α_a and PIx.

The absolute instant deviation from the average axis ($dDVC(i)$) was determined as

$$dDVC(i) = \sqrt{(\alpha(i) - \alpha_a)^2 + (\beta(i) - \beta_a)^2}. \quad (8)$$

$PIxy$ was calculated as

$$PIxy = \frac{1}{n}\sum_{i=1}^{n} dDVC(i). \quad (9)$$

Stability Index. A suitable index for ranking all kinds of performances from the highest (very narrow cone with complete autonomy) to the lowest level (very low autonomy) was needed, capable of classifying the performances in the transition zone where both Au and $PIxy$ decrease. To overcome the limits of Au and $PIxy$ in describing stability performances, it is necessary to consider the real contribution of each single sample. A sample performance value ($spv(i)$) was introduced by weighting the $dDVC$ (8) according to its value and its contact attribute:

without hand contact

$$\begin{cases} spv(i) = 10^{-dDVC(i)/25} & (dDVC(i) < 50^\circ) \\ spv(i) = 0.01 & (dDVC(i) \geq 50^\circ), \end{cases} \quad (10)$$

with hand contact

$$\begin{cases} spv(i) = 0 & (dDVC(i) < 2^\circ) \\ spv(i) = 10^{(dDVC(i)-32)/10} & \\ +0.0001(dDVC(i) - 12) & (2^\circ \leq dDVC(i) \leq 12^\circ) \\ spv(i) = 0.01 & (dDVC(i) > 12^\circ). \end{cases} \quad (11)$$

The different thresholds were defined after experiences in the field. They ensure that without contact spv is always higher than when contact is present. In the case of contact when $dDVC$ is less than 2°, spv equals 0, because it means that the subject is unable to widen the postural cone by activating the emergency responses (proprioceptive or vestibular). In fact the appropriate action to counteract a sudden risk of fall should be to break the vertical line of the body at hip level instead of relying on an immediate hand support. For $dDVC$ between 2° and 12°, spv rises as $dDVC$ grows, to reward the attempt to recover before using hand contact; then it saturates at 0.01. The sum of all spv gives the result of the whole trial. In the case of a virtually perfect trial (a standstill trial without hand contact, where also reading errors and measurement noise are nulled) each $dDVC$ equals 0 and each spv equals 1. Consequently the maximum possible spv sum of a trial will equal the number of samples. The stability index (SI) is the relation (in %) between the spv sum of the present trial and a virtually perfect one:

$$SI = \frac{100}{n}\sum_{i=1}^{n} spv(i), \quad (12)$$

where $spv(i)$ is the spv of the ith sample and n is the total number of samples. SI is a scalar number which makes it possible to rank different trials on a functional scale.

2.2.3. Double and Single Stance Tests. Double and single stance stability was tested with eyes open (EO) and closed (EC). The subject, barefooted, was asked to minimize $PIxy$ while staying in double or single stance on a stable wooden surface. The subject was looking at a display which showed the countdown before each trial, the eye condition requested, and in single stance which foot was to be used as support. No feedback on postural stability was given during the tests. The sequence proceeded automatically. Each trial lasted 20 seconds followed by a pause of 15 seconds. A red rectangle appeared on the display when the subject touched the sensorized bar: this warning urged the subject to touch the bar only when absolutely necessary to prevent falling and as briefly as possible. The double stance test (DT), with feet as close together as possible, consisted of 2 trials with eyes open and closed. It was performed twice: DT1 and DT2 (four trials in total). The single stance test (ST) consisted of four trials. Each leg performed a first trial with EO and a second trial with EC, in an alternated sequence of the left and the right limbs. It was performed twice: ST1 and ST2 (eight trials in total). The subject stood with the weight-bearing knee bent to 170° and the non-weight-bearing knee flexed to 45° (Figure 1). Prior to the ST, participants were provided with a propaedeutic test of shorter duration to familiarize with single stance. The average of the two limbs for all variables of ST was considered.

2.2.4. Basic Variables. *Au, SI,* and *PIxy* were the basic variables considered to analyze the eight trials of ST and the four trials of DT. The precautionary strategy (*Ps*) was represented by the complementary value of *Au* (100−*Au*).

2.2.5. Indicators of Proprioceptive Control and Emergency Responses in ST. The stability index of EO trials was taken as an indicator of postural control (all sensory channels open) while the stability index of EC trials was considered an indicator of proprioceptive control and of its effectiveness as primary stabilizer. High values of stability index in EC trials correspond to refined proprioceptive control (narrow cones), because they are the expression of effective proprioceptive reflexes able to rapidly stabilize the subject before the vestibular responses can be activated [44]. Intermediate values of stability index in EC trials may include the intervention of the vestibular system, but they are in any case the expression of rougher proprioceptive control. In fact, as the vestibular system has a higher threshold of intervention and takes longer before becoming active [45], it can intervene only if proprioceptive control is not refined and therefore permits a longer period for activation [44]. Low levels of stability index are characterized by a progressive increase in precautionary strategy and the decreasing probability of intervention of the vestibular responses.

The emergency responses are the compensatory countermovements which permit the management of a rougher vertical control without the intervention of the precautionary strategy. They are under the control of the vestibular and proprioceptive systems. The widening of *PIxy* to face a lack of stability was considered an indicator of the capability of activating the emergency responses.

2.2.6. Indicator of Visual Gain and Visual Dependence. The difference between EO and EC trials quantified the visual gain and the relative visual dependence of postural stability. Visual gain and visual dependence are two different ways of describing the same thing: the first quantifies the increase in stability due to the intervention of vision, and the latter quantifies the loss of stability due to the exclusion of vision.

2.3. Statistical Analysis. As it is known that the physical performance of older men differs from that of women, analyses were conducted separately for men and women [46, 47]. The means and the standard deviations of every test were measured, stratifying by sex and by age class within each gender. The *t*-test was used for comparing the performance of different subgroups of subjects (males versus females, 65–74 years versus 75–84 within each gender). The values of P were two tailed, and $P \leq 0.05$ was considered to indicate statistical significance. All analyses were performed using the SAS statistical software (version 9.2; SAS Institute Inc., Cary, NC, USA).

2.4. Test-Retest Reliability. In order to assess the test-retest reliability, each test was performed twice and the Pearson's correlation coefficient (r) was calculated [48]. When the variable showed a value greater than 0.80, the first trial of the test was considered. If the value was lower than 0.80, the better result of the two trials was chosen. For ST, in EO condition, the average between the left and right trials of the first test was considered in relation to its high test-retest reliability (ST1 versus ST2: $r = 0.86$). In EC the moderate test-retest reliability of the average between the left and right legs (ST1 versus ST2: $r = 0.76$) prompted the choice for each limb of the better trial between ST1 and ST2. The best trial, rather than the average between ST1 and ST2, is considered to express the real functional level of the subject, just as the value of an athlete is described by his/her best result (of an entire career, of a season). For DT the test-retest reliability was low in EO condition (DT1 versus DT2: $r = 0.38$) and moderate in EC condition ($r = 0.69$). Consequently in both conditions the better of the two trials was considered.

3. Results

The characteristics of the 597 participants in this study (319 males, 278 females) are summarized in Table 1. Since the health of Turin's population is related to socioeconomic factors [20], we tested whether the social class of the recruited subjects might have influenced the generalizability of the results: as would be expected, the educational level of respondents was similar to that of nonrespondents.

Single Stance Test. The results of ST are shown in Tables 2 and 3. Considering the eight trials of ST1 and ST2, the basic variables (*SI, Au* and its complementary value *Ps, PIxy*) were calculated from the following combinations of trials: the average between the two limbs of EO trials in ST1 and the average between the two limbs of the better EC trial for each limb in ST1 and ST2. Consequently each variable is identified by a compound name which includes the eye condition and the name of the basic variable. The *Au* and *SI* variables within each combination all showed a correlation coefficient (Pearson) greater than 0.97.

Age and Gender Relations (Table 2). All variables related to single stance stability were significantly better in the age group 65–74 years both for men ($P < 0.005$) and for women ($P < 0.001$). In the following parts of this paper, if not specified otherwise, *SI* will be the basic variable considered. Both performances in EO and EC showed that the differences between sexes were not significant in the younger subjects (Figure 2) but became highly significant in the older individuals (EO_*SI*: $w = 52.7$ versus $m = 60.8$, $P < 0.001$; EC_*SI*: $w = 29.0$ versus $m = 35.7$, $P <$

TABLE 1: Participant characteristics. Values are mean ± SD.

Age	Younger class (65–74)		Older class (75–84)	
Sex	Women	Men	Women	Men
Number of subjects	117	119	161	200
Age (years)	70.0 ± 2.5	69.8 ± 2.5	79.5 ± 2.6	79.4 ± 2.5
Height (cm)	160.3 ± 6.0	171.0 ± 6.4	160.0 ± 5.9	169.7 ± 6.3
Body mass (kg)	65.7 ± 10.6	78.6 ± 10.9	64.0 ± 10.9	75.0 ± 10.8
Body mass index (kg/m^2)	25.6 ± 4.3	26.9 ± 3.5	25.1 ± 4.5	26.0 ± 3.4
Instruction level				
High	35	57	31	61
Medium	51	38	59	77
Low	31	24	71	62

TABLE 2: The results of the single stance test (ST). Each variable in the first column is identified by a compound name which includes the eye condition and the name of the basic variable.

Variables	Eyes	Unit	Sex	Mean ± SD 65–74 yrs	Mean ± SD 75–84 yrs	P level*
EO_Au	Open	%	women	85.8 ± 20.0	62.6 ± 27.3	<0.001
			men	89.0 ± 17.4	73.6 ± 23.1	<0.001
			women	85.8 ± 20.0		ns
			men	89.0 ± 17.4		
			women		62.6 ± 27.3	<0.001
			men		73.6 ± 23.1	
EO_SI	Open	%	women	74.9 ± 20.4	52.7 ± 24.8	<0.001
			men	76.6 ± 17.5	60.8 ± 21.7	<0.001
			women	74.9 ± 20.4		ns
			men	76.6 ± 17.5		
			women		52.7 ± 24.8	<0.001
			men		60.8 ± 21.7	
EC_Au	Closed	%	women	50.5 ± 17.9	37.2 ± 19.0	<0.001
			men	53.2 ± 19.2	46.2 ± 21.2	<0.005
			women	50.5 ± 17.9		ns
			men	53.2 ± 19.2		
			women		37.2 ± 19.0	<0.001
			men		46.2 ± 21.2	
EC_SI	Closed	%	women	40.0 ± 14.6	29.0 ± 15.2	<0.001
			men	41.4 ± 15.8	35.7 ± 17.2	<0.005
			women	40.0 ± 14.6		ns
			men	41.4 ± 15.8		
			women		29.0 ± 15.2	<0.001
			men		35.7 ± 17.2	

EO: Eyes open; EC: Eyes closed; SI: Stability index; Au: Autonomy. The values are calculated considering the average between the two legs. *significance level according to t-test.

0.001). The EO performance decreased from 74.9 in younger women to 52.7 in older women ($P < 0.001$). In males the values were, respectively, 76.6 and 60.8 ($P < 0.001$). Among the younger subjects, 45.4% of males and 36.8% of females were able to perform the tests with EO on each leg without hand support to prevent fall. In the older individuals, the percentage dropped to 16.5% for males and 11.2% for females.

Visual Gain and Visual Dependence (Table 3). The difference between EO and EC trials quantified the visual gain and the relative visual dependence of postural stability. The visual

TABLE 3: The visual gain and the emergency responses in the single stance test (ST). Each variable in the first column is identified by a compound name which includes the eye condition and the name of the basic variable.

Variables	Eyes	Unit	Sex	Mean ± SD		P level*
				65–74 yrs	75–84 yrs	
Visual gain (EO-EC)_SI	Open closed	pp	Women	34.8 ± 15.7	23.8 ± 17.6	<0.001
			Men	35.2 ± 16.0	25.1 ± 17.4	<0.001
			Women	34.8 ± 15.7		ns
			Men	35.2 ± 16.0		
			Women		23.8 ± 17.6	ns
			Men		25.1 ± 17.4	
Emergency responses EO_PIxy	Open	Degrees	Women	2.2 ± 1.7	2.5 ± 1.2	ns
			Men	2.3 ± 1.6	2.8 ± 1.6	<0.05
Emergency responses EC_PIxy	Closed	Degrees	Women	3.3 ± 1.5	3.2 ± 1.3	ns
			Men	3.6 ± 1.6	3.4 ± 1.8	ns

EO: Eyes open; EC: Eyes closed; SI: Stability index; PIxy: Postural cone amplitude; pp: Percentage points. The values are calculated considering the worse leg in the EC trials. *significance level according to t-test.

gain and visual dependence in the younger subjects were high and similar for both sexes [(EO-EC)_SI: m = 35.2, pp; w = 34.9 pp; ns]. They decreased, instead, significantly in the older subjects, both in males (−10.1 pp, $P < 0.001$) and in females (−11.2 pp, $P < 0.001$), without significant gender differences (Figure 3(a)). To investigate this trend, we analyzed the visual gain of all ST. The visual gain of the tests where the EC trials showed a very low stability ($SI \leq 10$) was compared to the visual gain of the tests where the EC trials showed a less low stability ($10 < SI \leq 40$). The trials were selected considering both EC trials of each leg in ST1 and ST2. The visual gain (Figure 3(b)) was significantly lower in the case of very low EC stability (mean 34.1 ± 25.9 versus 38.4 ± 21.7; $P < 0.005$).

Emergency Responses (Tables 2 and 3). In EO condition (Figure 4(a)) both sexes aged 75–84 enhanced the emergency responses to face the increased instability by widening $PIxy$ (m: +20.3%, $P < 0.01$; w: +15.8%, ns), but females increased the use of Ps more than males (m: +15.5 pp, $P < 0.001$; w: +23.2 pp, $P < 0.001$). In EC trials the situation was different (Figure 4(b)): for both sexes, the older subjects narrowed $PIxy$ (m: −6.5%, w: −3.7%) with respect to the younger individuals and faced the higher instability by significantly increasing Ps (m: +7.1 pp, $P < 0.005$; w: +13.3 pp, $P < 0.001$) and weakening the emergency responses.

Double Stance Test. The results of DT are shown in Table 4. Considering the performances in both visual conditions, 97.6% of subjects showed complete autonomy. As in ST, the variable for the consideration of the autonomy and the postural cone was SI. No significant differences emerged between genders in each class of age. In EO condition the subjects aged 65–74 years were significantly more stable than the older ones, both for males ($P < 0.005$) and females ($P < 0.01$). In EC, comparing the younger to the older individuals, the stability decreased significantly both for males ($P < 0.05$) and females ($P < 0.05$). In EO, $PIxy$ and SI showed a correlation (Pearson) of 0.94 while in EC the correlation was lower (0.67). No significant correlation was present between DT and ST.

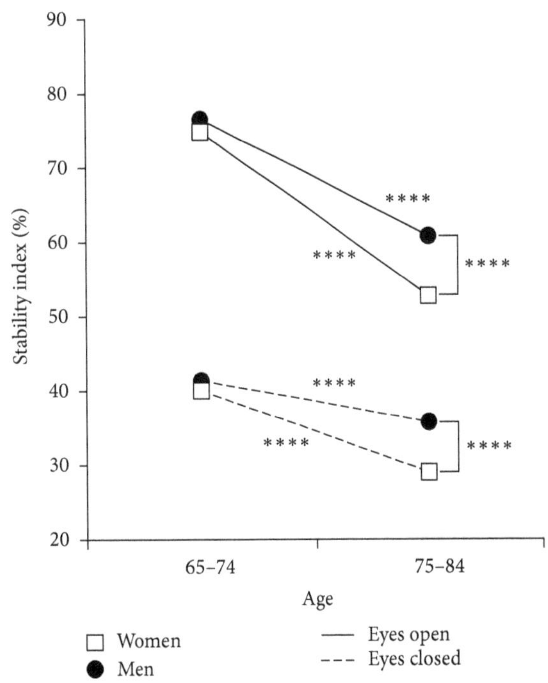

FIGURE 2: Single stance test: Stability index in men and women according to age. Values of stability index in eyes closed (indicator of proprioceptive control) and eyes open (all sensory channels open) conditions; ****$P < 0.001$.

4. Discussion

The main purpose of the present study was to describe the single stance stability in a representative sample of older subjects living at home, by means of a reliable instrumented

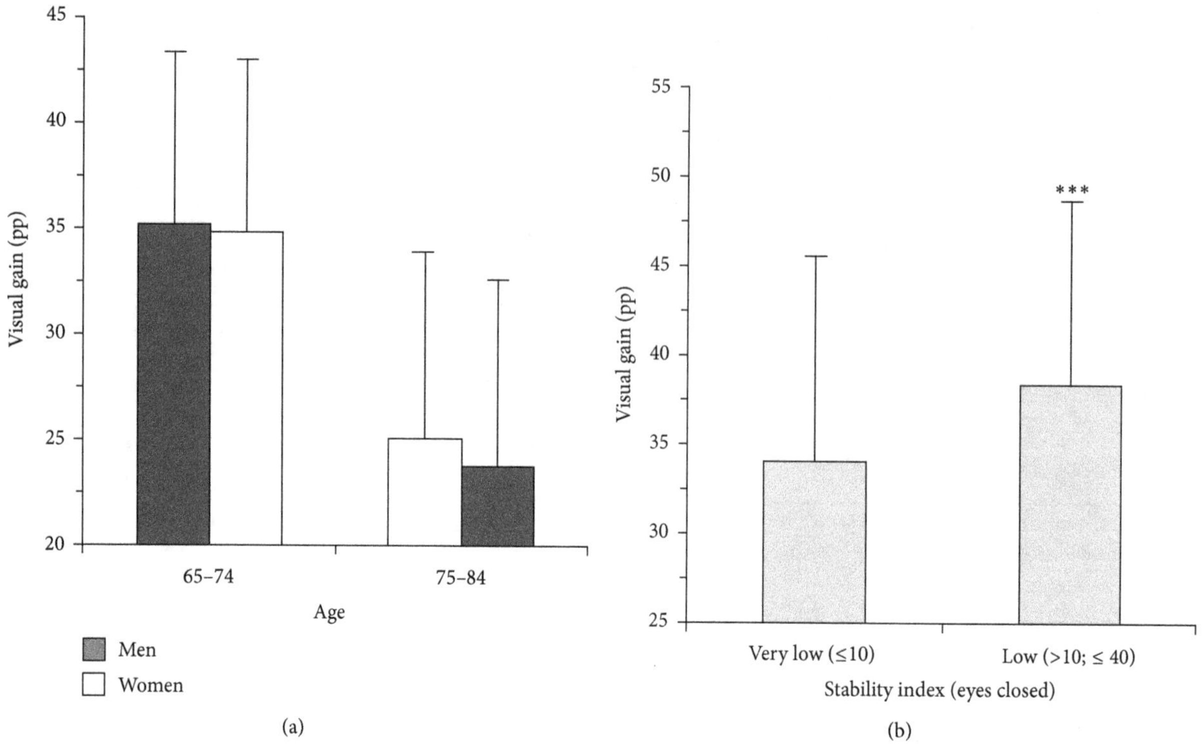

FIGURE 3: Single stance test (ST). The visual gain in supporting stability. (a) Visual gain according to sex and age: older women and older men showed a similar significant decrement of visual gain ($P < 0.001$) without gender differences. The greater decline of single stance stability in older women with respect to older men would be due to a more accentuated loss of proprioceptive control. (b) Visual gain according to different ranges of stability index in eyes closed; pp: Percentage points; $^{***}P < 0.005$.

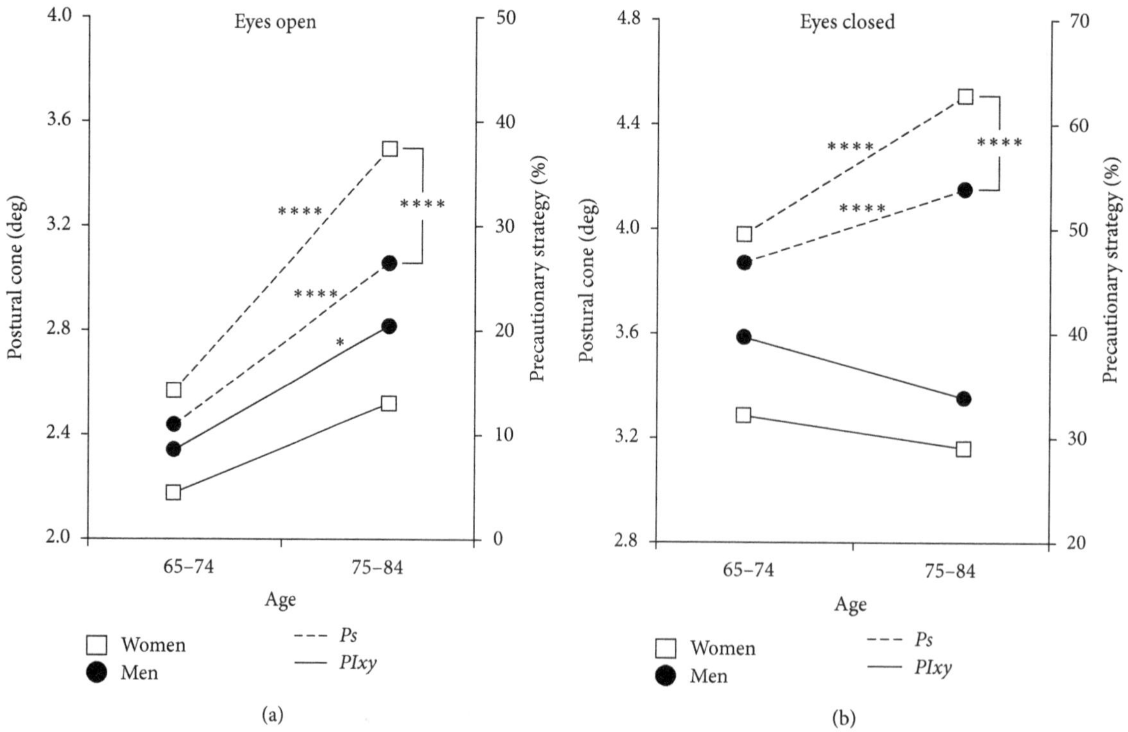

FIGURE 4: Single stance test: postural cone of instability (*PIxy*) and precautionary strategy (*Ps*) in males and females of different ages. (a) Eyes open. (b) Eyes closed. $^{****}P < 0.001$; $^{*}P < 0.05$.

TABLE 4: The results of the Double Stance Test (DT). Each variable in the first column is identified by a compound name which includes the eye condition and the name of the basic variable.

Variables	Eyes	Unit	Sex	Mean ± SD		P level*
				65–74 yrs	75–84 yrs	
EO_SI	Open	%	Women	95.87 ± 1.76	95.23 ± 1.95	<0.01
			Men	95.83 ± 1.20	95.41 ± 1.28	<0.005
EC_SI	Closed	%	Women	94.28 ± 6.00	92.79 ± 4.94	<0.05
			Men	94.23 ± 1.64	93.28 ± 4.04	<0.05
EO_PIxy	Open	Degrees	Women	0.45 ± 0.14	0.54 ± 0.22	<0.001
			Men	0.46 ± 0.13	0.51 ± 0.15	<0.005
EC_PIxy	Closed	Degrees	Women	0.58 ± 0.17	0.78 ± 0.47	<0.001
			Men	0.65 ± 0.19	0.73 ± 0.26	<0.01

EO: Eyes open; EC: Eyes closed; SI: Stability index; PIxy: Postural cone amplitude. The best trial, in the same eye condition, is considered. *significance level according to *t*-test.

test, highlighting and explaining the differences related to age and gender. Moreover, a fundamental goal was to quantify the primary role of proprioception, the compensatory intervention of the visual stabilizer, and the capability of activating the emergency responses.

4.1. Single Stance Stability. Single stance stability significantly worsened with age both in EO and EC conditions, showing significant gender differences in the older class of age. It worsened significantly more in older women than in older men. *SI* would emerge as the most important basic variable because, taking into consideration *Au* and *PIxy*, it is capable of ranking any level of performance. Instead, the timed tests in single stance, not considering the variations of the postural cone, can only measure the time before the subject touches the ground with the nonsupporting foot [35, 38–40].

4.1.1. Postural and Proprioceptive Control. In most cases proprioceptive control appeared inadequate, even in the presence of apparently sufficient postural control (adequate performance in EO trials).

Age Differences. The older subjects showed worse stability than the younger individuals ($P < 0.001$ for both sexes). These findings are consistent with previous literature [35, 38–40]; however, the methodology of the present study is able to quantify how this decline in single stance would be due to proprioceptive impairment (*m*: $P < 0.005$; *w*: $P < 0.001$) and to insufficient compensatory intervention of the visual stabilizer ($P < 0.001$ for both sexes). The consequences were a significant compensatory increase of *Ps* and less autonomous and frailer stability. Previous studies, all conducted in double stance, showed that the somatosensory component of postural stability increased its relative importance associated with age [8, 15, 36, 37] while vision reduced its contribution as postural stabilizer in the older subjects [8].

Gender Differences. Younger men performed slightly better than women, but the differences were not significant. In the older subjects (75–84 years), instead, women were significantly less stable than men, as a consequence of less effective proprioceptive control ($P < 0.001$) while visual gain was not significantly different between genders (the decrement of visual gain was similar in both sexes between the two classes of age). To our knowledge, age-related differences by gender of the proprioceptive component of single stance stability have not been shown in previous studies.

4.1.2. Visual Dependence. The compensatory intervention of the visual stabilizer would make the subject only apparently more stable.

In fact, previous studies showed that older fallers had a greater visual dependence than older nonfallers [21, 22]. The necessity of maintaining the eyes anchored to some points of the environment could explain why the stability depending on vision would be limited in range and poorly adaptable. This frail stability would lead to more and more simplified motor tasks. The results showed that very low proprioceptive control would limit partially or completely the visual gain in EO condition as compensatory postural stabilizer (Figure 3(b)). This situation would suggest that a minimum level of proprioceptive control is required to trigger the motor countermeasures activated by the other sensory systems. This hypothesis would be supported by our daily experience: in the subjects with very low proprioceptive control and deactivation of the visual gain, a moderate increase in proprioceptive control reactivates the visual gain, further enhancing single stance stability.

Some authors considered visual dependence as a response to the unavoidable proprioceptive and vestibular decline resulting from aging and chronic health problems [21, 22]. Other authors, instead, considered partially interchangeable the contribution of the different sensory components as an expression of the plasticity of the sensory systems [15]. Our results would suggest a different scenario where proprioceptive control plays a primary and conditioning role as postural stabilizer. The compensatory intervention of vision as postural stabilizer would be due to the impairment of proprioceptive control mainly because of disuse and could lead to further proprioceptive disengagement and to the deactivation of the emergency responses (Figure 5). Therefore, the primary function of vision should be to allow the

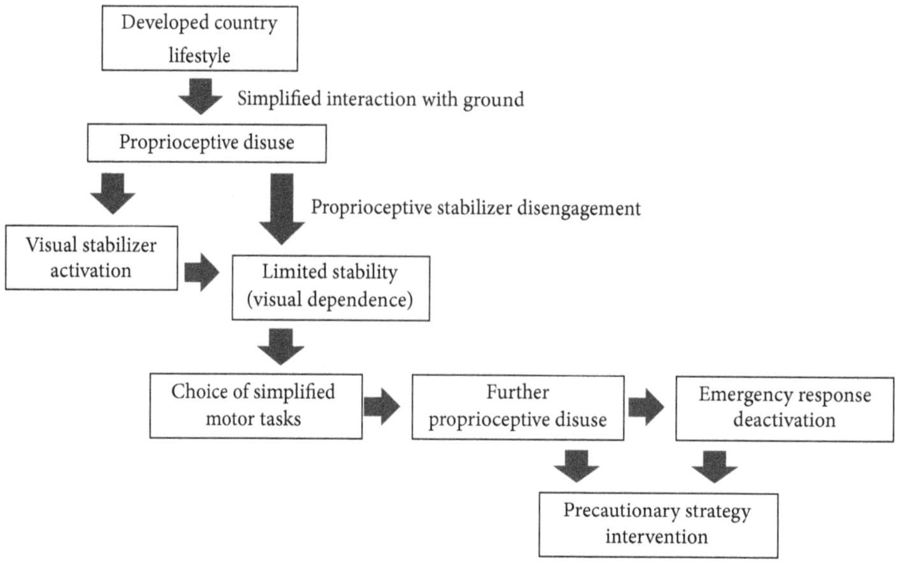

FIGURE 5: Causal chain of proprioceptive disuse and consequences. The sequence highlights how the intervention of vision as compensatory stabilizer leads to further proprioceptive disengagement.

best interaction with the environment and to avoid hazards [49]. This approach would not contrast with the studies which suggest that maximizing vision is an effective strategy for preventing falls [20, 50].

4.1.3. Emergency Responses

Age Differences. Despite rising instability, the narrowing of *PIxy* for both males and females in the older class of age (in EC) showed a change in the compensatory strategy between younger and older subjects. The results highlighted that the older subjects of both genders, even if more unstable than the younger individuals, presented a narrower *PIxy*, managing the increased instability with greater intervention of *Ps* (Figure 4(b)). To understand this change, the subject in single stance should be described as a broken line with multiple joints, instead of a straight vertical line tilting like an inverse pendulum. The capability of managing the body as a broken line is indispensable for maintaining the projection of the center of gravity in the area of support of the foot. The results would show that this capacity of breaking the line is progressively lost when proprioceptive control is impaired. In fact, subjects with high *Ps* generally present a narrow *PIxy* in EC situation, an expression of their incapacity to activate the emergency responses (Figure 6): they behave as rigid structures and tend to fall like a stick.

4.1.4. Consequences of Aging or Functional and Structural Disuse? The results suggest that the incapacity to activate compensatory intervention (visual stabilization and emergency responses) would be mostly consequent to the impairment of proprioceptive control. This decline could be firstly the consequence of disuse and only secondly the result of aging [51, 52]. In our opinion, this process would not compromise the potential of the functional reserve of the proprioceptive system. In fact the redundancy of its billions of receptors [53] would make it theoretically less sensitive to the effects of aging. The visual system, instead, is a postural stabilizer with significant anatomical and functional fragilities which favor its exposure to aging [54]. Consequently, postural control heavily based on this system can lead to a dramatic loss of stability in case of its decay. It may be hypothesized that the increasing intervention of the visual system in controlling single stance stability in the younger subjects (65–74 years) could contribute to the disengagement of the proprioceptive stabilizer leading to a more accentuated loss of stability in older age (Figure 5).

4.1.5. Gender Differences in the Older Subjects. The greater deterioration of single stance stability in older females would seem mainly due to more accentuated proprioceptive decay. In fact, the decrease in visual compensation and the reduction in the capacity of activating the emergency responses are similar in both sexes. It could be supposed that the more pronounced proprioceptive decay in women is due both to their muscle weakness which reaches a critical level earlier than in men [47, 55, 56] and to faster proprioceptive disuse (Figure 5) caused by more simplified interaction with the ground, consequent to the kind of shoes worn [57, 58], slower walking speed [47, 59], and so forth.

4.2. Double Stance Stability. Double stance stability significantly worsened with age in both EO and EC conditions but did not show significant gender differences. Age-related differences are consistent with all previous studies. Even if gender differences have been little studied and in small samples, our findings are consistent with most previous studies [36, 37]. The absence of a significant correlation between DT and ST would suggest that DT is not predictive of single stance stability and consequently of the effectiveness of

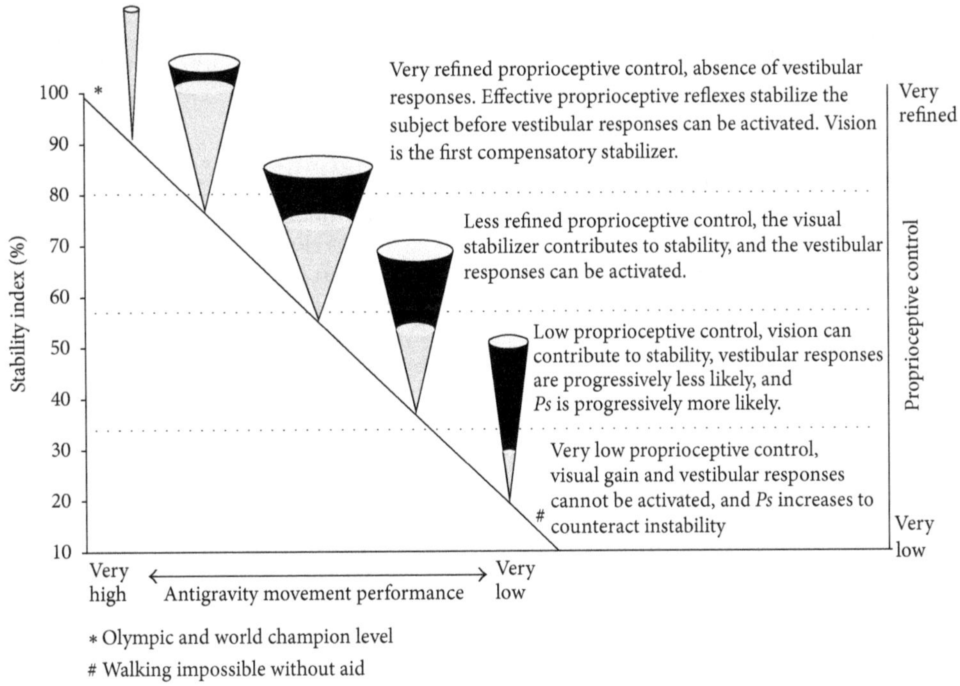

FIGURE 6: Single stance test (ST): model of interpretation. The impairment of stability is faced first by widening the postural cone (*PIxy*) and then by activating the precautionary strategy (*Ps*, black area of the cone in %). Then, if necessary, *Ps* increases further while *PIxy* tends progressively to become smaller. This behavior is observed both in eyes open and eyes closed (EC) conditions, even if in the latter condition it is more evident. The stability index of EC trials is an indicator of the effectiveness of proprioceptive control, even if the vestibular component is not excluded. From top to bottom higher values of stability index indicate more refined proprioceptive control. Didactically four functional zones can be identified (their dimensions are approximate). At the lower level of stability, the subject is unable to maintain the single stance without continuous hand support and cannot walk without aid. ST levels correspond to different antigravity movement performances.

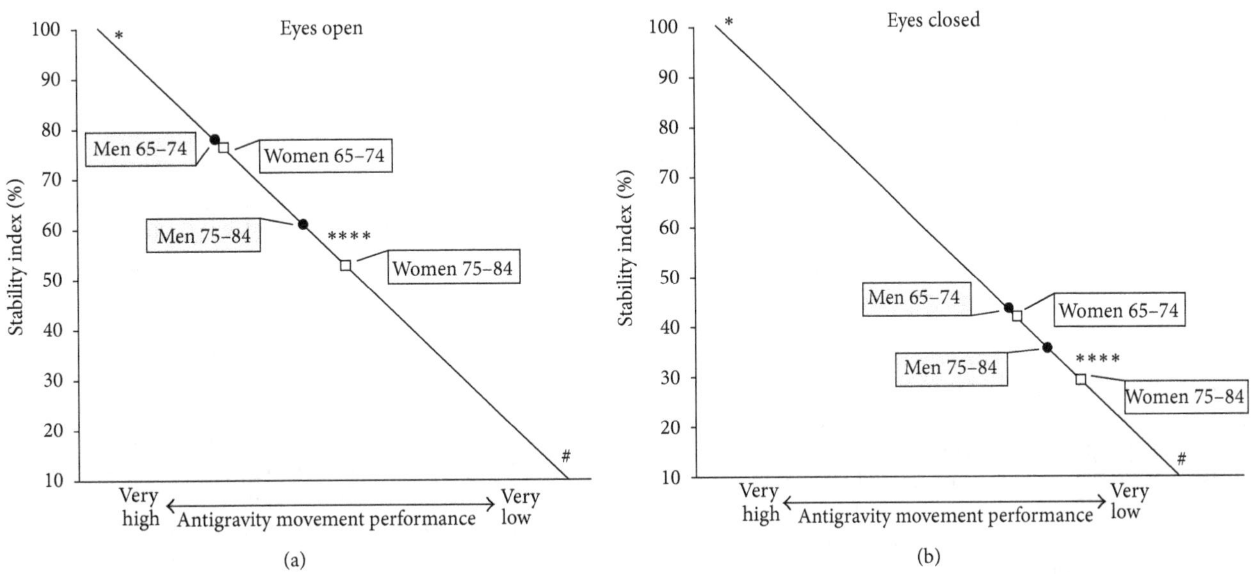

FIGURE 7: Single (ST). Postural and proprioceptive control: age and gender relations. The age groups of the study are positioned according to their ST level (a) in eyes open (indicator of postural control) and (b) in eyes closed (indicator of proprioceptive control). *Olympic and world champion level; #walking impossible without aid; $^{****}P < 0.001$.

the most critical phase of walking and of the other antigravity movements.

A possible limitation of the study could be the self-selection of the responders/attendees. It is known that the following subgroups tend to be underrepresented among the attendees: males, unmarried and separated/divorced subjects, immigrants, subjects with lower education, and low income receivers of disability benefit [60]. Although sampling methods, selection criteria, data collection, and purposes of the present study should minimize the problem of self-selection, a residual bias in the interpretation of the results could not be excluded completely.

5. Conclusions

The present study pointed out the characteristics of single stance stability in a large sample of older adults, highlighting the differences related to age and gender. Measurements obtained from the single stance test were used to quantify the primary role of proprioceptive control and the compensatory contribution of the visual stabilizer and of the emergency responses. The decline of single stance stability evidenced significant age-related gender differences (Figures 7(a) and 7(b)): while younger women aged 65–74 were not significantly different from men of the same age, women aged 75–84 were significantly less stable than men. This difference would appear to be the consequence of less effective proprioceptive control while the significant decrement in visual gain between the two classes of age was similar in both genders. The stabilizing action of the visual gain in the younger individuals, apparently positive, would guarantee limited and poorly adaptable stability. This frail stability would be a concurrent cause of proprioceptive decay because, leading to simplified motor tasks, it would accentuate proprioceptive disuse (Figure 5). Eyes closed condition was useful for simulating what happens when the visual stabilizer impairs its action or when visibility and luminosity are low in eyes closed: the emergency responses of the older subjects decreased in both sexes with respect to the younger subjects. The study showed that the higher instability of older subjects would be compensated neither by enhancing visual stabilization nor by the emergency responses, but by significantly increasing the precautionary strategy (Figure 6). Thus proprioceptive control would emerge as the real critical element in managing single stance stability. These findings are underlined by the observation that very low proprioceptive control would deactivate the compensatory action of the visual stabilizer and of the emergency responses. Single stance stability based on adequate proprioceptive control would appear to be a promising potential countermeasure which could mitigate the effects of all other intrinsic and extrinsic contributing causes of instability and risk of falling. The findings would suggest that the measurement of the sensory components of single stance stability could be an early predictor of functional decay in walking and antigravity movements, many years before the risk of falling becomes evident. As a development of the study, a follow-up of the participants is being carried out in order to assess the association between single stance stability and health outcomes. Considering that proprioceptive control in single stance would appear to be a key element of the safety and effectiveness of mobility, future research on the possibility of awakening its sleeping potential is suggested.

Abbreviations

Au: Autonomy
EC: Eyes closed
DVC: Delos vertical controller
dDVC: Absolute instant deviation of DVC measure from the average axis
DT: Double stance test
EO: Eyes open
PIx: Average postural instability in the frontal plane
PIxy: Average postural instability or amplitude of the postural cone
PIy: Average postural instability in the sagittal plane
Ps: Precautionary strategy (the complementary value of *Au*)
SI: Stability index
spv: Sample performance value
ST: Single stance test.

Conflict of Interests

Dario Riva is the scientific director of Delos, and he holds company equity. The other authors declare that they have no conflict of interest.

References

[1] C. Todd and D. Skelton, "What are the main risk factors for falls among older people and what are the most effective interventions to prevent these falls?" Health Evidence Network Report, WHO, Geneva, Switzerland, 2004, http://www.euro.who.int/document/E82552.pdf.

[2] S. Heinrich, K. Rapp, U. Rissmann, C. Becker, and H.-H. König, "Cost of falls in old age: a systematic review," *Osteoporosis International*, vol. 21, no. 6, pp. 891–902, 2010.

[3] T. Masud and R. O. Morris, "Epidemiology of falls," *Age and Ageing*, vol. 30, no. 4, pp. 3–7, 2001.

[4] J. M. Guralnik, L. Ferrucci, E. M. Simonsick, M. E. Salive, and R. B. Wallace, "Lower-extremity function in persons over the age of 70 years as a predictor of subsequent disability," *New England Journal of Medicine*, vol. 332, no. 9, pp. 556–561, 1995.

[5] S. Studenski, S. Perera, D. Wallace et al., "Physical performance measures in the clinical setting," *Journal of the American Geriatrics Society*, vol. 51, no. 3, pp. 314–322, 2003.

[6] M. Montero-Odasso, M. Schapira, E. R. Soriano et al., "Gait velocity as a single predictor of adverse events in healthy seniors aged 75 years and older," *Journals of Gerontology A*, vol. 60, no. 10, pp. 1304–1309, 2005.

[7] L. M. Nashner, F. O. Black, and C. Wall III, "Adaptation to altered support and visual conditions during stance: patients with vestibular deficits," *Journal of Neuroscience*, vol. 2, no. 5, pp. 536–544, 1982.

[8] S. R. Lord and J. A. Ward, "Age-associated differences in sensori-motor function and balance in community dwelling women," *Age and Ageing*, vol. 23, no. 6, pp. 452–460, 1994.

[9] S. R. Lord, D. G. Lloyd, and S. K. Li, "Sensori-motor function, gait patterns and falls in community-dwelling women," *Age and Ageing*, vol. 25, no. 4, pp. 292–299, 1996.

[10] H. Kobayashi, Y. Hayashi, K. Higashino et al., "Dynamic and static subjective visual vertical with aging," *Auris Nasus Larynx*, vol. 29, no. 4, pp. 325–328, 2002.

[11] M. L. Callisaya, L. Blizzard, J. L. McGinley, M. D. Schmidt, and V. K. Srikanth, "Sensorimotor factors affecting gait variability in older people-a population-based study," *Journals of Gerontology A*, vol. 65, no. 4, pp. 386–392, 2010.

[12] C. S. Sherrington, *The Integrative Action of the Nervous System*, Yale University Press, New Haven, Conn, USA, 1906.

[13] B. L. Riemann and S. M. Lephart, "The sensorimotor system, part I: the physiologic basis of functional joint stability," *Journal of Athletic Training*, vol. 37, no. 1, pp. 71–79, 2002.

[14] G. Moruzzi, *Physiology of Relational Life*, Utet, Turin, Italy, 1975.

[15] H. Cohen, L. G. Heaton, S. L. Congdon, and H. A. Jenkins, "Changes in sensory organization test scores with age," *Age and Ageing*, vol. 25, no. 1, pp. 39–44, 1996.

[16] S. R. Lord, "Visual risk factors for falls in older people," *Age and Ageing*, vol. 35, supplement 2, pp. ii42–ii45, 2006.

[17] A. L. Coleman, S. R. Cummings, F. Yu et al., "Binocular visual-field loss increases the risk of future falls in older white women," *Journal of the American Geriatrics Society*, vol. 55, no. 3, pp. 357–364, 2007.

[18] E. E. Freeman, A. T. Broman, K. A. Turano, and S. K. West, "Motion-detection threshold and measures of balance in older adults: the SEE project," *Investigative Ophthalmology and Visual Science*, vol. 49, no. 12, pp. 5257–5263, 2008.

[19] L. Salonen and S. L. Kivelä, "Eye diseased and impaired vision as possible risk factors for recurrent falls in the aged: a systematic review," *Current Gerontology and Geriatrics Research*, vol. 2012, Article ID 271481, 10 pages, 2012.

[20] S. R. Lord, S. T. Smith, and J. C. Menant, "Vision and falls in older people: risk factors and intervention strategies," *Clinics in Geriatric Medicine*, vol. 26, no. 4, pp. 569–581, 2010.

[21] J. S. Tobis, S. Reinsch, J. M. Swanson et al., "Visual perception dominance of fallers among community-dwelling older adults," *Journal of the American Geriatrics Society*, vol. 33, no. 5, pp. 330–333, 1985.

[22] S. R. Lord and I. W. Webster, "Visual field dependence in elderly fallers and non-fallers," *International Journal of Aging and Human Development*, vol. 31, no. 4, pp. 267–277, 1990.

[23] M. P. Murray, A. B. Drought, and R. C. Kory, "Walking patterns of normal men," *The Journal of Bone and Joint Surgery*, vol. 46, no. 2, pp. 335–360, 1964.

[24] M. M. Rodgers, "Dynamic biomechanics of the normal foot and ankle during walking and running," *Physical Therapy*, vol. 68, no. 12, pp. 1822–1832, 1988.

[25] D. A. Winter, *Biomechanics and Motor Control of Human Movement*, John Wiley & Sons, Hoboken, NJ, USA, 2009.

[26] M. P. Murray, R. C. Kory, and B. H. Clarkson, "Walking patterns in healthy old men," *Journals of Gerontology*, vol. 24, no. 2, pp. 169–178, 1969.

[27] R. J. Elble, S. S. Thomas, C. Higgins, and J. Colliver, "Stride-dependent changes in gait of older people," *Journal of Neurology*, vol. 238, no. 1, pp. 1–5, 1991.

[28] J. Woo, S. C. Ho, J. Lau, S. G. Chan, and Y. K. Yuen, "Age-associated gait changes in the elderly: pathological or physiological?" *Neuroepidemiology*, vol. 14, no. 2, pp. 65–71, 1995.

[29] M. E. Chamberlin, B. D. Fulwider, S. L. Sanders, and J. M. Medeiros, "Does fear of falling influence spatial and temporal gait parameters in elderly persons beyond changes associated with normal aging?" *Journals of Gerontology A*, vol. 60, no. 9, pp. 1163–1167, 2005.

[30] B. Maki, "Gait changes in older adults: predictors of falls or indicators of fear?" *Journal of the American Geriatrics Society*, vol. 45, no. 3, pp. 313–320, 1997.

[31] J. M. Hausdorff, B. R. Levy, and J. Y. Wei, "The power of ageism on physical function of older persons: reversibility of age-related gait changes," *Journal of the American Geriatrics Society*, vol. 47, no. 11, pp. 1346–1349, 1999.

[32] H. B. Menz, S. R. Lord, and R. C. Fitzpatrick, "Age-related differences in walking stability," *Age and Ageing*, vol. 32, no. 2, pp. 137–142, 2003.

[33] D. Riva, F. Rossitto, and L. Battocchio, "Postural muscle atrophy prevention and recovery and bone remodelling through high frequency proprioception for astronauts," *Acta Astronautica*, vol. 65, no. 5-6, pp. 813–819, 2009.

[34] P. W. Overstall, A. N. Exton Smith, F. J. Imms, and A. L. Johnson, "Falls in the elderly related to postural imbalance," *British Medical Journal*, vol. 1, no. 6056, pp. 261–264, 1977.

[35] R. W. Bohannon, P. A. Larkin, and A. C. Cook, "Decrease in timed balance test scores in aging," *Physical Therapy*, vol. 64, no. 7, pp. 1067–1070, 1984.

[36] N. R. Colledge, P. Cantley, I. Peaston, H. Brash, S. Lewis, and J. A. Wilson, "Ageing and balance: the measurement of spontaneous sway by posturography," *Gerontology*, vol. 40, no. 5, pp. 273–278, 1994.

[37] P. A. Hageman, J. M. Leibowitz, and D. Blanke, "Age and gender effects on postural control measures," *Archives of Physical Medicine and Rehabilitation*, vol. 76, no. 10, pp. 961–965, 1995.

[38] J. A. Balogun, K. A. Akindele, J. Nihinlola, and D. K. Marzouk, "Age-related changes in balance performance," *Disability and Rehabilitation*, vol. 16, no. 2, pp. 58–62, 1994.

[39] S. Morioka, T. Fukumoto, M. Hiyamizu, A. Matsuo, H. Takebayashi, and K. Miyamoto, "Changes in the equilibrium of standing on one leg at various life stages," *Current Gerontology and Geriatrics Research*, vol. 2012, Article ID 516283, 6 pages, 2012.

[40] B. A. Springer, R. Marin, T. Cyhan, H. Roberts, and N. W. Gill, "Normative values for the unipedal stance test with eyes open and closed," *Journal of Geriatric Physical Therapy*, vol. 30, no. 1, pp. 8–15, 2007.

[41] L. Wolfson, R. Whipple, C. A. Derby, P. Amerman, and L. Nashner, "Gender differences in the balance of healthy elderly as demonstrated by dynamic posturography," *Journals of Gerontology*, vol. 49, no. 4, pp. M160–M167, 1994.

[42] M. Cardano, G. Costa, and M. Demaria, "Social mobility and health in the Turin longitudinal study," *Social Science and Medicine*, vol. 58, no. 8, pp. 1563–1574, 2004.

[43] "Delos Postural Proprioceptive System," http://www.delos-international.com/prodotti.asp?sec=scheda&lang=eng, 2011.

[44] F. Baldissera, G. Bertocchi, P. Cavalari et al., *Neurosciences*, Poletto, Milan, Italy, 1999.

[45] A. M. Bacsi and J. G. Colebatch, "Evidence for reflex and perceptual vestibular contributions to postural control," *Experimental Brain Research*, vol. 160, no. 1, pp. 22–28, 2005.

[46] E. M. Simonsick, A. B. Newman, M. Visser et al., "Mobility limitation in self-described well-functioning older adults: importance of endurance walk testing," *Journals of Gerontology A*, vol. 63, no. 8, pp. 841–847, 2008.

[47] R. Cooper, R. Hardy, A. Sayer et al., "Age and gender differences in physical capability levels from mid-life onwards: the harmonisation and meta-analysis of data from eight UK cohort studies," *PLoS ONE*, vol. 6, no. 11, Article ID e27899, 2011.

[48] V. Rousson, T. Gasser, and B. Seifert, "Assessing intrarater, interrater and test-retest reliability of continuous measurements," *Statistics in Medicine*, vol. 21, no. 22, pp. 3431–3446, 2002.

[49] A. J. Campbell, M. J. Borrie, G. F. Spears, S. L. Jackson, J. S. Brown, and J. L. Fitzgerald, "Circumstances and consequences of falls experienced by a community population 70 years and over during a prospective study," *Age and Ageing*, vol. 19, no. 2, pp. 136–141, 1990.

[50] M. R. de Boer, S. M. F. Pluijm, P. Lips et al., "Different aspects of visual impairment as risk factors for falls and fractures in older men and women," *Journal of Bone and Mineral Research*, vol. 19, no. 9, pp. 1539–1547, 2004.

[51] R. S. Hutton and S. W. Atwater, "Acute and chronic adaptations of muscle proprioceptors in response to increased use," *Sports Medicine*, vol. 14, no. 6, pp. 406–421, 1992.

[52] S. W. Shaffer and A. L. Harrison, "Aging of the somatosensory system: a translational perspective," *Physical Therapy*, vol. 87, no. 2, pp. 193–207, 2007.

[53] D. Ian McCloskey, "Human proprioceptive sensation," *Journal of Clinical Neuroscience*, vol. 1, no. 3, pp. 173–177, 1994.

[54] R. Klein, "Age-related eye disease, visual impairment, and driving in the elderly," *Human Factors*, vol. 33, no. 5, pp. 521–525, 1991.

[55] W. R. Frontera, V. A. Hughes, K. J. Lutz, and W. J. Evans, "A cross-sectional study of muscle strength and mass in 45- to 78-yr-old men and women," *Journal of Applied Physiology*, vol. 71, no. 2, pp. 644–650, 1991.

[56] A. J. Campbell, M. J. Borrie, and G. F. Spears, "Risk factors for falls in a community-based prospective study of people of 70 years and older," *Journals of Gerontology*, vol. 44, no. 4, pp. M112–M117, 1989.

[57] J. C. Menant, J. R. Steele, H. B. Menz, B. J. Munro, and S. R. Lord, "Effects of footwear features on balance and stepping in older people," *Gerontology*, vol. 54, no. 1, pp. 18–23, 2008.

[58] N. J. Cronin, R. S. Barrett, and C. P. Carty, "Long-term use of high-heeled shoes alters the neuromechanics of human walking," *Journal of Applied Physiology*, vol. 112, no. 6, pp. 1054–1058, 2012.

[59] A. A. Butler, J. C. Menant, and A. C. Tiedemann, "Age and gender differences in seven tests of functional mobility," *Journal of NeuroEngineering and Rehabilitation*, vol. 6, no. 1, p. 31, 2009.

[60] A. J. Søgaard, R. Selmer, E. Bjertness, and D. Thelle, "The Oslo health study: the impact of self-selection in a large, population-based survey," *International Journal for Equity in Health*, vol. 3, no. 1, p. 3, 2004.

9

Falls Reduction and Exercise Training in an Assisted Living Population

Kimberly J. Alvarez,[1] Shannen Kirchner,[2] Serena Chu,[2] Sarah Smith,[2] Wendy Winnick-Baskin,[3] and Thelma J. Mielenz[1]

[1]*Department of Epidemiology, Mailman School of Public Health, Columbia University, 722 West 168th Street, New York, NY 10032, USA*
[2]*College of Physicians and Surgeons, Columbia University, New York, NY 10032, USA*
[3]*Atria Senior Living, Louisville, KY 40202, USA*

Correspondence should be addressed to Thelma J. Mielenz; tjm2141@columbia.edu

Academic Editor: Miriam Vollenbroek-Hutten

Multicomponent exercise programs are currently an efficacious fall prevention strategy among community dwelling older adults although research documents differential falls susceptibility among frail older adults. This study aimed to examine the association between the Boston FICSIT (Frailty and Injuries: Cooperative Studies of Intervention Techniques) exercise program (the original exercise program to demonstrate that nursing home residents can increase strength) and falls incidents in an assisted living community. A descriptive cross-sectional study matched exercise charts for frequency and duration of training with number of reported fall incidents. Among 39 participants, 33% (n = 13) reported a fall incident. Adults without a fall history reported more time in aerobic (26.30 versus 20.00, P value = 0.71) and strength (1.50 versus 0.50, P value = 0.01) training sessions compared to those with a fall history. Multivariate models adjusting for covariates illustrated a significant protective association between strength training and fall incidents (OR = 0.25; 95% CI = 0.07, 0.85). In this cross-sectional study, this progressive resistance exercise training program into an assisted living population was associated with a decrease in the number of fall incidents.

1. Introduction

In the US, 30% of older adults experience at least one fall annually, with a particularly higher rate (50%) over the age of 80 [1]. Falls not only are the leading cause of injury death, but also are the most common cause of nonfatal injuries and lead to chronic pain and disability [2]. An estimated $30 billion dollars was spent in 2010 on inpatient hospitalizations and outpatient medical costs related to falls [3]. Falls create an enormous economic burden and effective falls prevention will reduce health care costs and increase quality of life in older age [4].

The US Preventive Services Task Force states that multifactorial risk assessments offer a small benefit for falls prevention in community dwelling (CD) older adults [5]. Some risk factors can be modified using exercise (e.g., impaired balance and gait), whereas others require different intervention approaches (e.g., poor vision) [6]. On the other hand, exercise training programs for CD adults have considerable benefit and can be used as a stand-alone falls prevention intervention or as a component of a multifaceted program. Prior studies have established the fact that exercise interventions for falls reduction and injury prevention are effective in CD older adults [5–11]. However, high interindividual variability and differential falls susceptibility in CD versus frail older adults suggest falls prevention programs designed for CD older adults may not be translatable to more frail older adults in assisted living (AL) and nursing homes. AL communities are the fastest-growing noninstitutional long-term care alternative in the US for older adults [12]. As a result, AL communities are an extraordinarily diverse shelter and care alternative, and very frail older persons with serious chronic health conditions can be found in this setting [12]. Limited research has examined associations between exercise programs and falls among AL populations [13].

This exercise program was designed by exercise physiologists in the 1980s and 1990s from Tufts University School of Nutrition and Center for Healthy Aging (i.e., William J. Evans, Ph.D., and Miriam E. Nelson, Ph.D.). The aim of the program was to reverse bone loss and improve energy and balance among older adults by progressive resistance exercise training [14]. This exercise program laid the foundation for current evidence-based CD programs. Moreover, it was found to be efficacious by a randomized controlled trial conducted by Fiatarone and colleagues using data from the Boston Frailty and Injuries: Cooperative Studies of Intervention Techniques (FICSIT) study [15]. Results from the trial demonstrated that it was both feasible and effective in counteracting muscle weakness and physical frailty among nursing home residents [14, 15]. Progressive resistance exercise three days a week for ten weeks significantly improved the results of all muscle-strength tests. Specifically, among those who participated in exercise training, gait velocity increased by 11.8% and overall muscle strength increased by 111.3%, compared to nonexercisers [15]. While the exercise program was successful among frail adults in a nursing home, it is not clear whether this program would be efficacious among AL populations to reduce falls.

The goal of the present study was to evaluate the association of the aerobic and strength training exercise program, adopted from Fiatarone et al., to reduce falls incidents and falls-related injuries in an AL population [15].

2. Materials and Methods

Participants for this five-year period prevalence cross-sectional study (2007–2011) were ascertained from one community in a privately owned, for-profit senior housing company that provides independent living, assisted living, and memory care services. Inclusion criteria for participation in the exercise program included (1) being current community resident, (2) attending a meeting with the community activity director, and (3) having signed form submitted by participant's physician. The Columbia University Medical Center Institutional Review Board approved this retrospective study.

2.1. Exercise Intervention. Dr. Miriam E. Nelson, the Exercise Physiologist from Tufts, came to the AL communities in the late 1990s and helped to translate the Boston FICSIT program into several communities [15]. Exercise program guidelines advised AL residents to incorporate aerobic and strength training into their regular exercise routine three times a week using equipment available in the community's fitness center. Strength training was performed on Keiser Air Resistance Equipment, with supervision, and included shoulder press, seated row, leg extension, leg curl, and leg press machines. Aerobic training was performed on NuStep machines or treadmills. Residents also had the option of participating in chair exercise classes held six days a week for one hour; these sessions included stretching, hand weights, and resistance bands. Activity directors supervising the program assisted participants in the fitness center and followed up with those who failed to attend regular sessions.

The staff member on duty in the fitness center set up the equipment and recorded mode, frequency, and duration of each activity in participants' individual exercise chart. For strength training, staff documented exercise, machine resistance, and number of repetitions and sets. For aerobic training, time, speed, and resistance were recorded. The exercise chart remained with the participant throughout the program.

2.2. Falls Assessment. A fall was defined as unintentionally coming to rest on the ground, floor, or any other lower level [16]. Staff recorded the fall incident using a standard incident report form. Additional information collected about the fall incident included date, injury, location, cause (as stated by participant), reason for fall, and history of falls. Fall incident report data was merged with a participants' other study information.

2.3. Exercise Dose and Participation Assessment. Two primary measures of exercise were retrospectively obtained from exercise charts: aerobic training in minutes and number of strength training sessions. From these chart values, three variables were calculated: years of participation, number of aerobic and strength sessions attended each week, and minutes of participation in each aerobic session.

2.4. Statistical Analysis. Statistical analyses were performed using SAS Version 9.2. Descriptive analyses were used to report characteristics of the study population by falls history, including age, gender, and participation in the exercise program. Differences in participation history between those with a fall history and those without it were tested using t-tests. Logistic regression models were designed to assess the association between volume of exercise participation and falls incidents, adjusting for gender and age.

3. Results

In the 39 individuals in this analysis, a total of 13 (33.3%) reported a fall incident during the five-year period. The mean age in years was 87.4 at the beginning of the study; 74.4% (N = 29) were female. The mean participation in the exercise program was 2.2 years, with mean aerobic and strength training at 197.7 minutes and 136.1 sessions, respectively. Among those with a fall record, a total of 60 incidents were reported; of those, half reported at least two or more falls. Most common reported reason for fall incident was loss of balance.

Results comparing study population characteristics according to fall status are shown in Table 1. Negative associations for fall incidents were recorded with total exercise program participation, aerobic training, and strength training. Weekly descriptors of training illustrated similar results. Those with no reported fall incidents documented more time in aerobic training minutes per week (26.30 versus 20.00, P value = 0.71) and strength training sessions per week (1.50 versus 0.50, P value = 0.01) compared to those with a reported fall incident.

TABLE 1: Exercise participation in relation to fall status.

Characteristic	Fall history ($n = 13$) Mean ± SD	Range	No fall history ($n = 26$) Mean ± SD	Range	P for trend*
Fitness program participation, days	588.8 ± 648.4	1–1,834	886.7 ± 977.2	1–2,954	0.1389
Aerobic training					
Total aerobic training sessions	130.7 ± 190.6	1–567	231.2 ± 267.4	0–859	0.2201
Aerobic training minutes per week	20.0 ± 15.6	0–52	26.3 ± 14.4	0–49	0.7101
Strength training					
Total strength training sessions	81.5 ± 158.6	0–513	163.4 ± 248.5	0–831	0.1065
Strength training sessions per week	0.5 ± 0.2	0–2	1.5 ± 1.6	0–7	0.0054

*Results from t-test comparing means for fall history and no fall history groups.

Dose-dependent associations for fall incidents were seen with participation in the exercise program (Table 2). In adjusted models, aerobic and strength training were associated with decreased odds of a fall incident. Specifically, those who recorded a greater number of total strength training sessions were significantly less likely to experience a fall incident (OR = 0.25; 95% CI = 0.07, 0.85) than those with fewer total sessions.

TABLE 2: Multivariate logistic regression model of factors associated with fall history in an assisted living population.

Characteristic	Unadjusted OR(95% CI)	Adjusted OR* (95% CI)
Total program participation	1.00 (0.99, 1.00)	0.99 (0.99, 1.00)
Aerobic training	0.97 (0.93, 1.02)	0.97 (0.92, 1.03)
Strength training	0.42 (0.18, 0.96)	0.25 (0.07, 0.85)

*Adjusted for age and gender; $N = 39$.

4. Discussion

This study reports findings from a cross-sectional study investigating the association between the Boston FICSIT and fall incidents among older adults in one AL community. Our findings report a protective association between strength training and fall incidents; the odds of a fall incident among those who logged more time strength training were less compared to those who logged less time. More specifically, individuals with a greater number of strength training sessions per week had 75% reduced odds of a fall incident than those with fewer sessions.

Analysis of the Boston FICSIT cohort data by Fiatarone et al. reported this exercise training program significantly improved the results of all muscle-strength tests among exercise participants compared to controls [15]. Among those who participated in exercise training, gait velocity increased by 11.8% and overall muscle strength increased by 111.3%, compared to nonexercisers [15]. The present study attempts to investigate if this same exercise program is associated with falls reduction in the AL population. This study appears to provide additional evidence that progressive resistance exercise training, as first reported by Boston FICSIT exercise training study, is associated with reducing fall incidents in another frail older adult setting, the AL population [15].

Results of this study suggest that older adults who spent less time in the exercise program may be more susceptible to fall incidents than those with greater time spent. Our analysis is limited by the cross-sectional study design; caution in the interpretation of the observed associations must be taken into account. A second limitation was the inability to control for baseline health among participants and lack of screening for additional activity outside the prescribed exercise program. Third, incident reports, while standardized and structured, were used to enumerate the dependent variables and are likely to capture only falls requiring assistance from the facility staff. Therefore, fall incidents may be underreported in this population. Finally, there is no comparison group; this study assessed the association among only those who participated in the exercise program. Therefore, we do not have information about those who did not participate in the program and their fall incidents.

The findings of this study have important implications for AL populations and highlight the need for future research to identify specific exercise programs, specifically focusing on strength training protocols, to garner the best outcomes among this population. Future research should include the following topics: the amount of time spent in strength training to effectively reduce falls, the types of strength training exercises that are the most beneficial in reducing falls, and inclusion of both aerobic and strength training. This could facilitate interventions aimed at reducing falls incidents among vulnerable older adult populations.

Conflict of Interests

The authors declare that there is no conflict of interests regarding the publication of this paper.

Acknowledgments

This research was supported by the Atria Senior Living Group. It was supported in part by Grant 1 R49 CE002096-01 from the National Center for Injury Prevention and Control, Centers for Disease Control and Prevention, to the Center for Injury Epidemiology and Prevention at Columbia University.

Its contents are solely the responsibility of the authors and do not necessarily represent the official views of the Centers for Disease Control and Prevention.

References

[1] C. M. Arnold, M. M. Sran, and E. L. Harrison, "Exercise for fall risk reduction in community-dwelling older adults: a systematic review," *Physiotherapy Canada*, vol. 60, no. 4, pp. 358–372, 2008.

[2] Centers for Disease Control and Prevention, "Falls Among Older Adults: An Overview," 2013, http://www.cdc.gov/home-andrecreationalsafety/falls/adultfalls.html.

[3] N. V. Carroll, P. W. Slattum, and F. M. Cox, "The cost of falls among the community-dwelling elderly," *Journal of Managed Care Pharmacy*, vol. 11, no. 4, pp. 307–316, 2005.

[4] A. A. Bohl, E. A. Phelan, P. A. Fishman, and J. R. Harris, "How are the costs of care for medical falls distributed? The costs of medical falls by component of cost, timing, and injury severity," *The Gerontologist*, vol. 52, no. 5, pp. 664–675, 2012.

[5] V. A. Moyer, "Prevention of falls in community-dwelling older adults: U.S. Preventive Services Task Force recommendation statement," *Annals of Internal Medicine*, vol. 157, no. 3, pp. 197–204, 2012.

[6] C. Sherrington, J. C. Whitney, S. R. Lord, R. D. Herbert, R. G. Cumming, and J. C. T. Close, "Effective exercise for the prevention of falls: a systematic review and meta-analysis," *Journal of the American Geriatrics Society*, vol. 56, no. 12, pp. 2234–2243, 2008.

[7] A. Halvarsson, E. Olsson, E. Farén, A. Pettersson, and A. Ståhle, "Effects of new, individually adjusted, progressive balance group training for elderly people with fear of falling and tend to fall: a randomized controlled trial," *Clinical Rehabilitation*, vol. 25, no. 11, pp. 1021–1031, 2011.

[8] A. Barnett, B. Smith, S. R. Lord, M. Williams, and A. Baumand, "Community-based group exercise improves balance and reduces falls in at-risk older people: a randomised controlled trial," *Age and Ageing*, vol. 32, no. 4, pp. 407–414, 2003.

[9] J. C. Nitz and N. L. Choy, "The efficacy of a specific balance-strategy training programme for preventing falls among older people: a pilot randomised controlled trial," *Age and Ageing*, vol. 33, no. 1, pp. 52–58, 2004.

[10] S. R. Lord, S. Castell, J. Corcoran et al., "The effect of group exercise on physical functioning and falls in frail older people living in retirement villages: a randomized, controlled trial," *Journal of the American Geriatrics Society*, vol. 51, no. 12, pp. 1685–1692, 2003.

[11] J. Beling and M. Roller, "Multifactorial intervention with balance training as a core component among fall-prone older adults," *Journal of Geriatric Physical Therapy*, vol. 32, no. 3, pp. 125–133, 2009.

[12] S. M. Golant, "Do impaired older persons with health care needs occupy U.S. assisted living facilities? An analysis of six national studies," *Journals of Gerontology—Series B Psychological Sciences and Social Sciences*, vol. 59, no. 2, pp. S68–S79, 2004.

[13] M. Q. Vu, N. Weintraub, and L. Z. Rubenstein, "Falls in the nursing home: are they preventable?" *Journal of the American Medical Directors Association*, vol. 7, no. 3, supplement, pp. S53–S58, 2006.

[14] M. E. Nelson, M. A. Fiatarone, C. M. Morganti, I. Trice, R. A. Greenberg, and W. J. Evans, "Effects of high-intensity strength training on multiple risk factors for osteoporotic fractures: a randomized controlled trial," *Journal of the American Medical Association*, vol. 272, no. 24, pp. 1909–1914, 1994.

[15] M. A. Fiatarone, E. F. O'Neill, N. D. Ryan et al., "Exercise training and nutritional supplementation for physical frailty in very elderly people," *The New England Journal of Medicine*, vol. 330, no. 25, pp. 1769–1775, 1994.

[16] M. T. Hannan, M. M. Gagnon, J. Aneja et al., "Optimizing the tracking of falls in studies of older participants: comparison of quarterly telephone recall with monthly falls calendars in the MOBILIZE Boston study," *The American Journal of Epidemiology*, vol. 171, no. 9, pp. 1031–1036, 2010.

10

Decision Making Processes and Outcomes

Julie Hicks Patrick,[1] Jenessa C. Steele,[2,3] and S. Melinda Spencer[2,4]

[1] *Department of Psychology, West Virginia University, P.O. Box 6040, Morgantown, WV 26506-6040, USA*
[2] *Department of Psychology, West Virginia University, Morgantown, WV 26506-6040, USA*
[3] *Department of Psychology, Radford University, P.O. Box 6946, Radford, VA 24141, USA*
[4] *Department of Health Promotion Education and Behavior, University of South Carolina, Columbia, SC 2920, USA*

Correspondence should be addressed to Julie Hicks Patrick; julie.patrick@mail.wvu.edu

Academic Editor: Holly M. Brown-Borg

The primary aim of this study was to examine the contributions of individual characteristics and strategic processing to the prediction of decision quality. Data were provided by 176 adults, ages 18 to 93 years, who completed computerized decision-making vignettes and a battery of demographic and cognitive measures. We examined the relations among age, domain-specific experience, working memory, and three measures of strategic information search to the prediction of solution quality using a 4-step hierarchical linear regression analysis. Working memory and two measures of strategic processing uniquely contributed to the variance explained. Results are discussed in terms of potential advances to both theory and intervention efforts.

1. Introduction

1.1. Decision Making Processes and Outcomes. A significant body of research has examined problem solving and decision making performance in adulthood (see [1, 2] for reviews). Both problem solving and decision making are concerned with the ways in which people interpret problems, form goals, search information, and combine information to arrive at solutions. Researchers often employ think-aloud and other process-tracing techniques to investigate the processes governing information search and cessation [3, 4]. The extant literature demonstrates that relative to younger and middle-aged adults, older adults approach decision making with different goals, apply different heuristics, seek different amounts and types of information in the predecision phase, and offer different decisions (e.g., [4–6]).

Research has examined several possible mechanisms to explain this age difference, including the role of cognitive resources (e.g., [5, 7]), the social context and personal experience [8, 9], affective context [10], and the decision domain [11]. Sophisticated studies have examined these factors individually and in combination [12]. For many decision tasks, basic and intermediate cognitive skills such as working memory and speed of processing often are the strongest predictor of decision outcome [13].

Process-tracing techniques may allow a more thorough examination of task performance and strategic processing [3, 4, 14, 15]. In the standard decision making task, materials are structured to reflect those available in the real-world, similar to the ecologically-rich social vignettes used in the everyday problem solving approach. Although in actual real-world information searches, people are able to view all of the available information simultaneously, an advantage to the process-tracing technique is that one is able to directly examine how an adult: (a) selects important features, (b) combines the information obtained, (c) evaluates specific alternatives, and (d) arrives at an adequate decision [14–16]. Specifically, multiple measures are used to index task performance, including the amount of information searched and the order in which the information is searched. Indicators of the amount of information searched include time on task and the number of information cells viewed (i.e., thoroughness). Research shows that older adults often use less information than younger adults [4, 17].

Strategic search is also examined in the decision making task. The two main types of search strategies have been termed compensatory and noncompensatory [4, 18]. Compensatory search is an exhaustive strategy that relies on mathematical averaging of the features for each alternative. Thus, compensatory searches require significant effort as most or all of the available information is read, processed, evaluated, and combined. Noncompensatory strategies reduce the number of viable alternatives quickly when the information load exceeds a person's ability to attend to the information volume. Noncompensatory strategies accomplish this reduction by focusing exclusively on a few alternatives which have high or acceptable values on a set of key attributes. Thus, noncompensatory strategies are more resource-efficient than compensatory search strategies [14, 18].

One area that is often overlooked in decision making research concerns the value of the information participants choose to view. However, information quality has been studied in examinations of expert decisions [19]. For example, some studies of experts have shown that they search very little of the available information before making a decision, in some cases viewing only one or two pieces of highly relevant information [15]. The experts are able to "zero in" on the most critical pieces of information to make a high quality decision. If the value of any given piece of information is known, researchers can measure the selectivity with which decision makers choose information. Using search selectivity, the quality of information used can be separated from the amount used and from the order of search. Thus, selectivity allows one to interpret differences in thoroughness and strategy.

1.2. The Current Study. The current study extends investigations of strategic information search by focusing on both information quality and decision quality among a large sample of community-dwelling adults. By combining a focus on the contributions of individual characteristics of experience and working memory from the everyday problem solving literature with a focus on direct task performance measures from the decision making domain, the current study contributes to the literature by clarifying the roles of these predictors. By examining the ways in which differences in the information search process relate to differences in decision outcome, we can better understand age-related differences in decision making. Based on the everyday problem-solving literature, we expected to find age differences in decision quality, with older adults being less likely than younger and middle-aged adults to provide high quality decisions, as defined by agreement with expert rankings. However, similar to Queen et al. [14], we hypothesized that decision quality would be predicted by strategic processing measures rather than age or experience. We also expected that search selectivity would emerge as a significant predictor of decision quality, even when age, experience, working memory, and other strategic search measures were included in the model.

2. Methods

2.1. Sample. Data were provided by 176 adults who completed computerized decision making tasks and interviewer-administered surveys. Participants were recruited through published ads and posted fliers and received a cash honorarium for their participation. The adults ranged in age from 18 to 93 years, and about half (42.6%) were men. Reflecting the geographic region from which they were recruited, the majority of the sample (96%) were Caucasian. Most adults (97.6%) had completed high school, with 38.7% having a college degree. Participants completed a 90-minute test battery, including a variety of demographic, social, and cognitive measures; only those of interest to the current report are detailed below.

2.2. Task Materials and Procedure. All adults completed written informed consent before completing two practice trials. Participants then completed two computerized automobile purchasing decisions for hypothetical others whose needs were presented in short vignettes. The hypothetical vignettes were written such that the needs and resources of the target individuals were implied. Specifically, participants chose an automobile for a middle-aged professional couple who entertained clients regularly and they chose an automobile for a college student who commuted to school and work. The structured design of the scenarios enabled the determination of a correct response and helped to ensure that participants had the same goals for completing the task. The task materials accurately reflected automobiles available on the market, with information provided in a format similar to that found in published guides for consumers. Thus, each of the eight automobiles included information about price, style, appearance, safety, reliability, fuel economy, equipment, and performance. A panel of five experts, using all of the available information, rank ordered the alternatives for appropriateness for each of the vignettes. High interrater reliability was obtained (Kendall's coefficient of concordance, $W > .80$, $P < .01$). In addition, grammatical analyses showed that the reading level of each vignette was appropriate (Fleish index < grade 8.0). Finally, the order of presentation of the two scenarios was counterbalanced across participants to reduce the effects of practice and fatigue.

2.3. Variables and Measures

2.3.1. Individual Characteristics. For the regression analyses, age was used as a continuous variable, although mean age group comparisons were also conducted. Approximately equal numbers of younger adults ($M = 22.20$, SD = 3.44, $n = 54$), middle-aged adults ($M = 51.45$, SD = 11.14, $n = 60$), and older adults ($M = 76.82$, SD = 5.94, $n = 62$) participated. A dichotomous variable (1 = men, 2 = women) was used to index sex.

2.3.2. Cognitive Resources. Two indices of cognitive resources were used. Working memory span was measured using the digits backward test [20], with the standard administration and scoring procedures. The average backward working memory span for the current sample was 4.64 (SD = 1.11, range 2–7).

Three dichotomous items assessing experience with the task domain were combined to form a scale. The items included whether a participant had ever made an automobile purchase (70.1%), currently owned an automobile (87.4%),

Table 1: Descriptive statistics and correlations.

		Mean	SD	1	2	3	4	5	6	7	8
(1)	Age	51.41	23.45	1.0	.056	−.132	.164*	−.177*	−.396**	−.183*	−.175*
(2)	Gender (1 = men, 2 = women)	1.57	0.50	—	1.0	−.012	−.197**	.059	−.099	.050	−.073
(3)	Backward digit span	4.64	1.11	—	—	1.0	.022	.116	.016	.293**	.443**
(4)	Experience	2.06	0.89	—	—	—	1.0	−.108	.028	−.083	.036
(5)	Proportion of information viewed	0.42	0.24	—	—	—	—	1.0	−.194**	.618**	.196**
(6)	Noncompensatory search	0.38	0.28	—	—	—	—	—	1.0	−.088	−.013
(7)	Search selectivity	0.51	0.28	—	—	—	—	—	—	1.0	.525**
(8)	Decision quality	10.95	3.99	—	—	—	—	—	—	—	1.0

*$P < .05$, **$P < .01$.

and had ever been asked to give advice to another person considering an automobile purchase (47.9%). The scale ranged from 0 to 3; a mean of 2.06 (SD = .89) was obtained from the current sample.

2.3.3. Similarities across Vignettes. For each decision vignette, participants could view one piece of information at a time during their information search. They were permitted to review as much information as they desired, but were not allowed to take notes. The computer program recorded a variety of measures from which three information search measures were derived: proportion of information searched, order of information searched, and quality of information searched. Paired t-tests were used to examine differences across the two vignettes. No significant differences emerged for the amount of information viewed ($t(175) = 1.33$), order of information searched ($t(175) = 1.13$), or selectivity ($t(175) = 4.81$) across the two vignettes. When examining whether participants made one of the two best choices, 48.9% chose correctly in the college student scenario and 45.5% chose correctly in the couple scenario ($t(175) = .88$). Because no mean differences were found between the two vignettes, responses were combined to form a single, averaged index for each of the following measures.

2.3.4. Task Performance. Amount of information searched was assessed via the proportion of the total number of pieces of information viewed [4, 21]. On average, participants viewed less than half of the available information ($M = .419$, SD = .241).

Order of information search (noncompensatory search strategy) was indexed using a ratio of repetition (RR) measure. The RR was originally used in recall tasks to address category clustering, the phenomenon in which people tend to recall a list of randomly-presented words by regrouping the words into categories. Applied to the information matrices, the RR represents the order in which information is viewed. If a decision maker searched within a column of features to compare different alternatives on a single feature, the high RR for features would indicate a noncompensatory search. In the current sample, a mean noncompensatory strategy score of .38 (SD = .28) was obtained.

Finally, search selectivity was assessed. Search selectivity concerns which information is viewed, as contrasted with search order. Selectivity was operationalized as the proportion of relevant information the participant searched, with relevance determined by the individual value of a specific piece of information in relation to the needs of the target person. For example, in the college student vignette, the target had little income, no knowledge of autorepair, and needed to commute daily. Thus, the experts indicated that the most relevant features for the student were price, reliability, and fuel economy. For the middle-aged couple who entertained clients and needed an auto for pleasure use, the experts determined that style, safety, and reliability were most relevant. For each vignette, two automobiles were clearly superior, three were of medium quality, and three were inappropriate. Thus, for each vignette, six of the 64 pieces of information were especially relevant. If a participant viewed four of these six pieces of information, the selectivity score would equal .67. In the current sample, a mean selectivity score of .51 (SD = .28) was obtained.

2.3.5. Decision Quality. Each of the participant's choices were coded to reflect agreement with the rank ordering determined by the expert panels. Points were awarded such that the top choice received a total of 8 points and the least appropriate choice received one point. The points awarded for the two decisions were then combined to form a single index that ranged from 2 to 16 ($M = 10.95$; SD = 3.99).

3. Results

3.1. Preliminary Analyses. Means and correlations for the measures are presented in Table 1. To test our hypothesis that age differences would emerge, we conducted a series of one-way analysis of variance tests comparing the three age groups. As shown in Table 2, mean age differences in decision quality were observed. That is, middle-aged adults ($M = 12.38$) offered higher quality decisions than older adults ($M = 9.50$; $F(2, 173) = 8.68$, $P < .001$).

Mean age differences also emerged for strategic processing. Specifically, differences were observed for selectivity ($F(2, 173) = 4.72$, $P = .01$) and noncompensatory strategy ($F(2, 173) = 21.55$, $P < .001$). For both selectivity and noncompensatory strategy, younger and middle-aged adults scored higher than older adults. In terms of individual characteristics, differences in experience and working memory were

Table 2: Mean age group differences.

	Group A Younger (n = 54)	Group B Middle aged (n = 60)	Older (n = 62)	Group C F	Post Hoc
Age	22.20	51.45	76.82	737.22***	A < B < C
Experience	1.78	2.22	2.15	4.03*	A < B
Working memory	4.65	4.88	4.38	3.23*	B > C
Proportion viewed	0.47	0.42	0.37	2.97*	
Noncompensatory search	0.49	0.45	0.21	21.55***	A and B > C
Search selectivity	0.55	0.56	0.42	4.72**	A and B > C
Decision quality	11.03	12.38	9.50	8.68***	B > C

$^{*}P \le .05$, $^{**}P \le .01$, $^{***}P \le .001$.

observed. Younger adults had significantly less experience than middle-aged adults ($F(2, 173) = 4.03$, $P = .019$). Middle-aged adults had a higher mean working memory span than older adults ($F(2, 173) = 3.22$, $P = .042$). A nonsignificant age effect was observed for the amount of information viewed ($F(2, 173) = 2.97$, $P = .054$).

3.2. Hypothesis Testing. To examine our hypothesis regarding the relative contribution of individual characteristics and strategic task performance to the explanation of decision quality, we conducted a 4-step hierarchical linear regression analysis. Model 1 included the demographic indicators of age and gender, entered simultaneously. Model 2 added two individual characteristics, working memory span and domain-specific experience. Model 3 added two measures of strategic task performance, the amount of information viewed, and noncompensatory search strategy. Finally, Model 4 examined the unique contribution of search selectivity to the overall prediction of decision quality. Results for these analyses are presented in Table 3. The equation using only age and gender to explain variance in decision quality reached significance ($F(2, 173) = 3.12$, $P = .047$), but accounted for less than 3% of the variance. Age uniquely accounted for variance in Decision Quality.

The equation adding the two everyday problem solving predictors at Step 2 was significant ($F(4, 171) = 11.72$, $P < .001$). Together the four regressors accounted for 19.7% of the variance in Decision Quality. Of the four regressors, only working memory span uniquely contributed to the variance explained. That is, when everyday problem solving predictors were present in the model, age no longer uniquely contributed to the variance in Decision Quality. Adding the task performance measures at Step 3 resulted in an additional 2.0% of explained variance, although the step failed to reach significance ($F(2, 169) = 2.26$, $P = .11$). The model, however, continued to explain significant amounts of variance in decision quality ($F(6, 169) = 8.68$, $P < .001$; $R^2 = .208$). Again, only working memory span uniquely contributed to the explained variance.

Finally, Step 4 examined the contributions of search selectivity. Both the step ($F(1, 168) = 46.76$, $P < .001$) and the model ($F(7, 168) = 16.14$, $P < .001$) reached significance. Search selectivity accounted for an additional 16.6% of the variance beyond that explained by age, gender, working memory, experience, amount of information viewed, and noncompensatory search strategy. The final model accounted for 37.7% of the variance in Decision Quality. In the final model, larger working memory span, more information viewed, and higher search selectivity uniquely contributed to the variance accounted for in Decision Quality.

Table 3: Linear regression predicting decision quality (n = 176).

	b	SE_b	B
Step 1			
Age	−.029	.013	−.172*
Gender	−.513	.602	−.064
Step 2			
Age	−.021	.012	−.122
Gender	−.437	.558	−.054
Experience	161	.315	.036
Working memory	1.532	.246	.425***
Step 3			
Age	−.021	.013	−.124
Gender	−.517	.556	−.064
Experience	.222	.314	.050
Working memory	1.480	.246	.411***
Proportion of information viewed	2.077	1.192	.125
Noncompensatory search	−.752	1.108	−.052
Step 4			
Age	−.017	.012	−.099
Gender	−.597	.493	−.074
Experience	.256	.279	.057
Working memory	1.051	.227	.292***
Proportion of information viewed	−3.164	1.306	−.191*
Noncompensatory search	−.792	.983	−.055
Search selectivity	7.676	1.123	.543***

Step 1: $F(2, 173) = 3.12^{*}$; $R^2 = .027$. Step 2: $F(2, 171) = 19.65^{***}$; model $F(4, 171) = 11.72^{***}$; $R^2 = .197$. Step 3: $F(2, 169) = 2.26$; model $F(6, 169) = 8.68^{***}$; $R^2 = .208$. Step 4: $F(1, 168) = 46.76^{***}$; model $F(7, 168) = 16.14^{***}$; $R^2 = .377$.

A series of exploratory analyses was conducted to examine potential interactions with age and with working memory among the predictor set. Predictors were centered and entered into a first step of a hierarchical regression. The interaction terms were then entered in a second step. In no case did an interaction term add to the variance accounted for in Decision Quality.

4. Discussion

Our process-tracing technique and the known quality of information allows an examination of the adults' performance at multiple stages of decision making, including the selection of information and arriving at a solution. Our results show that the quality of the information one chooses directly affects the quality of the decisions one makes. While this finding is certainly intuitive, we empirically demonstrated this association. This is an important contribution because the finding can be used to guide training and intervention programs to increase the decision making competence of adults. Specifically, by being able to determine the relative value of a single piece of information, we can assess how selective a problem solver is in her search processes. Moreover, by knowing the value of each piece of information, we can determine decision quality.

In addition to the important role of search selectivity, our results show an important role for working memory span and search thoroughness. As an initial investigation into decision quality, we chose a consumer task in which identifying the relevance of the information and decision quality was somewhat straight-forward. Given previous findings in these domains [4, 14], it is surprising that mean age differences emerged. Interestingly, age contributed little to the explanation of decision quality. Together, these results suggest that we can begin to explore ways in which to improve decision making quality. Implications for each of these avenues, as well as how our results relate to current theoretical frameworks are discussed in the following sections.

4.1. Individual Characteristics. Several mean age differences were observed in the current study. Specifically, older adults had smaller working memory spans, searched less selectively, were less likely to use a noncompensatory strategy, and were less likely to choose one of the top two alternatives. Despite these mean differences, however, our regression results find no significant contribution of chronological age when additional measures are included in the equation. This result reaffirms the idea that chronological age is a poor proxy for cognitive ability.

Research demonstrates that decision making is affected by a variety of cognitive processes such as working memory and speed, which can be improved with training [13]. Our study adds to this literature by demonstrating that working memory is not only related to information search but also exerts direct effects on decision quality. Thus, it may be possible to improve decision making competence by intervening at the level of these cognitive processes.

The literature also suggests an important role for experience [9, 15, 17]. Among our community-dwelling nonexperts, experience did not contribute to decision quality. We suspect that our measure of experience was too crude to adequately assess the effects of experience on decision quality. Our index included three dichotomous items for which a large number of participants answered affirmatively. Thus, the failure of experience to relate to decision quality could be a function of ceiling effects on the measure. A second explanation for the failure of experience to explain variance in decision quality may relate to the nature of that experience. As Patrick and Strough [9] note, recency of experience may be particularly important. We encourage additional research that examines the role of prior experience in problem solving quality, particularly whether experience operates similarly across adulthood.

4.2. Task Performance. Decision making research often focuses on the thoroughness of information search. Typical results show that older adults use less information than younger or middle-aged adults [4]. In our analyses, no significant age differences in thoroughness emerged. Moreover, in the regressions, thoroughness only uniquely contributed to the variance in decision quality when selectivity was present in the equation. Although additional investigation is necessary, this relation may be due to potentially dual routes to acquiring the relevant information. People who are highly selective may view little of the total information, thus scoring lower on measures of thoroughness. However, through increased thoroughness, people increase the likelihood that they will view the relevant information. Thus, highly selective searchers may view less total information as they focus on the most relevant information. In contrast, highly thorough searchers are also likely to acquire the most important information. Overall, however, our results show that quantity is less important than the quality of the information. Additional investigation regarding the association between amount of information searched and the quality of that information is advised.

Both the age differences in search strategy and the relative importance of the use of a noncompensatory strategy in the regression analyses are intriguing. Together, these two sets of analyses suggest that age differences in problem solving efficiency may be a direct function of problem solving strategy. Such a conclusion is consistent with a range of everyday problem solving studies showing strong age differences in problem solving strategy [2]. The current data are able to link these strategic differences to differences in the quality of responses. Thus, the analyses demonstrate that age differences in strategic processing are important because they directly relate to age differences in solution quality.

The measure of strategic processing, drawn from the decision making literature, was a global summary of how much of an individual's search could be characterized as noncompensatory. Noncompensatory strategies are generally viewed as an adaptive response to working memory overload [4, 18]. It is interesting that older adults demonstrated smaller working memory spans but did not show a high use of noncompensatory search. Again, these results suggest two avenues for intervention: at the level of working memory capacity and at the level of task performance.

Finally, although the task offers several advantages to studying both problem solving process and outcome, it does have limitations. Specifically, participants could only view one piece of information at a time during their information search. They were permitted to review as much information as they desired, but were not allowed to take notes. In the real-world, consumers may adopt more external aids to facilitate their information search. However, the process tracing technique present in the current task offers sufficient advantages to offset this limitation. That is, the technique allows an examination of which information is viewed and in what order. These two aspects of information search are the essence of strategic processing.

4.3. Theoretical Implications and Future Directions. In our consumer problem, age contributed little to decision quality. This finding is consistent with previous research [4, 14] in this domain. A major contribution of our work rests with the computation of Decision Quality. Both Johnson [4] and Queen et al. [14] relied on the individuals' preferences as an outcome measure. Our conceptualization of decision quality focuses on making a decision for others with stated and implied needs. This difference is important in that it allows us to determine information quality and thus, search selectivity.

We strongly advocate for an extension of both the process-tracing approach and the information quality aspect to a wider range of domains. Significant newer research is examining the tradeoff between affective and logical goals [10], but because these domains may exhibit marked idiosyncrasies, it might be especially challenging to examine information quality in vignettes featuring an interpersonal problem [22]. Although work and wisdom [23] might inform such efforts. Such interpersonal expertise may be similar to the processes used by experts in instrumental domains and warrants additional research attention. Vignettes could be designed to include both emotion-laden and instrumental information. Investigators could then directly examine the type of information that adults use when making decisions in a variety of domains, including interpersonal, health [15], and financial [13].

In summary, it is important to develop tasks and measures that reflect the everyday competence of older adults [13] so that we can identify individuals in need of decision making support. Rather than cataloging age differences; however, it is necessary to link age differences in process to some difference in performance outcome. We present a task and measures that may significantly advance the field's progress toward that goal. By focusing on the quality of an adult's decision in a hypothetical vignette, differences in strategy become more meaningful. We encourage additional and independent investigation using this class of tasks, and we look forward to refinements of the measures of strategy, selectivity, and decision quality.

Acknowledgment

This work was supported by funding from the NIH (R03 AG19917).

References

[1] E. Peters and W. Bruine de Bruin, "Aging and decision skills," in *Judgment and Decision Making as a Skill: Learning, Development, and Evolution*, M. K. Dhami, A. Schlottmann, and M. Waldmann, Eds., chapter 5, pp. 113–1139, Cambridge University Press, 2012.

[2] W. J. L. Thornton and H. A. Dumke, "Age differences in everyday problem-solving and decision-making effectiveness: a meta-analytic review," *Psychology and Aging*, vol. 20, no. 1, pp. 85–99, 2005.

[3] J. Aschemann-Witzel and U. Hamm, "Measuring consumers' information acquisition and decision behavior with the computer-based information-display-matrix," *Methodology*, vol. 7, no. 1, pp. 1–10, 2011.

[4] M. M. S. Johnson, "Age differences in decision making: a process methodology for examining strategic information processing," *Journals of Gerontology*, vol. 45, no. 2, pp. P75–P78, 1990.

[5] H. Szrek and M. K. Bundorf, "Age and the purchase of prescription drug insurance by older adults," *Psychology and Aging*, vol. 26, no. 2, pp. 308–320, 2011.

[6] R. Mata and L. Nunes, "When less is enough: cognitive aging, information search, and decision quality in consumer choice," *Psychology and Aging*, vol. 25, no. 2, pp. 289–298, 2010.

[7] J. C. Allaire and M. Marsiske, "Everyday cognition: age and intellectual ability correlates," *Psychology and Aging*, vol. 14, no. 4, pp. 627–644, 1999.

[8] W. Bruine de Bruin, A. M. Parker, and B. Fishhoff, "Explaining adult age differences in decision-making competence," *Journal of Behavioral Decision Making*, vol. 25, no. 4, pp. 352–360, 2010.

[9] J. H. Patrick and J. Strough, "Everyday problem solving: experience, strategies, and behavioral intentions," *Journal of Adult Development*, vol. 11, no. 1, pp. 9–18, 2004.

[10] E. Peters, T. M. Hess, D. Västfjäll, and C. Auman, "Adult age difference in dual information processes: implications for the role of affective and deliberative processes in older adults' decision-making competence," *Psychology and Aging*, vol. 2, no. 1, pp. 1–23, 2007.

[11] W. J. L. Thornton, T. S. E. Paterson, and S. E. Yeung, "Age differences in everyday problem solving: the role of problem context," *International Journal of Behavioral Development*, vol. 37, pp. 13–20, 2013.

[12] M. L. Finucane, C. K. Mertz, P. Slovic, and E. S. Schemdit, "Task complexity and older adults decision-making competence," *Psychology and Aging*, vol. 20, no. 1, pp. 71–84, 2005.

[13] M. L. Finucane and C. M. Gullion, "Developing a tool for measuring the decision-making competence of older adults," *Psychology and Aging*, vol. 25, no. 2, pp. 271–288, 2010.

[14] T. L. Queen, T. M. Hess, G. E. Ennis, K. Dowd, and D. Gruhn, "Information search and decision making: effects of age and complexity on strategy use," *Psychology and Aging*, vol. 27, pp. 817–824, 2012.

[15] M. K. Dhami and C. Harries, "Information search in heuristic decision making," *Applied Cognitive Psychology*, vol. 24, no. 4, pp. 571–586, 2010.

[16] R. P. Bagozzi and U. Dholakia, "Goal setting and goal striving in consumer behavior," *Journal of Marketing*, vol. 63, pp. 19–32, 1999.

[17] S. L. Willis, M. M. Dolan, and R. M. Bertrand, "Problem solving on health-related tasks of daily living," in *Processing of Medical Information in Aging Patients: Cognitive and Human Factors Perspectives*, D. C. Park, R. W. Morrell, and K. Shifren, Eds., Erlbaum, New Jersey, NJ, USA, 1999.

[18] R. W. Olshavsky, "Task complexity and contingent processing in decision making: a replication and extension," *Organizational Behavior and Human Performance*, vol. 24, no. 3, pp. 300–316, 1979.

[19] J. F. Yates and A. L. Patalano, "Decision making and aging," in *Processing of Medical Information in Aging Patients: Cognitive and Human Factors Perspectives*, D. C. Park, R. W. Morrell, and K. Shifren, Eds., Erlbaum, New Jersey, NJ, USA, 1999.

[20] D. Wechsler, *WAIS-R Manual: Wechsler Adult Intelligence Scale-Revised*, Psychological Corporation, Cleveland, Ohio, USA, 1981.

[21] J. W. Payne, "Task complexity and contingent processing in decision making: an information search and protocol analysis," *Organizational Behavior and Human Performance*, vol. 16, no. 2, pp. 366–387, 1976.

[22] J. C. Allaire and M. Marsiske, "Well- and ill-defined measures of everyday cognition: relationship to older adults' intellectual ability and functional status," *Psychology and Aging*, vol. 17, no. 1, pp. 101–115, 2002.

[23] P. B. Baltes and U. M. Staudinger, "Wisdom: a metaheuristic (pragmatic) to orchestrate mind and virtue toward excellence," *American Psychologist*, vol. 55, no. 1, pp. 122–136, 2000.

11

Efficacy of Female Rat Models in Translational Cardiovascular Aging Research

K. M. Rice,[1] J. C. Fannin,[1,2] C. Gillette,[3] and E. R. Blough[1,2,4]

[1] *Center for Diagnostic Nanosystems and Robert C. Byrd Biotechnology Science Center, Marshall University, Room 241D, 1700 3rd Avenue, Huntington, WV 25755-1090, USA*
[2] *Department of Pharmacology, Physiology and Toxicology, Joan C. Edwards School of Medicine, Marshall University, Huntington, WV, USA*
[3] *Department of Pharmacy Practice, Administration, and Research, School of Pharmacy, Marshall University, Huntington, WV, USA*
[4] *Department of Pharmaceutical Sciences and Research, School of Pharmacy, Marshall University, Huntington, WV, USA*

Correspondence should be addressed to K. M. Rice; rice9@marshall.edu

Academic Editor: F. R. Ferraro

Cardiovascular disease is the leading cause of death in women in the United States. Aging is a primary risk factor for the development of cardiovascular disease as well as cardiovascular-related morbidity and mortality. Aging is a universal process that all humans undergo; however, research in aging is limited by cost and time constraints. Therefore, most research in aging has been done in primates and rodents; however it is unknown how well the effects of aging in rat models translate into humans. To compound the complication of aging gender has also been indicated as a risk factor for various cardiovascular diseases. This review addresses the systemic pathophysiology of the cardiovascular system associated with aging and gender for aging research with regard to the applicability of rat derived data for translational application to human aging.

1. Introduction

In 2005, cardiovascular disease (CVD) was the underlying cause of death in 864,480 of the approximately 2.5 million total deaths in the United States [1, 2]. CVD is the leading cause of death and the most costly disease in America and is expected to increase in costs to $1.48 trillion by 2030 [3]. Although the focus has been to reduce the modifiable risk factors for cardiovascular disease (such as lipid levels, diabetes, and sedentary lifestyle), the unmodifiable risk factor, aging, is a major risk factor for coronary disease, hypertension, congestive heart failure, and stroke [4]. The number of the aged in the United States is projected to increase by more than 20% by the year 2030. This growth in the elderly population is expected to significantly test our already overloaded health care system.

Although years of research have been conducted in regard to aging, we are still a long way from understanding the intricacies of age-related changes in human physiology, in particular the cardiovascular system. Whether aging in animal models mimics many of the cardiovascular changes seen in humans is not well understood. In addition, the process of delineating the effect gender has on aging provides yet another variable to be considered.

2. Discussion

2.1. Aging and Cardiovascular Disease. Aging is believed by some to be a progressive disorder that decreases an organism's ability to maintain reproductive capacity and "normostasis" [5]. Indeed a strong correlation exists between aging and higher incidence of several diseases including dementia, Parkinson's disease, diabetes, cancer, and Alzheimer's disease [5]. In the cardiovascular system, aging is positively correlated with an increasing risk of cardiac problems including arrhythmias and is a major independent risk factor for cardiovascular-related morbidity and mortality [6]. Indeed, more than 70% of males and females over 75 years of age present some clinically evident cardiovascular disease

(CVD) [7]. In addition to age, CVD risk also appears to vary with sex. CVD is the number one killer of women in Western nations [8]. Among women, more than 200,000 of the 454,613 total CVD deaths occurred in those above 85 years of age [2]. Although cardiovascular risk increases with age in both sexes, the increase in age-associated risk appears to be sharper in women [9]. Why CVD risk may differ between men and women is not well understood but may be related to differences in age-associated cardiovascular function [10]. Whereas congestive heart failure in men is oftentimes due to systolic insufficiencies, congestive heart failure in women is often related to diastolic dysfunction [10, 11]. The incidences of ischemia, cardiac failure, and cardiac rupture in addition to ventricular remodeling have also been shown to differ between genders with aging and often lead to worse outcomes in women [12–15]. Recent data suggests that premenopausal women have a decreased risk of CVD compared to men of comparable age [16, 17]. This cardioprotective benefit appears to be lost over time as the risk of developing cardiovascular disease in postmenopausal women increases to a rate that is similar to that observed in men [18]. The reason(s) for this increase in CVD risk following menopause is currently unclear; however, it is well known that early menopause is associated with an increased risk for coronary heart disease and cardiovascular disease death [19–21]. This finding is thought to be related, at least in part, to diminished estrogen exposure [22]. Consistent with this notion, each year of increasing age at natural menopause has been found to be associated with a 2% increase in total cardiovascular mortality [22, 23]. Whether differences in estrogen alone or changes in estrogen along with other factors can fully explain the sex related differences in age-related cardiovascular function is unknown and requires further investigation.

2.2. Aging Female Rat Models. Human aging research is limited due to cost, differences in lifestyle/history, and more importantly the time required for data collection as well as analysis of that particular system. Importantly, there are a number of different animal models that can be used to acquire information on how aging affects the female cardiovascular system. The most applicable aging female animals studied include primates. Primates are the closest in regard to female human aging due to the fact that they are the only species to undergo menstrual sloughing of the endometrial lining. Nonetheless, it is important to note that female primates do not experience menopause [25]. In addition, primate research is oftentimes ethically difficult to perform and costly.

Rats are widely used in aging research as they exhibit a relatively short lifespan and are genetically quite homogenous. Among the various strains of rats, the Wistar, F344, and F344/Brown Norway are the most common used aging female rat models [26–30]. Although rats do not experience menses, they do experience estrus cycling and ovarian aging. Table 1 presents the stages of ovarian aging in female rats. Reproductive maturity is reached at five months when there is an estrous cycle that lasts four to five days. Aging rats exhibit periods of persistent estrous cycle which consists of elevated and constant levels of estradiol, low levels of progesterone, and lack of luteinizing hormone (LH) surges, in addition to ovulation [24, 31, 32]. Ovarian decline occurs between six and eighteen months depending on the rodent strain and is characterized by low levels of estradiol and progesterone, with little or no developing follicles and increased prolactin secretion [24, 31, 32].

Comparisons between aging research in female rats models and humans can be complicated due to the differences in the mechanisms of ovarian/hormone aging in human females and its potential impact on cardiovascular disease. Though not fully understood, it is thought that the loss of the hormones estrogen and progesterone in aging human females is due to the decrease in the ovarian follicular reserve [33]. Conversely, aging female rats experience a persistent estrous cycle due to chronic anovulation which consist of pseudopregnant/disestrus estrogen levels as well as high progesterone levels from increased ovulation and the corpora lutea [33]. Therefore, reproductive senescence in female rats consists of alterations in the hypothalamic-pituitary axis while reproductive senescence in human females is classified as ovarian follicle depletion [33]. Due to these reasons and others, caution should be exercised in extrapolating the results from rodent studies to humans. Although estrogen secretion by the ovary promotes hypothalamic changes, the chronic administration of estrogen can damage neurons in the arcuate nucleus and medial basal hypothalamus. Therefore, it can be important to remember that the surgical removal of the ovaries can lead to neurological changes that may affect other organs during the aging process.

2.3. Ovariotoxicity and Ovariectomy on the Aging Cardiovascular System. The pharmacological acceleration of ovarian aging using 4-vinylcyclohexene diepoxide (VCD) (accelerated ovarian failure (AOF) [34] model) or ovariectomy (OVX) procedures are often performed due to the lack of natural menopause in rat research models because they are believed to better mimic the hormone milieu seen in aging human females. VCD has been shown to target the plasma membrane of the primordial and primary follicles through direct inhibition of autophosphorylation of the oocyte-associated receptor, Kit [35]. Kit acts as an antiapoptotic factor in primordial follicular survival [36, 37]. Although an effective model of chemical ovotoxicity limited research has been performed using female rat models [38–41] and to date no published data exist regarding VCD and rat cardiovascular aging. VCD in juvenile (1 month) and adult (3 months) Sprague-Dawley rats depleted follicles but had no effect on the duration or onset of persistent estrus. However, FSH levels were significantly high in VCD treated animals with no change in cyclicity or serum levels of 17β-estradiol [38]. The absence of a human based clinical menopausal hormone profile in the AOF model brings into question the ability to apply data derived from this model for translational relevant treatment of cardiovascular human based menopausal pathologies.

An ovariectomy is the removal of the ovaries which induces a surgical menopause characterized by the cessation

Table 1: Stages of ovarian aging in a female rat as described by Lu et al. (1979) [24].

Age (months)	Stages of ovarian aging in female rats
5 months	Reproductive maturity (i) Estrous cycle (4-5 days) (ii) Elevated and constant levels of estradiol (iii) Low levels of progesterone (iv) Lack of hormone surges and ovulation
6–8 months	Ovarian decline (i) Decreased levels of estradiol and progesterone (ii) Little or no follicles
10–12 months	Irregularity of estrous cycles
19 months	Constant estrous cycle (i) Low to medium levels of serum estradiol, estrone, testosterone, androstenedione, and progesterone (ii) Very low levels of 20α-hydroxyprogesterone (iii) No preovulatory release of gonadotropin and prolactin (iv) Increased levels of FSH
24 months	Prolactin (i) Increased levels of prolactin (abolished by ovariectomy) (ii) Retained ability to develop follicles and corpora (iii) Retained ability to secrete steroid hormones

of estrogen and progesterone, as well as reduced production of testosterone. Surgical menopause leads to more severe and sudden symptoms compared to that observed during the natural human menopause where ovaries produce lower levels of hormones over time. Like that seen in menopausal human females, ovariectomy in rats also increases cardiovascular risk [42, 43].

Studies have found that the majority of human females who undergo natural menopause exhibit different age-associated cardiovascular alterations than those who underwent ovariectomy-induced menopause [44]. Elective bilateral removal of the ovaries at a young age is associated with an increased risk for cardiovascular disease and premature death [43]. In addition to declines in well-being and sexual function, it is thought that elective oophorectomies are also associated with elevated risk of cognitive impairment, dementia, and Parkinsonism [43]. It is not known whether the increased risk to cardiovascular disease is due to alterations in hormones or the hypothalamic-pituitary axis [43]. As expected, bilateral oophorectomy is associated with different hormonal alterations including changes in estrogen production and reduced levels of progesterone and testosterone, as well as increases in gonadotropins (LH and follicle stimulating hormone (FSH)), compared to those that occur in human females who experience natural menopause [45, 46].

In rats, ovariectomy causes alterations to heart structure and function which include increases in cardiac interstitial space, cardiac fibrosis, heart weight, and left ventricular weight [47]. Ovariectomy in rats has been shown to reduce cardiac contractility [48]. Ovariectomized rats appear to exhibit increased evidence of oxidative stress and cardiac apoptosis [47–51]. In rats, cytokine expression (tumor necrosis factor-alpha (TNF-α) and interleukin-1 beta (IL-1β)) and angiotensin converting enzyme (ACE) and angiotensin II type 1 receptor gene expression also appear to be increased following ovariectomy [48, 50]. When estradiol treatment was given to ovariectomized rats, it prevented the reduction of cardiac contractility as well as the increase in apoptosis and cytokine expression [48, 51]. Research in other rats, namely, aging female Dahl salt-sensitive rats, has shown that female rats are more likely to develop hypertension after ovariectomy [52]. The researchers postulated that estrogen protects against the increased activity of the renin angiotensin system. However, in human females, research has shown that postmenopausal hypertension occurs approximately five to 10 years after menopause, not immediately after starting menopause. Therefore, other age-related causes must occur independently of estrogen loss that promotes CVD in postmenopausal human females, as is shown by the fact that estrogen replacement therapy is not cardioprotective after menopause [53, 54]. Interestingly, both natural and surgically induced reproductive senescence rats exhibit increased FSH as well as decreased levels of estradiol and inhibin (A/B) [55]. Surgically induced reproductive senescence in rats has also been shown to alter dopamine receptor affinity in the heart [55].

Alterations in cardiac structure and function are not the only alterations found after ovariectomy. Compared to aged controls, human females that underwent prophylactic bilateral salpingo-oophorectomy exhibit increased total and low-density lipoprotein cholesterol levels [56]. In light of the fact that within human females natural menopause and ovariectomy results altered hormonal profiles and cardiovascular risk, the data suggest that age-associated cardiovascular disease in human females may be associated with both time dependent hormone deprivation and age-associated changes in structure, function, and protein signaling. Of note is the fact that most studies have used ovariectomized female rats at young ages (6–12 weeks old) to examine the effects of hormone deprivation on the cardiovascular system which can lead to unreliable results given that the cardiovascular system has not yet "aged" [57].

2.4. Cardiac Structure and Function in the Aging Female Rat. The increased risk of CVD in human females may be due to differences in the type or magnitude of age-associated alterations in cardiac structure and function. Olivetti and colleagues have demonstrated a small decrease in human heart weight with aging in males but not females [58]. Additionally, no significant change was noted with myocardium, left ventricular, or right ventricular free wall weight in the aging human female heart with no underlying cardiovascular pathology nor were age associated changes detected in proportion, shapes, size, or number of mononucleated and binucleated cardiac myocytes [58]. Given this information, it appears that natural aging in human females is not associated with cardiac remodeling during or after menopause in the absence of preexisting pathologies or loading abnormalities [58]. Similar conclusions were reached from echocardiographic studies [59]. Although a limited number of studies have looked at how cardiac structure and function change with age in female rats, very few have directly investigated how sex may affect cardiac structure and function. Go demonstrated that cardiovascular aging in male and female rats demonstrated significant gender differences in LV size and function [60].

Boluyt and colleagues investigated how aging may affect cardiac structure and function in female F344 rats using echocardiography [61]. Aging female rat cardiac structural changes included a dilatation of the left ventricle between 13 and 22 months of age. This dilatation was characterized by increases in posterior and septal wall thickness during diastole at 22 and 30 months of age [61]. Aging in the female F344 was also associated with increases in collagen content and collagen cross-linking [62]. In addition, Boluyt and colleagues demonstrated mild systolic dysfunction (decline in left ventricle ejection fraction, fractional shortening, and velocity of circumferential fiber shortening) in female 22-month-old animals when compared to young adults and that these changes preceded the development of mild diastolic dysfunction [61, 63]. These authors suggested that this modest decline in systolic function was due, at least in part, to a shift in the amount of alpha and beta myosin heavy chains [61, 62], similar to what is seen in the human failing heart [64]. Additional work, perhaps using other rat models, is needed in order to truly distinguish if these alterations are due to increasing age or if they are simply specific to the F344 strain.

Fannin and colleagues found that increased age in the female F344xBN was associated with increases in oxidative stress and damage [65]. Age-related changes in cardiac structure were also found, such as increase in heart to body weight ratio, cardiomyocyte cross-sectional area, posterior wall thickening, and left ventricle chamber dilatation. Further, increased age was also associated with diastolic dysfunction, alterations in heart rhythm intervals, and alternations in connexin 43 expression [65]. The presence of age-associated cardiac structural changes in the F344 and F344xBN animal models calls into question the use of these strains for translational data, in light of the absence of age-associated change in human females reported by Olivetti et al. [58]. Additionally, the menstrual cycle induced hormonal changes have been shown to cause cardiac functional fluctuations [66]. This fact could indicate that the time at which functional measurements are taken may impact the results and must be a consideration in comparing all female derived cardiac functional data.

2.5. Cardiac Arrhythmias with Aging. Aging is considered a risk factor for ventricular arrhythmia [67, 68]. In addition, aging is also associated with an increase in the percentage of incidence of atrial fibrillation [60, 69]. In male rats, age-associated increases in cardiac fibrosis as well as the changes in gap junction morphology have been hypothesized to cause changes in cardiac conduction in addition to the incidence of arrhythmias and death [68, 70]. As humans age, there is an increase in the EKG abnormalities which are associated with increased mortality [71]. Men tend to experience more atrial fibrillation, early repolarizations, Brugada syndromes, and sudden cardiac death than women, while women are more likely to be at risk to develop long QT syndrome-based arrhythmias as well as bradycardia-induced torsades de pointes [72]. Although sex related differences in cardiac electrocardiogram parameters have been observed, electrocardiogram abnormalities seem to vary between studies. In men, there is an increase in QRS duration and sinus cycle length while women tended to a have a higher maximum heart rate [73, 74].

Electrocardiogram analysis in elderly men and women has demonstrated large or intermediate Q waves, left axis deviation, negative T-waves, and complete right bundle branch block as well as atrial fibrillation/flutter [75]. In aging men, the QRS complex has been found to be narrowed, while aged men and women have been shown to undergo a leftward shift of the QRS axis [75]. Another work has suggested that puberty in men is associated with a shortened QT interval which is not present in women [76] and that aging in men demonstrates an increase in PR intervals and a prolongation of the QT interval [74]. Conversely, another research found that aging did not appear to alter EKG tracings in either men or women [74].

Similar alterations in electrocardiogram parameters have also been found in aging rats. In male Wistar rats, the PR and corrected QT intervals were found to increase with age [70]. Alterations in aging electrocardiogram parameters have been shown to be rat strain dependent and could only be detected subsequently to heart failure as in male SHHF/Mcc-cp rat strain at 19 months of age [77]. Gonadectomy appears to decrease the number of arrhythmias in male but not female rats [78]. Though not fully understood, these differences in gender associated gonadectomy induced arrhythmia frequency have been attributed to higher heart rates in male animals and longer QT intervals, as well as gender differences in ion channel expression [79]. Very few studies have investigated electrocardiogram parameters in the aging female rat. Fannin and colleagues found that the arrhythmias were not significantly higher in older female F344xBN rats when compared with younger rats; however, the study did find that valvular dysfunction was increased in the older rats when compared to the younger ones [65].

The exact mechanisms of the gender associated reduction of arrhythmias in humans and the role estrogen may play are not fully understood but two potential indirect mechanisms have been proposed. One potential indirect mechanism may be related to the ability of estradiol to reduce the incidence of cardiac ischemia [80]. Other works have suggested that high levels of estradiol in female and male rats may directly reduce arrhythmias, possibly by causing slowing of the inward calcium current [80, 81]. Although multiple studies have investigated EKG changes in aging rats, these parameters have not been determined in the NIA approved aging F344xBN rat model. However, according to the ICH-S7B, the use of rats for the safety testing of drugs is not considered appropriate due to differences in the ionic mechanisms of repolarization [82]. Arrhythmia mechanisms [83], resting heart rate, Ca^+ homeostasis [84], and action potential configuration [85] are all important differences that limit the translational relevance of rat generated cardiovascular data for human application.

2.6. Aging Related Changes in Cardiac Oxidative Stress and ROS-Related Signaling. Aging in the male rat heart is associated with the accumulation of oxidative damage to lipids and proteins as well as decline in mitochondrial enzymes [86]. In addition, an increasing number of mutations in mitochondrial DNA (mtDNA) has been gradually observed during aging [87]. The level of 8-OHDG mtDNA adducts and deletions increase exponentially with age [87]. In human muscle, liver, and brain tissue, complex IV and mitochondrial oxidative phosphorylation enzyme activities decline with age. This decline in function is correlated with the accumulation of mtDNA mutations, including deletions, and base substitutions [87]. Similarly, aged male rat hearts exhibit an increase in superoxide, 4-hydroxynonenal (4-HNE), and nitrosative stress levels which appear to be highly correlated to increases in left ventricular thickness [88]. The exact role that increased levels of oxidative stress may play in the development and progression of age-associated cardiovascular disease remains to be determined.

Compared to that observed in females, the hearts of aging male rats exhibited increases in protein carbonylation, advanced oxidation protein products, nitrotyrosine, nonprotein thiol, reduced glutathione, and iron levels [89]. Although aging is associated with increases in oxidative stress in both male and female rat hearts, female rat hearts exhibited lower mitochondrial hydrogen peroxide production, oxidative damage, and a greater mitochondria differentiation compared to that seen in male animals [90]. It is thought that higher mitochondrial differentiation is a metabolic adaptation to increase energy efficiency as it is associated with their lower mitochondrial free radical production and oxidative damage [90]. In addition to differences with sex, it is also likely that reactive oxygen species (ROS) levels vary with animal strain as female Wistar and F344 rats exhibit lower ROS production and indices of oxidative damage than that seen in female Sprague-Dawley rats which may help to explain their greater mean lifespan [91, 92].

The mitogen-activated protein kinase (MAPK) cascades are evolutionary conserved serine/threonine protein kinases that regulate several important cellular functions including proliferation, differentiation, development, cell cycle, and cell death [93]. The major MAPK signaling pathways are the extracellular signal-regulated protein kinase cascade (p44/42), c-Jun amino-terminal kinase/stress-activated protein kinase cascade (JNK/SAPK), and the p38 cascade. Stimuli that include stress or injury typically activate the JNK and p38 MAPK kinases, while the p44/42 MAPKs are stimulated by mitogenic and growth factors [94, 95]. MAPK signaling is involved in many of the age-associated physiological changes (hypertrophy, oxidative stress, and apoptosis) as well as other cardiac pathologies. Works investigating MAPK signaling in aging human hearts have demonstrated reduced p38 MAPK activity/signaling in heart failure and impaired activation of MAPK target genes following increase in oxidative stress [96–98].

It is well recognized that increases in cellular stress cause the upregulation of the heat shock protein (Hsp) [99]. Hsps range in size from 10 to 150 kDa and function to prevent protein aggregation and assist in ensuring proper protein folding, as well as helping to mediate the translocation of damaged proteins [100]. Hsps are also involved in cardiac hypertrophy, in response to vascular wall injury, ischemic preconditioning, and aging [101]. During aging, there is an accumulation of damaged or misfolded proteins which may cause a burden on maintaining proteostasis [102–104]. An important function of heat shock proteins is to protect against age-related protein misfolding [103–105]. In aged male F344 rats (24 months), it appears that aging decreases Hsp70 upregulation following chronic exercise and heat stress [106–108].

Similar to the MAPK proteins, the nuclear factor-κB (NF-κB) pathway is thought to play a role in cardiac remodeling, apoptosis, acute ischemia and reperfusion, and unstable angina, as well as heart failure in both humans and rodents [109–112]. The NF-κB family consists of RelA (p65), c-Rel (Rel), RelB, NF-κB1 (p50), and NF-κB 2 (p52). Figure 1 presents the NF-κB signaling pathway. In the cytoplasm, the p50 and p65 are found as an inactive heterodimer due to the binding of the IκB kinase inhibitory proteins (IKKα and IKKβ). Cellular stimuli known to activate the NF-κB pathway include ROS, TNF-α, IL-1β, and bacterial lipopolysaccharides [113]. It has been shown that the IκBs must first become phosphorylated and degraded before p50/p65 activation can occur [113]. The p50/p65 when phosphorylated (activated) then translocates into the nucleus to induce the transcription of chemokines (IL-8, MCP-1), cytokines (TNF-α, IL-1, IL-2, IL-6), adhesion molecules (ICAM-1, VCAM-1, E-selectin), acute phase proteins, antimicrobial peptides, secondary inflammatory enzymes (COX-2, iNOS, PLA2, MnSOD), and antiapoptotic factors [114]. Upon termination of the NF-κB stimuli, p50/p65 binds to new IκBs and

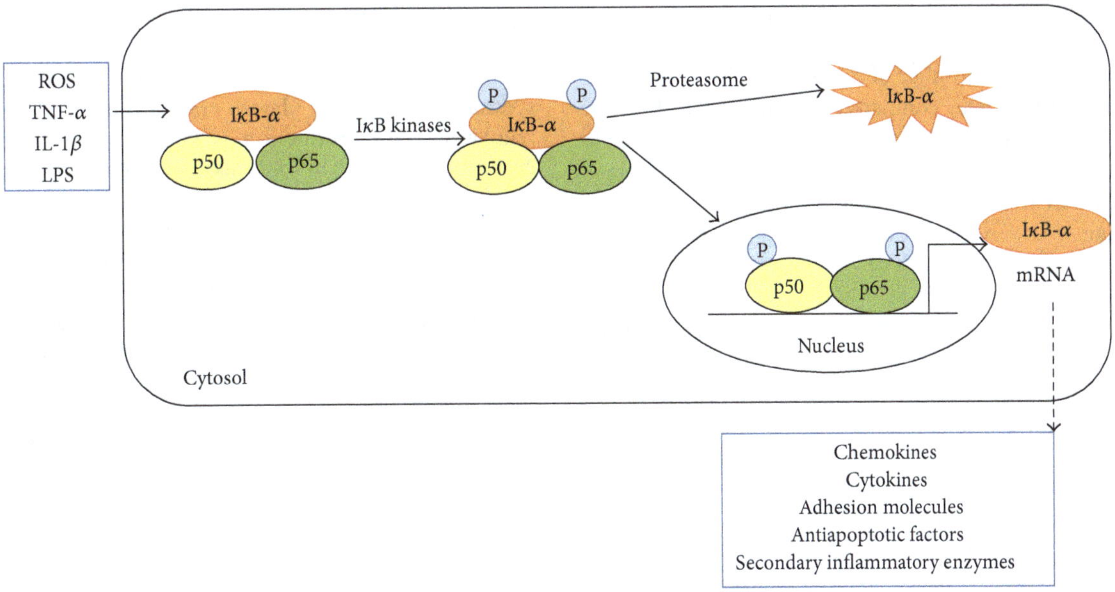

FIGURE 1: The NF-κB signaling pathway (see text for details).

the complex is translocated back to the cytoplasm. It is thought that the MAPK pathway works in concert with the NF-κB pathway to increase transcription of inflammatory genes [114]. Meldrum et al. extensively review the role of sex hormones in intracellular signaling mechanisms within the myocardial inflammation [66].

2.7. Activation of ROS-Related Signaling in the Female Aging Heart. Although the effects of estrogen on MAPK signaling have been studied in several pathological processes, for example, breast cancer, migraines, and polycystic ovarian syndrome, little is known regarding how this molecule affects MAPK signaling in the heart. It is thought that differences in MAPK activation between male and females may be regulated, at least in part, by the influence of estrogen [66, 115, 116]. Estrogen has been shown to stimulate the activation of p44/42 MAPK and JNK MAPK in different model systems including cardiomyocytes, mammary cancer cells, pituitary tumor cells, tissue slices of the hippocampus, and endometriotic stromal cells [117–119]. In males as well as ovariectomized females MAPK signaling is decreased after acute ischemia [115, 116]. In a model of cardiac pressure overload, estradiol treatment appeared to exhibit antihypertrophic effects by increasing the expression of atrial natriuretic peptide (ANP) and inhibiting p38-MAPK activation [120].

In addition to the regulation of MAPK proteins, there is evidence to suggest that gender also has an effect on the Hsp response. In hearts that were not exposed to increased cellular stress, male hearts have half as much Hsp72 expression compared to that observed in the female heart. Conversely, ovariectomy was found to reduce Hsp72 levels in female hearts [121]. Estradiol treatment has also been found to increase Hsp27, Hsp70, Hsp72, and Hsp90 expression in the heart [122–124]. To our knowledge, no studies have looked at Hsp27, Hsp70, and Hsp90 in the aging female heart.

Aging female and male hearts have shown increased apoptosis and inflammation, as well as age-associated gender differences in NF-κB signaling [125]. To our knowledge, only a few studies have investigated the changes in NF-κB expression and activity in the aging female rat heart. However, it has been reported that estradiol can decrease NF-κB binding activity [66].

2.8. Aging Heart Apoptosis. Apoptosis or programmed cell death is a highly conserved and regulated cell response to inhibit the abnormal proliferation of cells [126]. Cardiomyocytes are not capable of self-regeneration and are terminally differentiated but can undergo apoptosis, necrosis, or autophagy when unduly stressed [127]. Apoptosis is increased in many cardiovascular diseases such as dilated and ischemic cardiomyopathy, hypertrophic heart disease, and arrhythmias [126, 128, 129]. In rats, increased age has been shown to cause apoptotic susceptibility in the heart following oxidative injury [130, 131]. Aging in the male F344xBN heart is characterized by increases in the amount of cytochrome C, AIF, Bax, rate of permeability transition pore opening, and fragmented DNA [132]. The age-associated increase in apoptosis appears to be due not only to the activation of proapoptotic molecules but also to decreases in antiapoptotic NF-κB, Bcl-xL, and Grx1 signaling [130]. Another work has demonstrated that the aging male F344xBN rat heart is characterized by increases in TdT-mediated dUTP nick end labeling- (TUNEL-) positive nuclei, caspase-3 activation, caspase-dependent cleavage of alpha-fodrin, and diminished phosphorylation of protein kinase B/Akt (Thr308) [133]. The increase of apoptosis in the aging male F344xBN was highly correlated to age-associated increases in oxidative-nitrosative stress. Though not demonstrating cause and effect, these results suggest that increased cellular ROS and cardiomyocyte apoptosis may play a role in age-related cardiac remodeling.

The incidence of cells undergoing apoptosis in the heart has been shown to differ with sex in humans and rats. In humans, a higher number of TUNEL positive myocytes are seen in young males compared to females [58, 134]. In humans, aging appears to increase cardiac apoptosis in male but not female [58]; however, there was no gender difference in apoptosis in male and female F344 rat [92, 135]. These results suggest differences in apoptosis regulation between species.

2.9. Effects of Aging on Aorta Structure and Function. Cardiovascular disease affects not only the heart but the vasculature of the cardiovascular system. Structural changes found in the aging vasculature include an enlarged lumen, media-intimal thickening, irregularly shaped endothelial cells, migration and proliferation of vascular smooth muscle cells, increased deposition of extracellular matrix, increased expression of adhesion molecules, and alterations in the expression of metalloproteinases as well as cytokines [4, 136–138]. Functional changes with age in the vasculature consist of impaired distensibility, increased stiffness, increased endothelial permeability, attenuation of β 2-adrenoceptor vasodilator response to agonists, and diminished response to adrenergic receptor stimulation [4, 139]. Like humans, rats also appear to exhibit several age-associated changes in vascular structure and function including changes in intimal thickening, elevations in inflammation-associated molecule expression, and increased evidence of oxidative stress [4, 140].

Similar to that seen in other parts of the cardiovascular system, differences in aortic structure and function between genders have also been observed in the aging human and animals. In males, aortic wall and intimal-medial thickness are greater during aging than that observed in women; however, stiffness was not different between men and women [141]. Similarly, there were no differences in distensibility in the aging aorta between men and women [142]. Although the human aging aorta did not show increases in aortic stiffness, it has been documented that the increased vascular stiffness with aging is more prominent in male than female animal models [143, 144]. This may be due in part, to the lower total peripheral resistance and higher cardiac output seen in women compared to men of similar arterial pressure and age [58].

Abnormal proliferation and migration of vascular smooth muscle cells (VSMCs) play important roles in the pathophysiology of atherosclerotic diseases [145]. Previous studies have shown that VSMCs isolated from old animals replicate more actively than those obtained from young animals [145, 146]. Similarly, aging has been shown to be associated with an increased proliferative response of VSMCs after balloon angioplasty [147].

2.10. Effects of Aging on Aortic Endothelial Cell Function. Endothelial dysfunction is considered to be a common and early feature of vascular disease and impaired endothelium-dependent relaxation has been demonstrated in several rat models of hypertension, experimental diabetes, atherosclerosis, and high salt diet, as well as aging [148]. The factors regulating endothelial dysfunction are likely complex and may vary between models and with aging. Nitric oxide (NO) is a vasodilator that is produced by endothelial nitric oxide synthase (eNOS) that plays a crucial role in blood pressure regulation. NO production is stimulated by shear stress, cyclic strain, acetylcholine, vascular endothelial growth factor, bradykinin, estrogen, sphingosine-1 phosphate (S-1P), hydrogen peroxide, and angiotensin II [149]. It is thought that eNOS activity is regulated by eNOS phosphorylation at Serine 1177, Serine 635, and Serine 617 by phosphatidylinositol 3-kinase (PI3K)/Akt, adenosine monophosphate-activated protein kinase (AMPK), and cyclic AMP-dependent protein kinase signaling [149, 150]. Given its important role in regulating vascular function, it is not surprising that abnormalities in vascular NO production are thought to contribute to the pathogenesis of atherosclerosis and hypertension [151, 152]. Advanced age has been found to be associated with impaired endothelial NO synthesis and endothelial dysfunction [153, 154]. The mechanisms responsible [155] for age-associated alterations in NO synthesis are not fully known but may include changes in activity or expression of eNOS, increased breakdown of NO due to oxidative stress/oxidative injury, changes in antioxidant defense systems, and decreased availability of eNOS substrate, L-arginine [155], although the activity of eNOS is generally thought to be diminished with aging [156] in the aorta. In addition to changes in eNOS activity, decreased NO availability during aging can also be caused by oxidative stress [154] and alterations in eNOS structure [155, 156]. The regulation of eNOS function during aging may also differ with sex. Although estrogen (17-β estradiol) has been shown to activate eNOS [157], estrogen studies in rats have shown no effect [158] or increased eNOS expression following estrogen treatment [159]. Conversely, in humans, estrogen replacement appears to be largely ineffective as a means of decreasing CVD risk [159, 160].

2.11. Sex Related Differences in Aortic Vascular Smooth Muscle Cells with Aging. In women, the incidence of vascular dysfunction is thought to be related, at least in part, to the cessation of ovarian hormone production [161]. In vascular smooth muscle cells from young female Wistar Kyoto rats, estrogen inhibited VSMC proliferation following stimulation with fetal calf serum [162]. This effect was thought to be mediated by E2 receptors [162]. Similar decreases in VSMC proliferation with estrogen treatment following cell stimulation by growth factors or mechanical stress have also been noted [161, 163]. Like estrogen, progesterone is also thought to inhibit the proliferation of aortic VSMC, most likely via its ability to inhibit DNA synthesis [164]. Nonetheless, it should be noted that the effects of estrogen in vivo are likely more complex than those seen in cell culture. For example, in aortas from diabetic female rats, estrogen failed to reverse the impaired basal release of nitric oxide and the abnormal relaxation to histamine [165].

2.12. Aging Aorta Signaling. The MAPK signaling pathways function to regulate many processes in the aorta including VSMC proliferation, contraction, migration, differentiation, and cell survival [166–168]. Aging has also been shown to increase the activation (phosphorylation) of p44/42 and JNK MAPKs in the aorta [169] while another work has shown that aging affects the ability of the aged aorta to activate p38 and JNK MAPK signaling following mechanical loading [170]. In aged animals the activation of p44/42 MAPK in vascular smooth muscle was increased compared to young animals [145, 171].

Similar to that observed for the heart, age-associated changes in the expression/activity of NF-κB were found in the vascular smooth muscle cells of the aorta. Aging has been found to increase the sensitivity of NF-κB to glucose in aortic VSCM cells [172]. Another research has shown that VSCM proliferation and NF-κB activation stimulated by interleukin-1β were increased more in aged female rats than young female rats [173]. In premenopausal women, receiving hormone treatment appeared to reduce NF-κB activation [174] suggesting that estradiol reduces NF-κB activation. How estrogen may inhibit NF-κB activity is currently unclear but may be related to increased IκB levels or decreased levels of circulating TNF-α [174].

3. Conclusion

In summary, the loss of ovarian function during aging may influence cardiovascular structure and function. However, the fact that human females do not display cardiac hypertrophy or myocyte loss in the absence of loading abnormalities with aging may suggest the presence of estrogen prior to menopause acts to attenuate the cardiac response to pre-existing underlying pathologies. Due to the complexities of the aging process, more studies are needed to distinguish whether observed differences are due to aging alone, hormone deprivation, or a combination of both. In order to overcome the difficulties found in aging human research (ethics, cost, and long lifespan), rat models have been used to provide great insight in investigating age-related changes in cardiovascular structure and function. However, additional research examining how aging may affect cardiac structure and function in rats is needed to determine whether the alterations seen in rats mimic the changes seen in humans. Because of the systemic nature of reproductive senescence, the use of surgical practices to induce "pseudomenopause" or ovariotoxicity may be incomplete in the overall approach to female aging and cardiovascular changes. The global changes in the body with age may play a cumulative role in combination with the hormonal changes seen in reproductive senescence. Aging-associated increases in oxidative stress can lead to alterations in the cardiac cell signaling which may lead to deleterious changes in the heart. Because cardiac structure, function, signaling, and hormonal response appear to differ between male and female rats and humans with aging, care must be taken in evaluating current literature with regard to specific finding and gender. Studies investigating the details of cardiac signaling with gender and aging are likely to lead to a better understanding of the mechanisms responsible for cardiovascular diseases in both male and females. These findings may prove critical in the application of current prophylactic practices and pharmaceutical interventions in patient outcomes.

Conflict of Interests

The authors declare that there is no conflict of interests regarding the publication of this paper.

Authors' Contribution

K. M. Rice and J. C. Fannin contributed equally to the study.

Acknowledgment

This work was supported in part by DOE Grant (DE-PS02-09ER-01 to E. R. Blough).

References

[1] J. Johannes and C. N. Bairey Merz, "Is cardiovascular disease in women inevitable?: preparing for menopause and beyond," *Cardiology in Review*, vol. 19, no. 2, pp. 76–80, 2011.

[2] A. Yazdanyar and A. B. Newman, "The burden of cardiovascular disease in the elderly: morbidity, mortality, and costs," *Clinics in Geriatric Medicine*, vol. 25, no. 4, pp. 563–577, 2009.

[3] A. S. Go, D. Mozaffarian, V. L. Roger et al., "Heart disease and stroke statistics—2013 update: a report from the American Heart Association," *Circulation*, vol. 127, no. 1, pp. e6–e245, 2013.

[4] E. G. Lakatta, "Arterial and cardiac aging: major shareholders in cardiovascular disease enterprises: part III: cellular and molecular clues to heart and arterial aging," *Circulation*, vol. 107, no. 3, pp. 490–497, 2003.

[5] A. Anna, D. R. Riordon, and K. Boheler, "Molecular mechanisms of cardiomyocyte aging," *Clinical Science*, vol. 121, no. 8, pp. 315–329, 2011.

[6] F. Hatch, M. K. Lancaster, and S. A. Jones, "Aging is a primary risk factor for cardiac arrhythmias: disruption of intracellular Ca^{2+} regulation as a key suspect," *Expert Review of Cardiovascular Therapy*, vol. 9, no. 8, pp. 1059–1067, 2011.

[7] A. Karavidas, G. Lazaros, D. Tsiachris, and V. Pyrgakis, "Aging and the cardiovascular system," *Hellenic Journal of Cardiology*, vol. 51, no. 5, pp. 421–427, 2010.

[8] W. Rosamond, K. Flegal, K. Furie et al., "Heart disease and stroke statistics—2008 update: a report from the American Heart Association Statistics Committee and Stroke Statistics Subcommittee," *Circulation*, vol. 117, no. 4, pp. e25–e146, 2008.

[9] L. Mosca, J. E. Manson, S. E. Sutherland, R. D. Langer, T. Manolio, and E. Barrett-Connor, "Cardiovascular disease in women: a statement for healthcare professionals from the American Heart Association. Writing Group.," *Circulation*, vol. 96, no. 7, pp. 2468–2482, 1997.

[10] H. Okura, Y. Takada, A. Yamabe et al., "Age-and gender-specific changes in the left ventricular relaxation a doppler echocardiographic study in healthy individuals," *Circulation: Cardiovascular Imaging*, vol. 2, no. 1, pp. 41–46, 2009.

[11] C. G. Frazier, K. P. Alexander, L. K. Newby et al., "Associations of gender and etiology with outcomes in heart failure with systolic dysfunction: a pooled analysis of 5 randomized control trials," *Journal of the American College of Cardiology*, vol. 49, no. 13, pp. 1450–1458, 2007.

[12] C. D. Kimmelstiel and M. A. Konstam, "Heart failure in women," *Cardiology*, vol. 86, no. 4, pp. 304–309, 1995.

[13] I. Shapira, A. Isakov, and M. Burke, "Cardiac rupture in patients with acute myocardial infarction," *Chest*, vol. 92, no. 2, pp. 219–223, 1987.

[14] J. D. Carroll, E. P. Carroll, T. Feldman et al., "Sex-associated differences in left ventricular function in aortic stenosis of the elderly," *Circulation*, vol. 86, no. 4, pp. 1099–1107, 1992.

[15] C. S. Hayward, R. P. Kelly, and P. Collins, "The roles of gender, the menopause and hormone replacement on cardiovascular function," *Cardiovascular Research*, vol. 46, no. 1, pp. 28–49, 2000.

[16] M. Klein, C. Kortan, D. I. Kells, and K. J. Dorrington, "Equilibrium and kinetic aspects of the interaction of isolated variable and constant domains of light chain with the Fd' fragment of immunoglobulin G," *Biochemistry*, vol. 18, no. 8, pp. 1473–1481, 1979.

[17] P. Jousilahti, E. Vartiainen, J. Tuomilehto, and P. Puska, "Sex, age, cardiovascular risk factors, and coronary heart disease: a prospective follow-up study of 14 786 middle-aged men and women in Finland," *Circulation*, vol. 99, no. 9, pp. 1165–1172, 1999.

[18] S. D. Kafonek, "Postmenopausal hormone replacement therapy and cardiovascular risk reduction. A review," *Drugs*, vol. 47, supplement, no. 2, pp. 16–24, 1994.

[19] M. J. J. de Kleijn, Y. T. van der Schouw, A. L. M. Verbeek, P. H. M. Peeters, J.-D. Banga, and Y. van der Graaf, "Endogenous estrogen exposure and cardiovascular mortality risk in postmenopausal women," *American Journal of Epidemiology*, vol. 155, no. 4, pp. 339–345, 2002.

[20] B. K. Jacobsen, S. Nilssen, I. Heuch, and G. Kvåle, "Does age at natural menopause affect mortality from ischemic heart disease?" *Journal of Clinical Epidemiology*, vol. 50, no. 4, pp. 475–479, 1997.

[21] F. B. Hu, F. Grodstein, C. H. Hennekens et al., "Age at natural menopause and risk of cardiovascular disease," *Archives of Internal Medicine*, vol. 159, no. 10, pp. 1061–1066, 1999.

[22] V. L. Jacoby, D. Grady, and G. F. Sawaya, "Oophorectomy as a risk factor for coronary heart disease," *American Journal of Obstetrics & Gynecology*, vol. 200, no. 2, pp. 140.e1–140.e9, 2008.

[23] Y. T. van der Schouw, Y. van der Graaf, E. W. Steyerberg, M. J. C. Eijkemans, and J. D. Banga, "Age at menopause as a risk factor for cardiovascular mortality," *The Lancet*, vol. 347, no. 9003, pp. 714–718, 1996.

[24] K. H. Lu, B. R. Hopper, T. M. Vargo, and S. S. C. Yen, "Chronological changes in sex steroid, gonadotropin and prolactin secretion in aging female rats displaying different reproductive states," *Biology of Reproduction*, vol. 21, no. 1, pp. 193–203, 1979.

[25] S. C. Alberts, J. Altmannb, D. K. Brockman et al., "Reproductive aging patterns in primates reveal that humans are distinct," *Proceedings of the National Academy of Sciences of the United States of America*, vol. 110, no. 33, pp. 13440–13445, 2013.

[26] V. Ledvenyiova, D. Pancza, J. Matejiková, M. Ferko, I. Bernatova, and T. Ravingerova, "Impact of age and sex on response to ischemic preconditioning in the rat heart: differential role of the PI3K-AKT pathway," *Canadian Journal of Physiology and Pharmacology*, vol. 91, no. 8, pp. 640–647, 2013.

[27] G. C. S. V. Tezini, C. Becari, C. Z. Zanotto, M. C. O. Salgado, R. D. C. A. T. Passaglia, and H. C. D. Souza, "Ageing is the main determinant of haemodynamics and autonomic cardiac changes observed in post-menopausal female rats," *Autonomic Neuroscience: Basic and Clinical*, vol. 174, no. 1-2, pp. 36–41, 2013.

[28] S. G. Campbell, P. Haynes, W. K. Snapp, K. E. Nava, and K. S. Campbell, "Altered ventricular torsion and transmural patterns of myocyte relaxation precede heart failure in aging F344 rats," *American Journal of Physiology—Heart and Circulatory Physiology*, vol. 305, no. 5, pp. H676–H686, 2013.

[29] T. S. Lancaster, S. J. Jefferson, J. G. Hunter et al., "Quantitative proteomic analysis reveals novel mitochondrial targets of estrogen deficiency in the aged female rat heart," *Physiological Genomics*, vol. 44, no. 20, pp. 957–969, 2012.

[30] N. M. Tenõrio, S. Tufik, C. T. Bergamaschi et al., "Influence of acute sleep deprivation on cardiovascular parameters in female zucker obese and lean rats," *Obesity*, vol. 21, no. 3, pp. 510–515, 2013.

[31] J. W. Simpkins, H. H. Huang, J. P. Advis, and J. Meites, "Changes in hypothalamic NE and DA turnover resulting from steroid-induced LH and prolactin surges in ovariectomized rats," *Biology of Reproduction*, vol. 20, no. 3, pp. 625–632, 1979.

[32] J. P. Advis, J. W. Simpkins, H. T. Chen, and J. Meites, "Relation of biogenic amines to onset of puberty in the female rat," *Endocrinology*, vol. 103, no. 1, pp. 11–16, 1978.

[33] J. I. Acosta, L. Mayer, J. S. Talboom et al., "Transitional versus surgical menopause in a rodent model: etiology of ovarian hormone loss impacts memory and the acetylcholine system," *Endocrinology*, vol. 150, no. 9, pp. 4248–4259, 2009.

[34] T. A. Van Kempen, T. A. Milner, and E. M. Waters, "Accelerated ovarian failure: a novel, chemically induced animal model of menopause," *Brain Research*, vol. 1379, pp. 176–187, 2011.

[35] C. J. Kappeler and P. B. Hoyer, "4-vinylcyclohexene diepoxide: A model chemical for ovotoxicity," *Systems Biology in Reproductive Medicine*, vol. 58, no. 1, pp. 57–62, 2012.

[36] J. A. Parrott and M. K. Skinner, "Kit-ligand/stem cell factor induces primordial follicle development and initiates folliculogenesis," *Endocrinology*, vol. 140, no. 9, pp. 4262–4271, 1999.

[37] X. Jin, C.-S. Han, F.-Q. Yu, P. Wei, Z.-Y. Hu, and Y.-X. Liu, "Anti-apoptotic action of stem cell factor on oocytes in primordial follicles and its signal transduction," *Molecular Reproduction and Development*, vol. 70, no. 1, pp. 82–90, 2005.

[38] J. B. Frye, A. L. Lukefahr, L. E. Wright, S. L. Marion, P. B. Hoyer, and J. L. Funk, "Modeling perimenopause in sprague-dawley rats by chemical manipulation of the transition to ovarian failure," *Comparative Medicine*, vol. 62, no. 3, pp. 193–202, 2012.

[39] T. Kodama, J. Yoshida, T. Miwa, D. Hasegawa, and T. Masuyama, "Collaborative work on evaluation of ovarian toxicity. 4) Effects of fertility study of 4-vinylcyclohexene diepoxide in female rats," *Journal of Toxicological Sciences*, vol. 34, supplement 1, pp. SP59–SP63, 2009.

[40] A. Ito, N. Mafune, and T. Kimura, "Collaborative work on evaluation of ovarian toxicity 4) Two- or four-week repeated dose study of 4-vinylcyclohexene diepoxide in female rats," *The Journal of Toxicological Sciences*, vol. 34, no. 1, pp. SP53–SP58, 2009.

[41] F. S. Muhammad, A. K. Goode, N. D. Kock et al., "Effects of 4-vinylcyclohexene diepoxide on peripubertal and adult sprague-dawley Rats: ovarian, clinical, and pathologic outcomes," *Comparative Medicine*, vol. 59, no. 1, pp. 46–59, 2009.

[42] R. A. Lobo, "Surgical menopause and cardiovascular risks," *Menopause*, vol. 14, no. 3, part 2, pp. 562–566, 2007.

[43] L. T. Shuster, B. S. Gostout, B. R. Grossardt, and W. A. Rocca, "Prophylactic oophorectomy in premenopausal women and long-term health," *Menopause International*, vol. 14, no. 3, pp. 111–116, 2008.

[44] E. Özkaya, E. Çakr, E. Okuyan, C. Çakr, G. Üstün, and T. Küçüközkan, "Comparison of the effects of surgical and natural menopause on carotid intima media thickness, osteoporosis, and homocysteine levels," *Menopause*, vol. 18, no. 1, pp. 73–76, 2011.

[45] J. H. Morrison, R. D. Brinton, P. J. Schmidt, and A. C. Gore, "Estrogen, menopause, and the aging brain: how basic neuroscience can inform hormone therapy in women," *The Journal of Neuroscience*, vol. 26, no. 41, pp. 10332–10348, 2006.

[46] W. A. Rocca, B. R. Grossardt, and L. T. Shuster, "Oophorectomy, menopause, estrogen, and cognitive aging: the timing hypothesis," *Neurodegenerative Diseases*, vol. 7, no. 1–3, pp. 163–166, 2010.

[47] S. D. Lee, W.-W. Kuo, Y.-J. Ho et al., "Cardiac Fas-dependent and mitochondria-dependent apoptosis in ovariectomized rats," *Maturitas*, vol. 61, no. 3, pp. 268–277, 2008.

[48] J. P. Stice, L. Chen, S.-C. Kim et al., "17β-estradiol, aging, inflammation, and the stress response in the female heart," *Endocrinology*, vol. 152, no. 4, pp. 1589–1598, 2011.

[49] I. Baeza, J. Fdez-Tresguerres, C. Ariznavarreta, and M. de la Fuente, "Effects of growth hormone, melatonin, oestrogens and phytoestrogens on the oxidized glutathione (GSSG)/reduced glutathione (GSH) ratio and lipid peroxidation in aged ovariectomized rats," *Biogerontology*, vol. 11, no. 6, pp. 687–701, 2010.

[50] B. Fabris, R. Candido, M. Bortoletto et al., "Stimulation of cardiac apoptosis in ovariectomized hypertensive rats: potential role of the renin-angiotensin system," *Journal of Hypertension*, vol. 29, no. 2, pp. 273–281, 2011.

[51] C.-M. Liou, A.-L. Yang, C.-H. Kuo, H. Tin, C.-Y. Huang, and S.-D. Lee, "Effects of 17beta-estradiol on cardiac apoptosis in ovariectomized rats," *Cell Biochemistry and Function*, vol. 28, no. 6, pp. 521–528, 2010.

[52] C. Hinojosa-Laborde, T. Craig, W. Zheng, H. Ji, J. R. Haywood, and K. Sandberg, "Ovariectomy augments hypertension in aging female Dahl salt-sensitive rats," *Hypertension*, vol. 44, no. 4, pp. 405–409, 2004.

[53] J. F. Reckelhoff, "Sex steroids, cardiovascular disease, and hypertension: unanswered questions and some speculations," *Hypertension*, vol. 45, no. 2, pp. 170–174, 2005.

[54] J. P. Stice, J. S. Lee, A. S. Pechenino, and A. A. Knowlton, "Estrogen, aging and the cardiovascular system," *Future Cardiology*, vol. 5, no. 1, pp. 93–103, 2009.

[55] O. M. Kharchilava and L. A. Valeeva, "Effects of surgical ovariectomy on dopamine receptors of the heart and brain," *Patologicheskaia Fiziologiia i Èksperimental'naia Terapiia*, no. 4, pp. 21–23, 2008.

[56] M. O. Verhoeven, M. J. Van Der Mooren, T. Teerlink, R. H. M. Verheijen, P. G. Scheffer, and P. Kenemans, "The influence of physiological and surgical menopause on coronary heart disease risk markers," *Menopause*, vol. 16, no. 1, pp. 37–49, 2009.

[57] C. M. Wong, X. Yao, C. L. Au et al., "Raloxifene prevents endothelial dysfunction in aging ovariectomized female rats," *Vascular Pharmacology*, vol. 44, no. 5, pp. 290–298, 2006.

[58] G. Olivetti, G. Giordano, D. Corradi et al., "Gender differences and aging: effects on the human heart," *Journal of the American College of Cardiology*, vol. 26, no. 4, pp. 1068–1079, 1995.

[59] A. L. Danneberg, D. Levy, and R. J. Garrison, "Impact of age on echocardiographic left ventricular mass in a healthy population (the Framingham Study)," *American Journal of Cardiology*, vol. 64, no. 16, pp. 1066–1068, 1989.

[60] A. S. Go, "The epidemiology of atrial fibrillation in elderly persons: the tip of the iceberg," *The American Journal of Geriatric Cardiology*, vol. 14, no. 2, pp. 56–61, 2005.

[61] M. O. Boluyt, K. Converso, H. S. Hwang, A. Mikkor, and M. W. Russell, "Echocardiographic assessment of age-associated changes in systolic and diastolic function of the female F344 rat heart," *Journal of Applied Physiology*, vol. 96, no. 2, pp. 822–828, 2004.

[62] M. O. Boluyt, S. T. Devor, J. A. Opiteck, and T. P. White, "Regional variation in cardiac myosin isoforms of female F344 rats during aging," *Journals of Gerontology Series A: Biological Sciences and Medical Sciences*, vol. 54, no. 8, pp. B313–B317, 1999.

[63] M. O. Boluyt, J. A. Opiteck, K. A. Esser, and T. P. White, "Cardiac adaptations to aortic constriction in adult and aged rats," *The American Journal of Physiology—Heart and Circulatory Physiology*, vol. 257, no. 2, pp. H643–H648, 1989.

[64] S. Miyata, W. Minobe, M. R. Bristow, and L. A. Leinwand, "Myosin heavy chain isoform expression in the failing and nonfailing human heart," *Circulation Research*, vol. 86, no. 4, pp. 386–390, 2000.

[65] J. Fannin, K. M. Rice, S. Thulluri et al., "Age-associated alterations of cardiac structure and function in the female F344xBN rat heart," *AGE*, vol. 36, article 9684, 2014.

[66] D. R. Meldrum, M. Wang, B. M. Tsai et al., "Intracellular signaling mechanisms of sex hormones in acute myocardial inflammation and injury," *Frontiers in Bioscience*, vol. 10, no. 2, pp. 1835–1867, 2005.

[67] A. K. Gupta, A. Maheshwari, D. D. Tresch, and R. K. Thakur, "Cardiac arrhythmias in the elderly," *Cardiac Electrophysiology Review*, vol. 6, no. 1-2, pp. 120–128, 2002.

[68] S. Rossi, S. Baruffi, A. Bertuzzi et al., "Ventricular activation is impaired in aged rat hearts," *The American Journal of Physiology: Heart and Circulatory Physiology*, vol. 295, no. 6, pp. H2336–H2347, 2008.

[69] S. Xing, S.-W. Tsaih, R. Yuan et al., "Genetic influence on electrocardiogram time intervals and heart rate in aging mice," *American Journal of Physiology: Heart and Circulatory Physiology*, vol. 296, no. 6, pp. H1907–H1913, 2009.

[70] V. J. D. da Silva, E. F. Neto, H. C. Salgado, and R. F. Júnior, "Chronic converting enzyme inhibition normalizes QT interval in aging rats," *Brazilian Journal of Medical and Biological Research*, vol. 35, no. 9, pp. 1025–1031, 2002.

[71] U. Molander, D. K. Dey, V. Sundh, and B. Steen, "ECG abnormalities in the elderly: prevalence, time and generation trends and association with mortality," *Aging Clinical and Experimental Research*, vol. 15, no. 6, pp. 488–493, 2003.

[72] A. F. James, S. C. M. Choisy, and J. C. Hancox, "Recent advances in understanding sex differences in cardiac repolarization," *Progress in Biophysics and Molecular Biology*, vol. 94, no. 3, pp. 265–319, 2007.

[73] P. W. Macfarlane, S. C. McLaughlin, B. Devine, and T. F. Yang, "Effects of age, sex, and race on ECG interval measurements," *Journal of Electrocardiology*, vol. 27, pp. 14–19, 1994.

[74] T. Taneja, B. W. Mahnert, R. O. D. Passman, J. Goldberger, and A. Kadish, "Effects of sex and age on electrocardiographic and cardiac electrophysiological properties in adults," *PACE-Pacing and Clinical Electrophysiology*, vol. 24, no. 1, pp. 16–21, 2001.

[75] D. Levy, J. J. Bailey, R. J. Garrison et al., "Electrocardiographic changes with advancing age. A cross-sectional study of the association of age with QRS axis, duration and voltage," *Journal of Electrocardiology*, vol. 20, pp. 44–47, 1987.

[76] P. Rautaharju, S. H. Zhou, S. Wong et al., "Sex differences in the evolution of the electrocardiographic QT interval with age," *Canadian Journal of Cardiology*, vol. 8, no. 7, pp. 690–695, 1992.

[77] R. J. Pocchiari, R. L. Hamlin, and S. A. McCune, "Electrocardiographic findings in rats with cardiomyopathy," *The American Journal of Veterinary Research*, vol. 54, no. 4, pp. 607–611, 1993.

[78] I. Netuka, O. Szárszoi, J. Malý et al., "Late effect of early hypoxic disturbance in the rat heart: gender differences," *Physiological Research*, vol. 59, no. 1, pp. 127–131, 2010.

[79] J. A. Wasserstrom, S. Kapur, S. Jones et al., "Characteristics of intracellular Ca^{2+} cycling in intact rat heart: a comparison of sex differences," *American Journal of Physiology-Heart and Circulatory Physiology*, vol. 295, no. 5, pp. H1895–H1904, 2008.

[80] K. L. Philp, M. Hussain, N. F. Byrne, M. J. Diver, G. Hart, and S. J. Coker, "Greater antiarrhythmic activity of acute 17β-estradiol in female than male anaesthetized rats: correlation with Ca^{2+} channel blockade," *British Journal of Pharmacology*, vol. 149, no. 3, pp. 233–242, 2006.

[81] C. Jiang, P. A. Poole-Wilson, P. M. Sarrel, S. Mochizuki, P. Collins, and K. T. MacLeod, "Effect of 17β-oestradiol on contraction, Ca^{2+} current and intracellular free Ca^{2+} in guinea-pig isolated cardiac myocytes," *British Journal of Pharmacology*, vol. 106, no. 3, pp. 739–745, 1992.

[82] ICH, "Guidance for industry: S7B nonclinical evaluation of the potential for delayed ventricular repolarization (QT interval prolongation) by human pharmaceuticals," in *Proceedings of the International Conference on Harmonisation of Technical Requirements for Registration of Pharmaceuticals for Human Use (ICH '05)*, U.S. Department of Health and Human Services, Food and Drug Administration, Center for Drug Evaluation and Research (CDER), and Center for Biologics Evaluation and Research (CBER), Eds., pp. 1–10, Rockville, Md, USA, 2005.

[83] L. K. Bhatt, K. Nandakumar, and S. L. Bodhankar, "Experimental animal models to induce cardiac arrhythmias," *Indian Journal of Pharmacology*, vol. 37, no. 6, pp. 348–357, 2005.

[84] W. E. Louch, M. K. Stokke, I. Sjaastad, G. Christensen, and O. M. Sejersted, "No rest for the weary: diastolic calcium homeostasis in the normal and failing myocardium," *Physiology*, vol. 27, no. 5, pp. 308–323, 2012.

[85] S. J. Shipsey, S. M. Bryant, and G. Hart, "Effects of hypertrophy on regional action potential characteristics in the rat left ventricle: a cellular basis for T-wave inversion?" *Circulation*, vol. 96, no. 6, pp. 2061–2068, 1997.

[86] Z. Tatarková, S. Kuka, P. Račay et al., "Effects of aging on activities of mitochondrial electron transport chain complexes and oxidative damage in rat heart," *Physiological Research*, vol. 60, no. 2, pp. 281–289, 2011.

[87] H. Huang and K. G. Manton, "The role of oxidative damage in mitochondria during aging: a review," *Frontiers in Bioscience*, vol. 9, pp. 1100–1117, 2004.

[88] S. Asano, K. M. Rice, S. Kakarla et al., "Aging influences multiple indices of oxidative stress in the heart of the Fischer 344/NNia x Brown Norway/BiNia rat," *Redox Report*, vol. 12, no. 4, pp. 167–180, 2007.

[89] R. Kayali, U. Çakatay, H. Uzun, and H. Genç, "Gender difference as regards myocardial protein oxidation in aged rats: male rats have increased oxidative protein damage," *Biogerontology*, vol. 8, no. 6, pp. 653–661, 2007.

[90] B. Colom, J. Oliver, P. Roca, and F. J. Garcia-Palmer, "Caloric restriction and gender modulate cardiac muscle mitochondrial H_2O_2 production and oxidative damage," *Cardiovascular Research*, vol. 74, no. 3, pp. 456–465, 2007.

[91] C. Borrás, J. Sastre, D. García-Sala, A. Lloret, F. V. Pallardó, and J. Viña, "Mitochondria from females exhibit higher antioxidant gene expression and lower oxidative damage than males," *Free Radical Biology & Medicine*, vol. 34, no. 5, pp. 546–552, 2003.

[92] Y. M. Jang, S. Kendaiah, B. Drew et al., "Doxorubicin treatment in vivo activates caspase-12 mediated cardiac apoptosis in both male and female rats," *FEBS Letters*, vol. 577, no. 3, pp. 483–490, 2004.

[93] M. Strniskova, M. Barancik, and T. Ravingerova, "Mitogen-activated protein kinases and their role in regulation of cellular processes," *General Physiology and Biophysics*, vol. 21, no. 3, pp. 231–255, 2002.

[94] T. P. Garrington and G. L. Johnson, "Organization and regulation of mitogen-activated protein kinase signaling pathways," *Current Opinion in Cell Biology*, vol. 11, no. 2, pp. 211–218, 1999.

[95] S. L. House, B. E. House, B. Glascock et al., "Fibroblast growth factor 2 mediates isoproterenol-induced cardiac hypertrophy through activation of the extracellular regulated kinase," *Molecular and Cellular Pharmacology*, vol. 2, no. 4, pp. 143–154, 2010.

[96] L. E. Lemke, L. J. Bloem, R. Fouts, M. Esterman, G. Sandusky, and C. J. Vlahos, "Decreased p38 MAPK activity in end-stage failing human myocardium: p38 MAPK α is the predominant isoform expressed in human heart," *Journal of Molecular and Cellular Cardiology*, vol. 33, no. 8, pp. 1527–1540, 2001.

[97] C. Communal, W. S. Colucci, A. Remondino et al., "Reciprocal modulation of mitogen-activated protein kinases and mitogen-activated protein kinase phosphatase 1 and 2 in failing human myocardium," *Journal of Cardiac Failure*, vol. 8, no. 2, pp. 86–92, 2002.

[98] J. N. Peart, E. R. Gross, J. P. Headrick, and G. J. Gross, "Impaired p38 MAPK/HSP27 signaling underlies aging-related failure in opioid-mediated cardioprotection," *Journal of Molecular and Cellular Cardiology*, vol. 42, no. 5, pp. 972–980, 2007.

[99] A. A. Knowlton, P. Brecher, and C. S. Apstein, "Rapid expression of heat shock protein in the rabbit after brief cardiac ischemia," *Journal of Clinical Investigation*, vol. 87, no. 1, pp. 139–147, 1991.

[100] S. Storti, S. Vittorini, M. R. Iascone et al., "Analysis of the variation in the hsp70-1 and hsp90alpha mRNA expression in human myocardial tissue that has undergone surgical stress," *Cell Stress Chaperones*, vol. 8, no. 1, pp. 18–25, 2003.

[101] I. J. Benjamin and D. R. McMillan, "Stress (heat shock) proteins: molecular chaperones in cardiovascular biology and disease," *Circulation Research*, vol. 83, no. 2, pp. 117–132, 1998.

[102] M. Tatar, A. A. Khazaeli, and J. W. Curtsinger, "Chaperoning extended life," *Nature*, vol. 390, no. 6655, p. 30, 1997.

[103] W. E. Balch, R. I. Morimoto, A. Dillin, and J. W. Kelly, "Adapting proteostasis for disease intervention," *Science*, vol. 319, no. 5865, pp. 916–919, 2008.

[104] W. R. Swindell, M. M. Masternak, J. J. Kopchick, C. A. Conover, A. Bartke, and R. A. Miller, "Endocrine regulation of heat shock protein mRNA levels in long-lived dwarf mice," *Mechanisms of Ageing and Development*, vol. 130, no. 6, pp. 393–400, 2009.

[105] S. D. Westerheide and R. I. Morimoto, "Heat shock response modulators as therapeutic tools for diseases of protein conformation," *The Journal of Biological Chemistry*, vol. 280, no. 39, pp. 33097–33100, 2005.

[106] J. W. Starnes, A. M. Choilawala, R. P. Taylor, M. J. Nelson, and M. D. Delp, "Myocardial heat shock protein 70 expression in young and old rats after identical exercise programs," *Journals of Gerontology—Series A Biological Sciences and Medical Sciences*, vol. 60, no. 8, pp. 963–969, 2005.

[107] J. M. Lawler, H.-B. Kwak, J.-H. Kim, and M.-H. Suk, "Exercise training inducibility of MnSOD protein expression and activity

is retained while reducing prooxidant signaling in the heart of senescent rats," *American Journal of Physiology: Regulatory Integrative and Comparative Physiology*, vol. 296, no. 5, pp. R1496–R1502, 2009.

[108] K. C. Kregel, P. L. Moseley, R. Skidmore, J. A. Gutierrez, and V. Guerriero Jr., "HSP70 accumulation in tissues of heat-stressed rats is blunted with advancing age," *Journal of Applied Physiology*, vol. 79, no. 5, pp. 1673–1678, 1995.

[109] B. Chandrasekar and G. L. Freeman, "Induction of nuclear factor κB and activation protein 1 in postischemic myocardium," *FEBS Letters*, vol. 401, no. 1, pp. 30–34, 1997.

[110] C. Li, W. Browder, and R. L. Kao, "Early activation of transcription factor NF-kappaB during ischemia in perfused rat heart," *American Journal of Physiology-Heart and Circulatory Physiology*, vol. 276, no. 2, pp. H543–H552, 1999.

[111] S. C. Y. Wong, M. Fukuchi, P. Melnyk, I. Rodger, and A. Giaid, "Induction of cyclooxygenase-2 and activation of nuclear factor-κB in myocardium of patients with congestive heart failure," *Circulation*, vol. 98, no. 2, pp. 100–103, 1998.

[112] S. Frantz, D. Fraccarollo, H. Wagner et al., "Sustained activation of nuclear factor kappa B and activator protein 1 in chronic heart failure," *Cardiovascular Research*, vol. 57, no. 3, pp. 749–756, 2003.

[113] M. J. May and S. Ghosh, "Signal transduction through NF-κB," *Immunology Today*, vol. 19, no. 2, pp. 80–88, 1998.

[114] G. Bonizzi and M. Karin, "The two NF-κB activation pathways and their role in innate and adaptive immunity," *Trends in Immunology*, vol. 25, no. 6, pp. 280–288, 2004.

[115] M. Wang, P. Crisostomo, G. M. Wairiuko, and D. R. Meldrum, "Estrogen receptor-α mediates acute myocardial protection in females," *American Journal of Physiology: Heart and Circulatory Physiology*, vol. 290, no. 6, pp. H2204–H2209, 2006.

[116] M. Wang, B. M. Tsai, K. M. Reiger, J. W. Brown, and D. R. Meldrum, "17-β-Estradiol decreases p38 MAPK-mediated myocardial inflammation and dysfunction following acute ischemia," *Journal of Molecular and Cellular Cardiology*, vol. 40, no. 2, pp. 205–212, 2006.

[117] W. Cheng, L. Chen, S. Yang et al., "Puerarin suppresses proliferation of endometriotic stromal cells partly via the MAPK signaling pathway induced by 17ss-estradiol-BSA," *PLoS ONE*, vol. 7, no. 9, Article ID e45529, 2012.

[118] S. Nuedling, S. Kahlert, K. Loebbert, R. Meyer, H. Vetter, and C. Grohé, "Differential effects of 17β-estradiol on mitogen-activated protein kinase pathways in rat cardiomyocytes," *FEBS Letters*, vol. 454, no. 3, pp. 271–276, 1999.

[119] C. S. Watson, A. M. Norfleet, T. C. Pappas, and B. Gametchu, "Rapid actions of estrogens in GH3/B6 pituitary tumor cells via a plasma membrane version of estrogen receptor-α," *Steroids*, vol. 64, no. 1-2, pp. 5–13, 1999.

[120] M. van Eickels, C. Grohé, J. P. M. Cleutjens, B. J. Janssen, H. J. J. Wellens, and P. A. Doevendans, "17β-estradiol attenuates the development of pressure-overload hypertrophy," *Circulation*, vol. 104, no. 12, pp. 1419–1423, 2001.

[121] M. R. Voss, J. N. Stallone, M. Li, R. N. M. Cornelussen, P. Knuefermann, and A. A. Knowlton, "Gender differences in the expression of heat shock proteins: the effect of estrogen," *American Journal of Physiology-Heart and Circulatory Physiology*, vol. 285, no. 2, pp. H687–H692, 2003.

[122] A. A. Knowlton and L. Sun, "Heat-shock factor-1, steroid hormones, and regulation of heat-shock protein expression in the heart," *American Journal of Physiology: Heart and Circulatory Physiology*, vol. 280, no. 1, pp. H455–H464, 2001.

[123] K. Rayner, J. Sun, Y.-X. Chen et al., "Heat shock protein 27 protects against atherogenesis via an estrogen-dependent mechanism: role of selective estrogen receptor beta modulation," *Arteriosclerosis, Thrombosis, and Vascular Biology*, vol. 29, no. 11, pp. 1751–1756, 2009.

[124] A. S. Al-Madhoun, Y.-X. Chen, L. Haidari et al., "The interaction and cellular localization of HSP27 and ERβ are modulated by 17β-estradiol and HSP27 phosphorylation," *Molecular and Cellular Endocrinology*, vol. 270, no. 1-2, pp. 33–42, 2007.

[125] C. Borras, J. Gambini, M. C. Gómez-Cabrera et al., "17beta-oestradiol up-regulates longevity-related, antioxidant enzyme expression via the ERK1 and ERK2[MAPK]/NFkappaB cascade," *Aging Cell*, vol. 4, no. 3, pp. 113–118, 2005.

[126] G. W. Dorn II, "Apoptotic and non-apoptotic programmed cardiomyocyte death in ventricular remodelling," *Cardiovascular Research*, vol. 81, no. 3, pp. 465–473, 2009.

[127] R. S. Hotchkiss, A. Strasser, J. E. McDunn, and P. E. Swanson, "Cell death," *The New England Journal of Medicine*, vol. 361, no. 16, pp. 1570–1583, 2009.

[128] G. Olivetti, R. Abbi, F. Quaini et al., "Apoptosis in the failing human heart," *The New England Journal of Medicine*, vol. 336, no. 16, pp. 1131–1141, 1997.

[129] S. Hein, E. Arnon, S. Kostin et al., "Progression from compensated hypertrophy to failure in the pressure-overloaded human: heart structural deterioration and compensatory mechanisms," *Circulation*, vol. 107, no. 7, pp. 984–991, 2003.

[130] M. M. Gallogly, M. D. Shelton, S. Qanungo et al., "Glutaredoxin regulates apoptosis in cardiomyocytes via NFκb targets Bcl-2 and Bcl-xl: implications for cardiac aging," *Antioxidants and Redox Signaling*, vol. 12, no. 12, pp. 1339–1353, 2010.

[131] S. K. Kakarla, J. C. Fannin, S. Keshavarzian et al., "Chronic acetaminophen attenuates age-associated increases in cardiac ROS and apoptosis in the Fischer Brown Norway rat," *Basic Research in Cardiology*, vol. 105, no. 4, pp. 535–544, 2010.

[132] V. Ljubicic, K. J. Menzies, and D. A. Hood, "Mitochondrial dysfunction is associated with a pro-apoptotic cellular environment in senescent cardiac muscle," *Mechanisms of Ageing and Development*, vol. 131, no. 2, pp. 79–88, 2010.

[133] S. K. Kakarla, K. M. Rice, A. Katta et al., "Possible molecular mechanisms underlying age-related cardiomyocyte apoptosis in the F344XBN rat heart," *The Journals of Gerontology A: Biological Sciences and Medical Sciences*, vol. 65, no. 2, pp. 147–155, 2010.

[134] Z. Mallat, P. Fornes, R. Costagliola et al., "Age and gender effects on cardiomyocyte apoptosis in the normal human heart," *Journals of Gerontology Series A: Biological Sciences and Medical Sciences*, vol. 56, no. 11, pp. M719–M723, 2001.

[135] G. G. L. Biondi-Zoccai, A. Baldi, L. M. Biasucci, and A. Abbate, "Female gender, myocardial remodeling and cardiac failure: are women protected from increased myocardiocyte apoptosis?" *Italian Heart Journal*, vol. 5, no. 7, pp. 498–504, 2004.

[136] M. Challah, S. Nadaud, M. Philippe et al., "Circulating and cellular markers of endothelial dysfunction with aging in rats," *American Journal of Physiology*, vol. 273, no. 4, part 2, pp. H1941–H1948, 1997.

[137] S. S. Najjar, A. Scuteri, and E. G. Lakatta, "Arterial aging: is it an immutable cardiovascular risk factor?" *Hypertension*, vol. 46, no. 3, pp. 454–462, 2005.

[138] D. H. O'Leary, J. F. Polak, R. A. Kronmal, T. A. Manolio, G. L. Burke, and S. K. Wolfson Jr., "Carotid-artery intima and media thickness as a risk factor for myocardial infarction and stroke

in older adults," *The New England Journal of Medicine*, vol. 340, no. 1, pp. 14–22, 1999.

[139] A. U. Ferrari, A. Radaelli, and M. Centola, "Aging and the cardiovascular system," *Journal of Applied Physiology*, vol. 95, no. 6, pp. 2591–2597, 2003.

[140] S. J. Miller, W. C. Watson, K. A. Kerr et al., "Development of progressive aortic vasculopathy in a rat model of aging," *The American Journal of Physiology—Heart and Circulatory Physiology*, vol. 293, no. 5, pp. H2634–H2643, 2007.

[141] W. Zhang, X. Zhang, and Y. Zhang, "Evaluation of thoracic aortic anatomy and function with transesophageal echocardiography," *Zhonghua Yi Xue Za Zhi*, vol. 78, no. 9, pp. 666–669, 1998.

[142] J. J. van der Heijden-Spek, J. A. Staessen, R. H. Fagard, A. P. Hoeks, H. A. Struijker Boudier, and L. M. Van Bortel, "Effect of age on brachial artery wall properties differs from the aorta and is gender dependent: a population study," *Hypertension*, vol. 35, no. 2, pp. 637–642, 2000.

[143] P. Albaladejo, P. Laurent, B. Pannier, A. Achimastos, M. Safar, and A. Benetos, "Influence of sex on the relation between heart rate and aortic stiffness," *Journal of Hypertension*, vol. 21, no. 3, pp. 555–562, 2003.

[144] H. Qiu, B. Tian, R. G. Resuello et al., "Sex-specific regulation of gene expression in the aging monkey aorta," *Physiological Genomics*, vol. 29, no. 2, pp. 169–180, 2007.

[145] G. Gennaro, C. Ménard, E. Giasson et al., "Role of p44/p42 MAP kinase in the age-dependent increase in vascular smooth muscle cell proliferation and neointimal formation," *Arteriosclerosis, Thrombosis, and Vascular Biology*, vol. 23, no. 2, pp. 204–210, 2003.

[146] E. Porreca, R. Ciccarelli, C. Di Febbo, and F. Cuccurullo, "Protein kinase C pathway and proliferative responses of aged and young rat vascular smooth muscle cells," *Atherosclerosis*, vol. 104, no. 1-2, pp. 137–145, 1993.

[147] R. J. Hariri, D. R. Alonso, D. P. Hajjar, D. Coletti, and M. E. Weksler, "Aging and arteriosclerosis. I. Development of myointimal hyperplasia after endothelial injury," *Journal of Experimental Medicine*, vol. 164, no. 4, pp. 1171–1178, 1986.

[148] V. Sagach, A. Bondarenko, O. Bazilyuk, and A. Kotsuruba, "Endothelial dysfunction: possible mechanisms and ways of correction," *Experimental & Clinical Cardiology*, vol. 11, no. 2, pp. 107–110, 2006.

[149] T. Hayashi and A. Iguchi, "Possibility of the regression of atherosclerosis through the prevention of endothelial senescence by the regulation of nitric oxide and free radical scavengers," *Geriatrics and Gerontology International*, vol. 10, no. 2, pp. 115–130, 2010.

[150] D. M. Dudzinski and T. Michel, "Life history of eNOS: partners and pathways," *Cardiovascular Research*, vol. 75, no. 2, pp. 247–260, 2007.

[151] F. M. Ho, W. W. Lin, B. C. Chen et al., "High glucose-induced apoptosis in human vascular endothelial cells is mediated through NF-κB and c-Jun NH2-terminal kinase pathway and prevented by PI3K/Akt/eNOS pathway," *Cellular Signalling*, vol. 18, no. 3, pp. 391–399, 2006.

[152] Y. C. Boo and H. Jo, "Flow-dependent regulation of endothelial nitric oxide synthase: role of protein kinases," *The American Journal of Physiology—Cell Physiology*, vol. 285, no. 3, pp. C499–C508, 2003.

[153] Y. Dohi, M. Kojima, K. Sato, and T. F. Luscher, "Age-related changes in vascular smooth muscle and endothelium," *Drugs and Aging*, vol. 7, no. 4, pp. 278–291, 1995.

[154] J. Hoffmann, J. Haendeler, A. Aicher et al., "Aging enhances the sensitivity of endothelial cells toward apoptotic stimuli: important role of nitric oxide," *Circulation Research*, vol. 89, no. 8, pp. 709–715, 2001.

[155] R. P. Brandes, I. Fleming, and R. Busse, "Endothelial aging," *Cardiovascular Research*, vol. 66, no. 2, pp. 286–294, 2005.

[156] J. H. Kim, L. J. Bugaj, J. O. Young et al., "Arginase inhibition restores NOS coupling and reverses endothelial dysfunction and vascular stiffness in old rats," *Journal of Applied Physiology*, vol. 107, no. 4, pp. 1249–1257, 2009.

[157] S. Chakrabarti, O. Lekontseva, A. Peters, and S. T. Davidge, "17β-Estradiol induces protein S-nitrosylation in the endothelium," *Cardiovascular Research*, vol. 85, no. 4, pp. 796–805, 2010.

[158] J. P. Stice, J. P. Eiserich, and A. A. Knowlton, "Role of aging versus the loss of estrogens in the reduction in vascular function in female rats," *Endocrinology*, vol. 150, no. 1, pp. 212–219, 2009.

[159] J. Widder, T. Pelzer, C. von Poser-Klein et al., "Improvement of endothelial dysfunction by selective estrogen receptor-α stimulation in ovariectomized SHR," *Hypertension*, vol. 42, no. 5, pp. 991–996, 2003.

[160] P. Angerer, S. Störk, W. Kothny, P. Schmitt, and C. Von Schacky, "Effect of oral postmenopausal hormone replacement on progression of atherosclerosis: a randomized, controlled trial," *Arteriosclerosis, Thrombosis, and Vascular Biology*, vol. 21, no. 2, pp. 262–268, 2001.

[161] S. Ling, A. Dai, R. J. Dilley et al., "Endogenous estrogen deficiency reduces proliferation and enhances apoptosis-related death in vascular smooth muscle cells: insights from the aromatase-knockout mouse," *Circulation*, vol. 109, no. 4, pp. 537–543, 2004.

[162] E. Espinosa, E. Espinosa, B. S. Oemar, B. S. Oemar, T. F. Luscher, and T. F. Lüscher, "17β-estradiol and smooth muscle cell proliferation in aortic cells of male and female rats," *Biochemical and Biophysical Research Communications*, vol. 221, no. 1, pp. 8–14, 1996.

[163] A. Suzuki, K. Mizuno, Y. Ino et al., "Effects of 17β-estradiol and progesterone on growth-factor-induced proliferation and migration in human female aortic smooth muscle cells *in vitro*," *Cardiovascular Research*, vol. 32, no. 3, pp. 516–523, 1996.

[164] W.-S. Lee, J. A. Harder, M. Yoshizumi, M.-E. Lee, and E. Haber, "Progesterone inhibits arterial smooth muscle cell proliferation," *Nature Medicine*, vol. 3, no. 9, pp. 1005–1008, 1997.

[165] C. Bolego, A. Cignarella, V. Zancan, C. Pinna, R. Zanardo, and L. Puglisi, "Diabetes abolishes the vascular protective effects of estrogen in female rats," *Life Sciences*, vol. 64, no. 9, pp. 741–749, 1999.

[166] Q.-W. Chen, L. Edvinsson, and C.-B. Xu, "Role of ERK/MAPK in endothelin receptor signaling in human aortic smooth muscle cells," *BMC Cell Biology*, vol. 10, article 52, 2009.

[167] T. Zou, W. Yang, Z. Hou, and J. Yang, "Homocysteine enhances cell proliferation in vascular smooth muscle cells: Role of p38 MAPK and p47phox," *Acta Biochimica et Biophysica Sinica*, vol. 42, no. 12, pp. 908–915, 2010.

[168] I. Bhattacharya, M. Damjanović, A. Perez Dominguez, and E. Haas, "Inhibition of activated ERK1/2 and JNKs improves vascular function in mouse aortae in the absence of nitric oxide," *European Journal of Pharmacology*, vol. 658, no. 1, pp. 22–27, 2011.

[169] K. M. Rice, E. M. Walker, S. K. Kakarla et al., "Fluprostenol-induced MAPK signaling is independent of aging in Fischer 344/NNiaHSd x Brown Norway/BiNia rat aorta," *Annals of Clinical and Laboratory Science*, vol. 40, no. 1, pp. 26–31, 2010.

[170] K. M. Rice, R. S. Kinnard, R. Harris, G. L. Wright, and E. R. Blough, "Effects of aging on pressure-induced MAPK activation in the rat aorta," *Pflügers Archiv*, vol. 450, no. 3, pp. 192–199, 2005.

[171] A. J. Lusis, "Atherosclerosis," *Nature*, vol. 407, no. 6801, pp. 233–241, 2000.

[172] N. K. Fukagawa, M. Li, C. R. Timblin, and B. T. Mossman, "Modulation of cell injury and survival by high glucose and advancing age," *Free Radical Biology & Medicine*, vol. 31, no. 12, pp. 1560–1569, 2001.

[173] R. V. Sharma, M. V. Gurjar, and R. C. Bhalla, "Selected contribution: estrogen receptor-alpha gene transfer inhibits proliferation and NF-kappaB activation in VSM cells from female rats," *Journal of Applied Physiology*, vol. 91, no. 5, pp. 2400–2389, 2001.

[174] D. Xing, S. Nozell, Y. F. Chen, F. Hage, and S. Oparil, "Estrogen and mechanisms of vascular protection," *Arteriosclerosis, Thrombosis, and Vascular Biology*, vol. 29, no. 3, pp. 289–295, 2009.

12

Does Sensory Function Decline Independently or Concomitantly with Age? Data from the Baltimore Longitudinal Study of Aging

Shekhar K. Gadkaree,[1] Daniel Q. Sun,[1] Carol Li,[1] Frank R. Lin,[1] Luigi Ferrucci,[2] Eleanor M. Simonsick,[2] and Yuri Agrawal[1]

[1]*Department of Otolaryngology-Head & Neck Surgery, Johns Hopkins University School of Medicine, Baltimore, MD, USA*
[2]*National Institute on Aging, National Institutes of Health, Baltimore, MD, USA*

Correspondence should be addressed to Yuri Agrawal; yagrawa1@jhmi.edu

Academic Editor: F. R. Ferraro

Objectives. To investigate whether sensory function declines independently or in parallel with age within a single individual. *Methods.* Cross-sectional analysis of Baltimore Longitudinal Study of Aging (BLSA) participants who underwent vision (visual acuity threshold), proprioception (ankle joint proprioceptive threshold), vestibular function (cervical vestibular-evoked myogenic potential), hearing (pure-tone average audiometric threshold), and Health ABC physical performance battery testing. *Results.* A total of 276 participants (mean age 70 years, range 26–93) underwent all four sensory tests. The function of all four systems declined with age. After age adjustment, there were no significant associations between sensory systems. Among 70–79-year-olds, dual or triple sensory impairment was associated with poorer physical performance. *Discussion.* Our findings suggest that beyond the common mechanism of aging, other distinct (nonshared) etiologic mechanisms may contribute to decline in each sensory system. Multiple sensory impairments influence physical performance among individuals in middle old-age (age 70–79).

1. Introduction

The peripheral sensory systems—including the visual, proprioceptive, auditory, and vestibular systems—provide feedback from the environment, facilitating interaction and engagement with the external world. Each sensory system may become impaired with age, contributing to increased isolation from the outside world. Age-related reductions in visual function, including in visual acuity, field of view, and contrast sensitivity, are universal in older individuals [1–3]. Additionally, proprioceptive function declines with age, with studies reporting differences in proprioceptive ability of around 50% in metrics such as joint deviation thresholds between older and younger adults [4–6]. Hearing is also well known to decline with age, with presbycusis a widespread phenomenon among individuals aged 80 and above [2, 7, 8]. A decline in vestibular physiologic function associated with age has also been well documented in a number of studies [9–12].

Although age-related decline in each of these peripheral sensory systems has been well established in the literature, it is unknown whether these systems tend to lose function concomitantly with age within a single individual. This is an important consideration as parallel decline in these systems would suggest a common pathophysiology, perhaps related to the biology of aging [13]. A few studies have examined the prevalence and impact of dual sensory impairments, typically involving hearing and vision and hearing and vestibular function [14–18]. One study that observed the common cooccurrence of vision and hearing loss found that these sensory impairments act multiplicatively and increase the risk of adverse health outcomes and mortality [2, 19]. Another study observed an association between hearing loss and vestibular loss and postulated that the inner ear cochlear and vestibular structures may have shared vulnerabilities to toxic exposures such as noise [20]. However, whether individuals with impairment in one peripheral sensory system have higher than expected risk of also developing impairment in other sensory systems is unknown.

In this study, we use data from the Baltimore Longitudinal Study of Aging (BLSA) to evaluate visual, proprioceptive, hearing, and vestibular function in relation to age and with respect to one another. We also explored how the presence of multiple sensory impairments influences physical performance across age categories. The BLSA is a large, prospective cohort of community-dwelling individuals spanning a wide age range that rigorously assesses each of these peripheral sensory systems. Findings from this study will provide insight into how changes in sensory function accrue with age, and the impact of multiple sensory impairments on physical disability.

2. Methods

2.1. Participants. Participants are enrolled in the BLSA, a prospective cohort study of the normative aging process conducted by the National Institute on Aging (NIA) Intramural Research Program. Healthy community-dwelling adults age ≥20 years are eligible to enroll in the BLSA [21]. At each visit, participants undergo a broad array of assessments and are followed longitudinally through the end of life. A total of 276 BLSA participants underwent tests of all four sensory systems: vision, proprioceptive, auditory, and vestibular between February 2013 and June 2014. The analytic sample was limited based on vestibular testing, which was only fully implemented on all participants in the BLSA in late 2013. Olfaction and taste are not measured in BLSA and therefore could not be evaluated in this study. Informed consent was obtained from all participants, and the study protocol has an ongoing approval with the institutional review board of the National Institute of Environmental Health Science, National Institutes of Health.

Trained interviewers administered detailed questionnaires on demographic and health-related data. Each participant underwent sensory evaluation as detailed below.

2.2. Visual Acuity Testing. A trained examiner conducted visual acuity testing using the Contrast Sensitivity Viewer-1000 Halogen Glare Test (CSV-1000 HGT) Early Treatment Diabetic Retinopathy Study (ETDRS) acuity chart (VectorVision, Greenville, OH). Participants were seated eight feet from the chart and a calibrated light at a constant level of 85 cd/m^2 (candela per square meter) highlighted the row participants were prompted to read. Corrective lenses were permitted. Participants started reading a row where they could see all five letters clearly and progressed down the chart towards rows with smaller letters until they could correctly identify just two letters. This last line was considered to be their visual acuity level and was recorded as a Logarithm of the Minimal Angle of Resolution (LogMAR) score, where each line on the chart corresponds to a difference of 0.1 LogMAR. Standard visual acuity measurements of 20/10, 20/20, 20/40, and 20/200 correspond to LogMAR scores of −0.3, 0, 0.3, and 1.0 [21, 22]. For the sensory impairment analyses involving dichotomous measures, visual impairment was defined as any corrected LogMAR score greater than or equal to 0.3, corresponding to a 20/40 visual acuity [23].

2.3. Proprioceptive Testing. Trained examiners used customized equipment to quantitatively test proprioception [24]. The equipment consisted of two pedals: the right pedal controlled by a motor (BALDOR, Ft. Smith, AZ, USA) and the left pedal moved freely by the participant. Both pedals measured angle deviation from a baseline using potentiometers. For testing, participants were blindfolded and had their bare or stocking feet placed on the pedals, which were set at a neutral ankle angle of 100 degrees that would serve as the baseline for testing. The minimal angular displacement (degrees) of ankle deviation in the motorized pedal foot that could be detected by the participant was determined and recorded as the ankle proprioceptive threshold. The motorized pedal was moved at an angular speed of 0.3 degrees/second and followed a preset pattern of four trials. The lowest ankle threshold deviation angle (in degrees) from the four trials was considered the best threshold and was used as the measure of proprioception for this study [24]. For the sensory impairment analyses involving dichotomous measures, abnormal proprioception was defined as 2 standard deviations above the population average thresholds for men (1.00 degrees) and women (1.11 degrees) established previously in the BLSA [24]. This yielded cutoffs of >1.12 degrees for men and >1.25 degrees for women.

2.4. Audiometric Testing. Audiometric testing was performed by a trained examiner with the participant in a sound attenuating booth using an Interacoustics AD629 audiometer with ER3A insert earphones. Audiometric thresholds were obtained at frequencies 500 Hz to 8000 Hz. Pure-tone averages (PTA) were calculated as the mean thresholds in decibels Hearing Level (dB HL) at the frequencies of 0.5 KHz, 1 KHz, 2 KHz, 4 KHz, and 8 KHz in both ears [25]. The hearing threshold for each participant was calculated by averaging the mean thresholds across all frequencies in both ears, and those with an averaged hearing threshold of greater than 25 dB were considered to have impaired sensory function.

2.5. Vestibular Function Testing. Cervical vestibular-evoked myogenic potential (cVEMP) testing was used to assess vestibular function, specifically the function of the saccular end-organ of the vestibular system [26–28]. Participants were asked to lie at a 30-degree angle from the horizontal on the testing chair. Alcohol was used to cleanse the skin overlying the upper sternal area and both sternocleidomastoid (SCM) muscles, and electrodes were placed at these sites. A noninverting electrode was placed at the midpoint of the SCM muscle, an inverting electrode was placed at the sternoclavicular joint, and a ground electrode was placed at the upper sternum. Prior to applying the stimulus, participants were asked to lift their heads to provide a sample of background SCM activity. Audible stimuli were delivered through Audiocups noise canceling headphones from Amplivox (Eden Prairie, MN, USA). The stimulus was a 500 Hz, 125 dB Sound Pressure Level (SPL) tone burst, with a repetition rate of 5 Hz, a 1 ms rise/fall time, and a 2 ms plateau. In order for a cVEMP tracing to be valid, the background electromyography (EMG) signal was required to reach at least 30 mV over the 10 ms prior to the applied stimulus.

The cVEMP waveform consisted of a positive initial deflection followed by a negative deflection. The peak-to-peak amplitude was the voltage difference between the peak of the first positive deflection and the peak of the following negative deflection. The peak-to-peak cVEMP amplitude was divided by the background EMG signal to obtain the "corrected" peak-to-peak amplitude, which accounted for background level of muscle activity. Subjects with EMG recordings that lacked the initial characteristic positive deflection of the waveform were considered to have an absent cVEMP response and vestibular impairment for the purposes of this study.

The Health ABC Physical Performance Battery (PPB) score is a validated predictor of functional capacity, particularly useful for distinguishing higher levels of function [29, 30]. PPB testing consists of repeated chair stands, a six-meter normal walk, a six-meter narrow walk, and a standing series of balance testing (semi-tandem, full tandem, and single legged) [30]. Chair stand rate, average velocity for the normal walk, average velocity for the narrow walk, and the summed time held in each of the three balance stance tests were recorded and each result was divided by the maximal possible performance on the respective test, as determined by other studies [30–34]. Specifically, for chair stands, the maximal possible performance (MPP) value was 1 chair stand/second; for normal and narrow walks, the MPP was 2 m/s; for balance stance testing, the MPP was 90 seconds [30]. The ratios from each of these four domains, which ranged from 0 to 1, were summed for an ultimate score of 0 to 4, where 0 implied that none of the tests were performed successfully and 4 represented a perfect score [30]. In evaluating physical performance in this study, we used a cutoff score of 2.9, corresponding to the lowest third of physical performance tests, to indicate diminished physical performance.

2.6. Statistical Analysis. Simple linear regression models were used to evaluate the association between each sensory system and aging and between each of the sensory systems. For each bivariate association, a linear trend line and loess trend line were fitted to the graphical data. The loess trend line was created using loess regression, a locally weighted regression technique that provides a more detailed weighted trend line for grouped data segments [35]. Multiple linear regression analyses were used to evaluate the associations between sensory systems adjusted for age. Standardized regression coefficients were determined by calculating z scores in order to normalize each variable to be included in regression analysis. Estimating expected percentages of sensory impairments for multiple systems was calculated by multiplying the corresponding observed ratios of individual sensory impairments for a particular age category together. p values of less than 0.05 were considered statistically significant. All statistical analyses were performed using STATA 12.0 Statistical Software (College Station, TX, USA).

Table 1: Demographic characteristics and baseline sensory function, Baltimore Longitudinal Study of Aging 2013-4.

Characteristics	No (%)/mean (±SD[a])
Total participants	276
Age (years)	70.3 (±13.7)
Sex	
Male	116 (42.0%)
Female	160 (58.0%)
Race	
White, non-Hispanic	168 (60.9%)
Black, non-Hispanic	79 (28.6%)
Asian or Pacific Islander	17 (6.2%)
Other	12 (6.4%)
Best proprioception threshold (degrees)	1.4 (±1.6)
Visual acuity (LogMAR[b])	0.06 (±0.14)
Hearing threshold (dB)	33.8 (±17.8)
cVEMP[c] amplitude (μV)	1.2 (±1.1)

[a]SD: standard deviation.
[b]LogMAR: Logarithm of the minimal angle of resolution.
[c]cVEMP: cervical vestibular-evoked myogenic potential.

3. Results

Between February 2013 and June 2014, 276 participants underwent visual, vestibular, hearing, and proprioceptive testing in the BLSA. Sociodemographic characteristics and mean sensory function of the study participants are presented in Table 1. The participants had a mean (SD) age of 70.3 (13.7) years, ranging from 26 to 93 years. Fifty-eight percent of study participants were female, and the distribution by race was 60.9% white, 28.6% black, 6.2% Asian or Pacific Islander, and 6.4% other race. Mean (SD) visual acuity for the study population was 0.06 (0.14) LogMAR. The mean (SD) ankle threshold to detect movement in the joint was 1.2 (1.1) degrees. The mean (SD) pure-tone average hearing threshold was 33.8 (17.8) dB. The mean (SD) cVEMP amplitude was 1.2 (1.1) μV. We evaluated the associations between each of the peripheral sensory systems and age. As expected, we observed decline in sensory function with age, although these associations were only statistically significant for the visual, hearing, and vestibular systems (Figure 1). Visual acuity worsened with age (0.004 increase in LogMAR per year, $p < 0.001$). Hearing PTA thresholds increased with age (0.95 dB increase per year, $p < 0.001$), and cVEMP amplitude decreased with age (0.03 μV per year, $p < 0.001$).

Next, we considered the mutual associations between each of the sensory systems in unadjusted and age-adjusted analyses (Table 2(a)). The unadjusted analyses indicate whether pairs of sensory systems decline concomitantly, and age-adjusted analyses suggest whether the observed associations in unadjusted analyses can be explained by a shared association with age. Visual acuity and vestibular

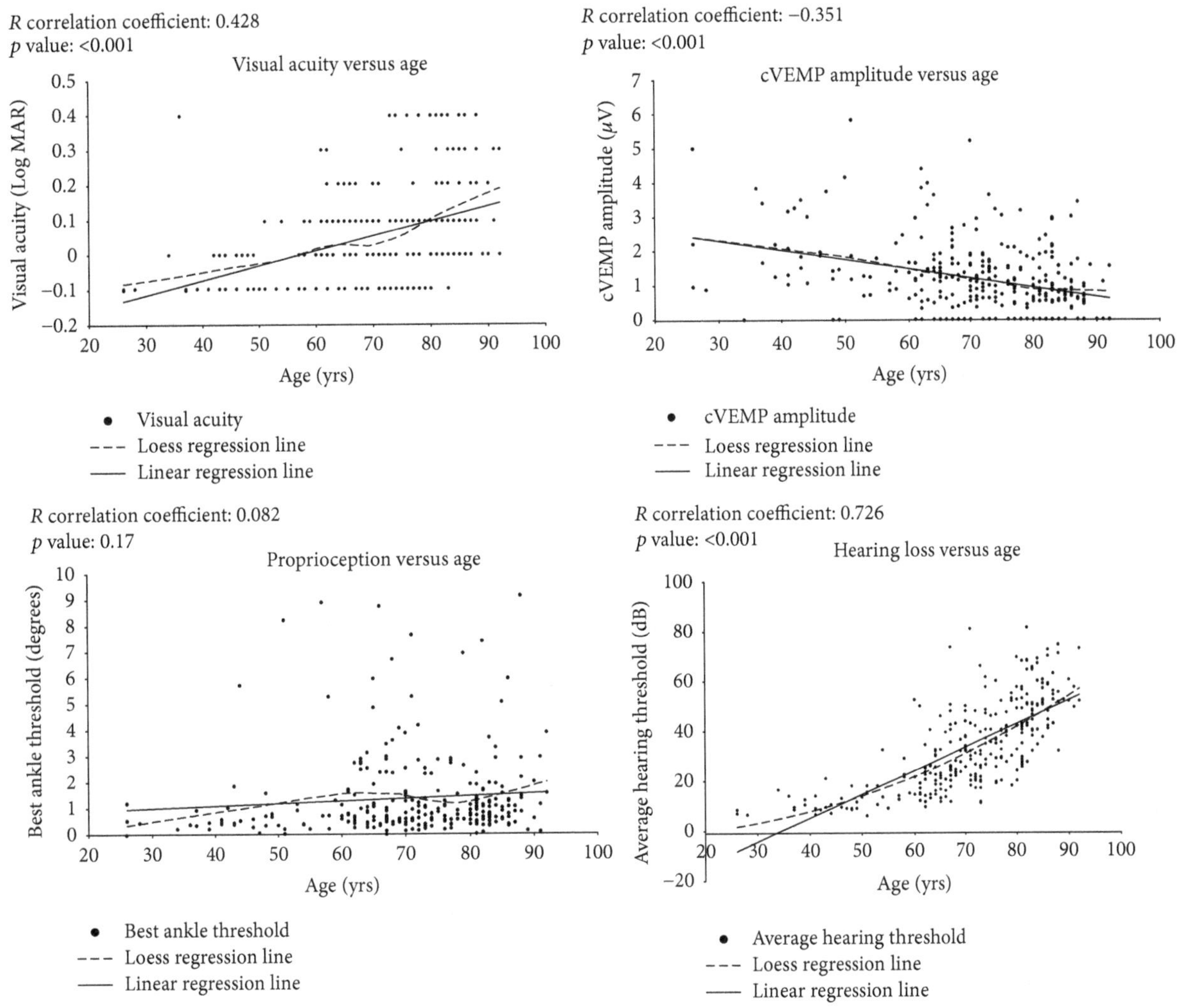

FIGURE 1: Individual associations between sensory system and age.

function were associated with one another ($p = 0.01$), although neither system was associated with proprioceptive function in unadjusted analyses. Additionally, we observed a positive association between poorer hearing thresholds and both poorer visual acuity ($p < 0.001$) and poorer vestibular function ($p < 0.001$). In multivariate models that adjusted for age, none of the associations retained their statistical significance (Table 2(b)). This indicates that the functions of the sensory systems decline with age, but they do so independently of one another.

Further, we evaluated the proportion of individuals with multiple (2–4) concurrent sensory impairments across age categories in participants aged 60 or older (Table 3). We compared the observed prevalence of multiple sensory impairment with the expected prevalence based on compounded probabilities of multiple impairments under the assumption of independence (i.e., sensory impairments occur independently). Overall, we observed an increase in the prevalence of multiple sensory impairments with increasing age category. Among the participants aged 80 years or older, 43.6% had dual sensory impairment and the most prevalent dual sensory impairment was hearing and vestibular loss (17.2%). Eighteen percent of participants aged 80 years and older had triple sensory impairment and the most prevalent triple sensory impairment was vision, proprioception, and hearing loss (8.0%). Only two participants had quadruple sensory impairments and both were over age 80. Notably, observed probabilities for dual sensory impairments were often lower than expected under an assumption of independence.

Finally, we explored the physical performance associated with single versus multiple sensory impairments across age categories in participants aged 60 or older (Table 3). Overall, we observed that participants aged 60–69 had normal Health ABC physical performance scores, while participants aged ≥80 had the lowest tertile Health ABC performance scores. Sensory impairments influenced physical performance in the middle old-age category (age 70–79). Individuals with single vision or proprioceptive impairments had poor physical performance, whereas individuals with single hearing or vestibular impairments had normal physical performance. Dual vision and proprioceptive, vestibular and hearing, and vision and hearing impairments were associated with poor

TABLE 2: (a) Bivariate associations between peripheral sensory systems. (b) Bivariate associations between peripheral sensory systems adjusted for age.

(a)

	Vestibular function	Proprioceptive threshold	Visual acuity	Hearing threshold
Vestibular function		−0.02 (−0.14, 0.10) $p = 0.73^{\dagger}$	−0.13 (−0.25, −0.02) $p = 0.026^{\dagger}$	−0.24 (−0.36, −0.13) $p < 0.001^{\dagger}$
Proprioceptive threshold	−0.01 (−0.09, 0.07) $p = 0.78$		−0.02 (−0.14, 0.09) $p = 0.68^{\dagger}$	0.06 (−0.06, 0.18) $p = 0.32^{\dagger}$
Visual acuity	−1.21 (−2.1, −0.28) $p = 0.01^{\ddagger}$	−0.29 (−1.7, 1.1) $p = 0.68$		0.33 (0.22, 0.44) $p < 0.001^{\dagger}$
Hearing threshold	−0.014 (−0.02, −0.01) $p < 0.001^{\ddagger}$	0.005 (−0.01, 0.02) $p = 0.32$	0.002 (0.001, 0.003) $p < 0.001^{\ddagger}$	

Regression coefficients refer to change in the column variable associated with 1 unit change in row variable for bottom half of table. † represents normalized regression coefficients corresponding to bottom half of table. 95% confidence intervals are included in parentheses. The units for the variables are vestibular function (VOR gain ratio), proprioceptive threshold (degrees), visual acuity (LogMAR), and hearing threshold (dB).
‡ = p value < 0.05.

(b)

	Vestibular function	Proprioceptive threshold	Visual acuity	Hearing threshold
Vestibular function		0.008 (−0.10, 0.12) $p = 0.89^{\dagger}$	0.018 (−0.11, 0.14) $p = 0.77^{\dagger}$	0.019 (−0.14, 0.18) $p = 0.82^{\dagger}$
Proprioceptive threshold	0.009 (−0.07, 0.08) $p = 0.82$		−0.074 (−0.20, 0.06) $p = 0.27^{\dagger}$	0.001 (−0.17, 0.17) $0.99^{\dagger}$
Visual acuity	−0.005 (−0.99, 0.98) $p = 0.99$	−0.86 (−2.4, 0.67) $p = 0.27$		0.036 (−0.12, 0.19) $p = 0.65^{\dagger}$
Hearing threshold	0.001 (−0.01, 0.01) $p = 0.83$	0.001 (−0.02, 0.02) $p = 0.99$	0.001 (−0.001, 0.001) $p = 0.65$	

Regression coefficients refer to the change in the column variable associated with 1 unit change in row variable for bottom half of table. † represents normalized regression coefficients corresponding to bottom half of table. 95% confidence intervals are included in parentheses. The units for the variables are vestibular function (VOR gain ratio), proprioceptive threshold (degrees), visual acuity (LogMAR), and hearing threshold (dB).

physical performance, and all triple sensory impairments were associated with poor physical performance.

4. Discussion

Our results demonstrate that while visual acuity, proprioceptive function, hearing, and vestibular function all decline with age, these sensory systems also decline through other mechanisms unique to each sensory system. After adjustment for age in regression models, there were no significant associations between any of the sensory systems. This observation suggests that, beyond the common mechanism of aging, other distinct (nonshared) etiologic mechanisms may contribute to the decline in each of these sensory systems. For instance, low antioxidant levels and vitamin deficiencies may disproportionately contribute to vision loss, while noise exposure and ototoxic medications may uniquely affect hearing [36–39]. The vestibular system may be specifically targeted by certain viral infections and aminoglycoside antibiotics, while proprioception may be particularly affected by diabetes [4, 40, 41]. Our findings suggest that the probability that sensory impairments cooccur within an individual is not greater than that expected by chance; however, an alternate explanation for these findings is that age itself may explain all variability in sensory impairment.

This study is among the first to evaluate the multiple sensory decline that occurs with aging. Growing evidence suggests that progressive loss of sensory input leads to increased isolation from the external world and presages important geriatric outcomes such as declining physical and social activity, mobility disability, falls, and dementia [42, 43]. Although sensory impairments appear to occur through independent age-related mechanisms, multiple impairments are more likely to accrue in older individuals because the prevalence of each impairment increases with age.

We also observed that single versus multiple sensory impairments impact physical performance among participants in "middle" old-age (age 70–79). Younger participants had normal physical performance and older participants had impaired physical performance regardless of sensory function. This suggests that other key factors, such as muscle strength and reaction time, contribute to physical performance and decline with age. Our findings suggest the particular importance of vision and proprioception in physical performance, given that single impairments in these sensory

Table 3: Number of impaired sensory systems in study participants by age and Health ABC score.

Number of impairments	Sensory system	Age categories 60–69 (N = 68) Observed N (%)‡	60–69 (N = 68) Expected N (%)	70–79 (N = 78) Observed N (%)‡	70–79 (N = 78) Expected N (%)	80+ (N = 87) Observed N (%)‡	80+ (N = 87) Expected N (%)
Any	Hearing (Hear)	25/68 (36.8)†		60/78 (76.9)†		84/87 (97.0)#	
	Vestibular (Vest)	11/68 (16.2)†		14/78 (17.9)†		27/87 (31.0)#	
	Vision (Vis)	3/68 (4.4)†		5/78 (6.4)#		20/87 (23.0)#	
	Proprioceptive (Pro)	24/68 (35.3)†		25/78 (32.1)#		30/87 (34.5)#	
Two	Vest + Vis	0/68 (0)‡	<1/68 (0.71)	1/78 (1.3)†	<1/78 (1.1)	0/87 (0)‡	6.2/87* (7.1)
	Vest + Prop	3/68 (4.4)†	3.9/68 (5.7)	0/78 (0)‡	4.5/78* (5.7)	1/87 (1.1)#	9.3/87 (10.7)
	Vis + Prop	1/68 (1.5)†	1.1/68 (1.6)	1/78 (1.3)#	1.6/78 (2.1)	0/87 (0)‡	6.9/87** (7.9)
	Vest + Hear	3/68 (4.4)†	4.1/68 (6.0)	6/78 (7.7)#	11/78 (13.8)	15/87 (17.2)#	26/87* (30.1)
	Vis + Hear	0/68 (0)‡	1.1/68 (1.6)	1/78 (1.3)#	3.8/78 (4.9)	8/87 (9.2)†	19/87* (22.3)
	Prop + Hear	5/68 (7.4)#	8.8/68 (13.0)	17/78 (21.8)†	19/78 (24.7)	14/87 (16.1)#	29/87* (33.5)
Three	Vest+ Vis + Prop	0/68 (0)‡	<1/68 (0.25)	0/78 (0)‡	<1/78 (0.36)	0/87 (0)‡	2.1/87 (2.5)
	Vest + Vis + Hear	0/68 (0)‡	<1/68 (0.26)	0/78 (0)‡	<1/78 (0.88)	3/87 (3.4)#	6/87 (6.9)
	Vis + Prop + Hear	0/68 (0)‡	<1/68 (0.57)	2/78 (2.6)#	1.2/78 (1.6)	7/87 (8.0)#	6.7/87 (7.7)
	Prop + Hear + Vest	2/68 (2.9)†	1.4/68 (2.1)	3/78 (3.8)#	3.4/78 (4.4)	6/87 (6.9)#	9.0/87 (10.4)
Four	Vest + Vis + Prop + Hear	0/68 (0)‡	<1/68 (0.09)	0/78 (0)‡	<1/78 (0.28)	2/87 (2.3)#	2.1/87 (2.4)

Greater than or equal to Health ABC score of 2.9 marked as †; below cutoff marked as #.
Single or double asterisk signifies observed and expected probabilities being significantly different using Chi-squared analysis (* $p < 0.05$) (** $p < 0.01$).

systems were associated with impaired physical performance. Most dual sensory impairments and all triple sensory impairments among 70–79-year-olds were associated with poor physical performance. Further studies in larger samples will be needed to establish which thresholds and combinations of sensory impairments result in poorer physical and functional status.

Very few studies have investigated multiple sensory impairments. One nationally representative study of the US population found that 11.3% of adults aged 80 or older had concurrent vision and hearing loss, similar to the 9.2% prevalence of dual vision and hearing impairment observed in this sample [2]. A longitudinal study in women found that individuals with dual vision and hearing loss were significantly more likely to experience incident cognitive decline [14]. Another population-based longitudinal study in Australia found that dual vision and hearing impairment at baseline was associated with a significantly increased risk of 10-year all-cause mortality [19]. Of note, in both studies, individuals with single impairments did not have increased risk of either cognitive decline or death relative to individuals with no sensory impairments. These data underscore the hazards of multiple sensory impairments with respect to adverse geriatric outcomes. Future studies will be needed to also consider how multiple impairments including vestibular and proprioceptive function affect morbidity and mortality risk. Interestingly, we observed that the prevalence of multiple sensory impairments (specifically dual) was lower than expected based on calculated probabilities. Whether enhancement in a modality of sensory function may occur in the context of loss of another sensory modality remains to be explored.

This study has several limitations. For the sake of simplicity, only a single measure was used to represent each of the sensory systems. However, each of the sensory systems has multiple dimensions; for example, vision encompasses not only visual acuity but also visual fields and contrast sensitivity, and vestibular function includes not only saccular function but also the function of the semicircular canals. Further studies involving larger cohorts will be needed to evaluate the parallel versus interrelated trajectories of each of these subdomains of sensory function. Moreover, we did not consider olfaction or taste sensation, given that these systems are not evaluated in the BLSA. Finally, the BLSA cohort is a highly selected sample that is healthier than the general US population. As such, findings from this analysis may not be applicable to other populations with higher rates of disease burden. For example, while this study suggests that there is no concomitant sensory decline of multiple sensory systems beyond the effects of aging in healthy individuals, cohorts with significant neuropathology, such as Alzheimer's Disease, are known to have linked impairment in olfaction loss, hearing loss, and vision loss [25, 44, 45]. Further data collection will be required to evaluate how the chemical sensory systems are impaired with age relative to the other sensory systems in participants with significant disease pathology.

5. Conclusion

In conclusion, we observed that while peripheral sensory function declines with age, once the effect of age is accounted for sensory decline occurs through independent mechanisms. Nevertheless the probability of multiple sensory impairments increases with age, given that each impairment is more likely to occur at older ages. Further investigation is needed to evaluate whether different combinations of sensory impairments confer specific risks and how these risks can be mitigated.

Disclosure

There are no other significant contributors to this manuscript who are not listed as authors. Funding had no direct impact on study design/conduct of the study/data collection, management/analysis/interpretation of the data, and preparation/review/or approval of the manuscript.

Competing Interests

None of the authors have conflict of interests regarding the content of this manuscript.

Acknowledgments

This study was funded with Grant no. K23 DC013056/DC/ NIDCD, NIH HHS/United States.

References

[1] N. S. Gittings and J. L. Fozard, "Age related changes in visual acuity," *Experimental Gerontology*, vol. 21, no. 4-5, pp. 423–433, 1986.

[2] B. K. Swenor, P. Y. Ramulu, J. R. Willis, D. Friedman, and F. R. Lin, "The prevalence of concurrent hearing and vision impairment in the United States," *JAMA Internal Medicine*, vol. 173, no. 4, pp. 312–313, 2013.

[3] D. E. Warren, M. J. Thurtell, J. N. Carroll, and M. Wall, "Perimetric evaluation of saccadic latency, saccadic accuracy, and visual threshold for peripheral visual stimuli in young compared with older adults," *Investigative Ophthalmology & Visual Science*, vol. 54, no. 8, pp. 5778–5787, 2013.

[4] S. Robbins, E. Waked, and J. McClaran, "Proprioception and stability: foot position awareness as a function of age and footwear," *Age and Ageing*, vol. 24, no. 1, pp. 67–72, 1995.

[5] S. H. You, "Joint position sense in elderly fallers: a preliminary investigation of the validity and reliability of the SENSERite measure," *Archives of Physical Medicine and Rehabilitation*, vol. 86, no. 2, pp. 346–352, 2005.

[6] H. B. Skinner, R. L. Barrack, and S. D. Cook, "Age-related decline in proprioception," *Clinical Orthopaedics and Related Research*, no. 184, pp. 208–211, 1984.

[7] F. R. Lin, J. K. Niparko, and L. Ferrucci, "Hearing loss prevalence in the United States," *Archives of Internal Medicine*, vol. 171, no. 20, pp. 1851–1852, 2011.

[8] D. J. Genther, K. D. Frick, D. Chen, J. Betz, and F. R. Lin, "Association of hearing loss with hospitalization and burden of disease in older adults," *The Journal of the American Medical Association*, vol. 309, no. 22, pp. 2322–2324, 2013.

[9] Y. Agrawal, M. G. Zuniga, M. Davalos-Bichara et al., "Decline in semicircular canal and otolith function with age," *Otology & Neurotology*, vol. 33, no. 5, pp. 832–839, 2012.

[10] M. A. Schrager, V. E. Kelly, R. Price, L. Ferrucci, and A. Shumway-Cook, "The effects of age on medio-lateral stability during normal and narrow base walking," *Gait and Posture*, vol. 28, no. 3, pp. 466–471, 2008.

[11] Y. Tang, I. Lopez, and R. W. Baloh, "Age-related change of the neuronal number in the human medial vestibular nucleus: a stereological investigation," *Journal of Vestibular Research: Equilibrium and Orientation*, vol. 11, no. 6, pp. 357–363, 2001.

[12] Y. Agrawal, J. P. Carey, C. C. Della Santina, M. C. Schubert, and L. B. Minor, "Disorders of balance and vestibular function in US adults: data from the National Health and Nutrition Examination Survey, 2001–2004," *Archives of Internal Medicine*, vol. 169, no. 10, pp. 938–944, 2009.

[13] B. K. Kennedy, S. L. Berger, A. Brunet et al., "Geroscience: linking aging to chronic disease," *Cell*, vol. 159, no. 4, pp. 709–713, 2014.

[14] M. Y. Lin, P. R. Gutierrez, K. L. Stone et al., "Vision impairment and combined vision and hearing impairment predict cognitive and functional decline in older women," *Journal of the American Geriatrics Society*, vol. 52, no. 12, pp. 1996–2002, 2004.

[15] K. J. Anstey, S. M. Hofer, and M. A. Luszcz, "A latent growth curve analysis of late-life sensory and cognitive function over 8 years: evidence for specific and common factors underlying change," *Psychology and Aging*, vol. 18, no. 4, pp. 714–726, 2003.

[16] K. M. Kiely, K. J. Anstey, and M. A. Luszcz, "Dual sensory loss and depressive symptoms: the importance of hearing, daily functioning, and activity engagement," *Frontiers in Human Neuroscience*, vol. 7, article 837, 2013.

[17] U. Lindenberger and P. Ghisletta, "Cognitive and sensory declines in old age: gauging the evidence for a common cause," *Psychology and Aging*, vol. 24, no. 1, pp. 1–16, 2009.

[18] M. I. Wallhagen, W. J. Strawbridge, S. J. Shema, J. Kurata, and G. A. Kaplan, "Comparative impact of hearing and vision impairment on subsequent functioning," *Journal of the American Geriatrics Society*, vol. 49, no. 8, pp. 1086–1092, 2001.

[19] B. Gopinath, J. Schneider, C. M. McMahon, G. Burlutsky, S. R. Leeder, and P. Mitchell, "Dual sensory impairment in older adults increases the risk of mortality: a population-based study," *PLoS ONE*, vol. 8, no. 3, Article ID e55054, 2013.

[20] M. G. Zuniga, R. E. Dinkes, M. Davalos-Bichara et al., "Association between hearing loss and saccular dysfunction in older individuals," *Otology & Neurotology*, vol. 33, no. 9, pp. 1586–1592, 2012.

[21] National Institutes of Health, *Baltimore Longitudinal Study of Aging*, 2014, http://www.blsa.nih.gov/participate.

[22] VectorVision, *ETDRS Acuity*, 2014, http://www.vectorvision.com/clinical-use-etdrs-acuity.

[23] D. Robaei, S. C. Huynh, A. Kifley, and P. Mitchell, "Correctable and non-correctable visual impairment in a population-based sample of 12-year-old Australian children," *American Journal of Ophthalmology*, vol. 142, no. 1, pp. 112–118, 2006.

[24] S.-U. Ko, E. Simonsick, N. Deshpande, and L. Ferrucci, "Sex-specific age associations of ankle proprioception test performance in older adults: results from the Baltimore Longitudinal Study of Aging," *Age and Ageing*, vol. 44, no. 3, pp. 485–490, 2015.

[25] F. R. Lin, E. J. Metter, R. J. O'Brien, S. M. Resnick, A. B. Zonderman, and L. Ferrucci, "Hearing loss and incident dementia," *Archives of Neurology*, vol. 68, no. 2, pp. 214–220, 2011.

[26] C. Li, A. J. Layman, J. P. Carey, and Y. Agrawal, "Epidemiology of vestibular evoked myogenic potentials: data from the Baltimore Longitudinal Study of Aging," *Clinical Neurophysiology*, vol. 126, no. 11, pp. 2207–2215, 2015.

[27] K. D. Nguyen, M. S. Welgampola, and J. P. Carey, "Test-retest reliability and age-related characteristics of the ocular and cervical vestibular evoked myogenic potential tests," *Otology & Neurotology*, vol. 31, no. 5, pp. 793–802, 2010.

[28] K. L. Janky and N. Shepard, "Vestibular Evoked Myogenic Potential (VEMP) testing: normative threshold response curves and effects of age," *Journal of the American Academy of Audiology*, vol. 20, no. 8, pp. 514–522, 2009.

[29] S. Perera, S. Studenski, A. Newman et al., "Are estimates of meaningful decline in mobility performance consistent among clinically important subgroups? (Health ABC study)," *Journals of Gerontology, Series A: Biological Sciences and Medical Sciences*, vol. 69, no. 10, pp. 1260–1268, 2014.

[30] E. M. Simonsick, A. B. Newman, M. C. Nevitt et al., "Measuring higher level physical function in well-functioning older adults: expanding familiar approaches in the health ABC study," *Journals of Gerontology—Series A: Biological Sciences and Medical Sciences*, vol. 56, no. 10, pp. M644–M649, 2001.

[31] R. W. Bohannon, "Comfortable and maximum walking speed of adults aged 20–79 years: reference values and determinants," *Age and Ageing*, vol. 26, no. 1, pp. 15–19, 1997.

[32] J. M. Guralnik, E. M. Simonsick, L. Ferrucci et al., "A short physical performance battery assessing lower extremity function: association with self-reported disability and prediction of mortality and nursing home admission," *Journals of Gerontology*, vol. 49, no. 2, pp. M85–M94, 1994.

[33] J. M. Guralnik, T. E. Seeman, M. E. Tinetti, M. C. Nevitt, and L. F. Berkman, "Validation and use of performance measures of functioning in a non-disabled older population: MacArthur studies of successful aging," *Aging Clinical and Experimental Research*, vol. 6, no. 6, pp. 410–419, 1994.

[34] C. H. Hirsch, L. P. Fried, T. Harris, A. Fitzpatrick, P. Enright, and R. Schulz, "Correlates of performance-based measures of muscle function in the elderly: the Cardiovascular Health Study," *The Journals of Gerontology, Series A: Biological Sciences and Medical Sciences*, vol. 52, no. 4, pp. M192–M200, 1997.

[35] N. J. Cox, "Speaking Stata: smoothing in various directions," *Stata Journal*, vol. 5, pp. 574–593, 2005.

[36] C. L. Koay, D. K. Patel, I. Tajunisah, V. Subrayan, and V. C. Lansingh, "A comparative analysis of avoidable causes of childhood blindness in Malaysia with low income, middle income and high income countries," *International Ophthalmology*, vol. 35, no. 2, pp. 201–207, 2015.

[37] M. A. Muhit, S. P. Shah, C. E. Gilbert, and A. Foster, "Causes of severe visual impairment and blindness in Bangladesh: a study of 1935 children," *British Journal of Ophthalmology*, vol. 91, no. 8, pp. 1000–1004, 2007.

[38] W. E. Fee, "Aminoglycoside ototoxicity in the human," *The Laryngoscope*, vol. 90, no. 10, part 2, supplement 24, pp. 1–19, 1980.

[39] E. Daniel, "Noise and hearing loss: a review," *Journal of School Health*, vol. 77, no. 5, pp. 225–231, 2007.

[40] R. E. Ariano, S. A. Zelenitsky, and D. A. Kassum, "Aminoglycoside-induced vestibular injury: maintaining a sense of balance," *Annals of Pharmacotherapy*, vol. 42, no. 9, pp. 1282–1289, 2008.

[41] S. R. Lord, G. A. Caplan, R. Colagiuri, S. Colagiuri, and J. A. Ward, "Sensori-motor function in older persons with diabetes," *Diabetic Medicine*, vol. 10, no. 7, pp. 614–618, 1993.

[42] S. W. van Landingham, J. R. Willis, S. Vitale, and P. Y. Ramulu, "Visual field loss and accelerometer-measured physical activity in the United States," *Ophthalmology*, vol. 119, no. 12, pp. 2486–2492, 2012.

[43] F. R. Lin, K. Yaffe, J. Xia et al., "Hearing loss and cognitive decline in older adults," *JAMA Internal Medicine*, vol. 173, no. 4, pp. 293–299, 2013.

[44] D. P. Devanand, S. Lee, J. Manly et al., "Olfactory deficits predict cognitive decline and Alzheimer dementia in an urban community," *Neurology*, vol. 84, no. 2, pp. 182–189, 2014.

[45] M. F. Mendez, R. L. Tomsak, and B. Remler, "Disorders of the visual system in Alzheimer's disease," *Journal of Clinical Neuro-Ophthalmology*, vol. 10, no. 1, pp. 62–69, 1990.

13

Health Status and Health Determinants of Older Immigrant Women in Canada

Sepali Guruge,[1] Birpreet Birpreet,[1] and Joan A. Samuels-Dennis[2]

[1]*School of Nursing, Ryerson University, 350 Victoria Street, Toronto, ON, Canada M5B 2K3*
[2]*School of Health Science, Humber College ITAL, 205 Humber College Boulevard, Toronto, ON, Canada M9W 5L7*

Correspondence should be addressed to Sepali Guruge; sguruge@ryerson.ca

Academic Editor: Wojtek Chodzko-Zajko

Increasing international migration in the context of aging populations makes a comprehensive understanding of older immigrant women's health status and determinants of their health particularly urgent. Using Arksey and O'Malley's framework, we conducted a scoping review to examine the available literature on the health of older immigrant women in Canada. We searched CINAHL, PsycINFO, Embase, Medline, and Cochrane databases for the period of 1990 to 2014 for Canadian-based, peer-reviewed studies on the topic. A total of 20 articles met the inclusion criteria. These articles were divided into six areas of focus: physical health; mental health; abuse; health promotion and chronic disease prevention; barriers to healthcare access and utilization; and health beliefs, behaviours, and practices. Our results show that the health of older immigrant women is affected by the interplay of various social determinants of health including the physical and social environment; economic conditions; cultural beliefs; gendered norms; and the healthcare delivery system. Our results also revealed that older immigrant women tend to have more health problems, underutilize preventive services, such as cancer screening, and experience more difficulties in accessing healthcare services.

1. Background

Aging and international migration are two prevailing global trends that have changed the age and ethnic composition of populations in countries worldwide, particularly Canada, the United States, the United Kingdom, and Australia. The global share of older people (aged 60 years or over) increased from 9.2% in 1990 to 11.7% in 2013 and will continue to grow, reaching 21.1% by 2050 [1]. Between 1990 and 2013, the number of older immigrants increased from 26 to 37 million worldwide [1]. This trend that is being observed in nearly all countries around the globe is the result of several factors including declining fertility rates as well as advances in medical care and technology and public health initiatives that have reduced mortality and morbidity rates for both chronic and acute illnesses [1]. These demographics demand changes in policies and service delivery systems that address the health and illness concerns of older immigrants [2].

The number of older women exceeds that of older men in most countries worldwide. In 2013, globally, there were 85 men per 100 women in the age group 60–79 years and 61 men per 100 women in the age group 80 years or older [3]. This phenomenon is referred to as the "feminization of aging" [3]. Older men and women have different health and illness experiences: women tend to experience more illnesses, more years of disability, and more stress than men, but they tend to live longer [4]. These gender disparities have been attributed partly to genetic predisposition, physiological and hormonal differences, and socioeconomic factors [4]. Research suggests that the family roles and responsibilities (such as caregiving) of older women often reduce their ability to make decisions regarding their own health and limit their access to and use of healthcare services [5]. Clarifying what is known about the health status of older women and the factors that affect their health is important to meet the health needs of this population. Building on our current and previous work, we focused on this topic in Canada.

Older adults are the fastest-growing age group in Canada. In 2011, an estimated 5.0 million individuals in Canada were 65 years or older, and this number is expected to double in the next 25 years to 10.4 million by 2036. By 2051, approximately one in four (25%) Canadians is expected to be 65 years or older [6]. The health of Canada's older immigrant population is of great interest to clinicians, health care managers, and policymakers because older immigrants' health is an important measure of population health and is directly related to issues, such as the cost and adequacy of the Canadian healthcare system [7]. For example, Gee et al. [5] reported that recent older immigrants are usually healthier than their Canadian-born counterparts or older immigrants who have been in Canada for many years, but over time their health may decline to a level that is worse than that of Canadian-born older adults. This phenomenon, the "healthy immigrant effect," has also been documented in Australia [8], the United Kingdom [9], and the United States [10]. It has been reported that this deterioration applied only to "non-European" immigrants [11]. Overall, this topic has begun to receive attention from health sciences researchers.

We conducted a scoping review to examine the existing literature about the health of older immigrant women in Canada. Our objectives were to (1) summarize the current knowledge about the health status of older immigrant women in Canada; (2) identify gaps in the existing knowledge; and (3) highlight implications for research, practice, and policy.

2. Methods

We followed the five-stage process that was proposed by Arksey and O'Malley [12] for conducting a scoping review: to identify a research question; identify studies relevant to the research question; review and select a subset of studies for inclusion in the final review; chart the information and data for the selected studies; and collate, summarize, and present the results.

Our research question for the scoping review was as follows: what is known from the existing literature about the health of older immigrant women in Canada? With the help of an experienced librarian, we searched CINAHL, Embase, Cochrane, Medline, and PsycINFO databases from January 1990 to 2014 using the following combinations of keywords: old age OR senior, elder, and older; AND immigrant, refugees, precarious, ethnic minority, visible minority, racial, and racialized; AND health AND Canada, Canadian. Inclusion criteria for articles were (1) peer-reviewed research findings; (2) being published in English or French; (3) focusing on older immigrant women's health; and (4) being based on studies conducted in Canada.

In most developed countries, including Canada, an "older adult" is defined as someone aged 65 years or older [13]. However, in many low-income countries with relatively shorter life expectancies, this definition may be expanded to include individuals aged 55 years or older [14]. For the purposes of this scoping review, we defined older adults as individuals aged 55 and older, because this is the definition generally used among our target population, which consists of a large proportion of older immigrants from low- and middle-income countries. We included studies that did not focus primarily on older women if their sample mean or median age range was 55 years or older and if at least half of the participants were women and separate results were available for this group. We defined "immigrants" as individuals who were born outside Canada (to non-Canadian parents), at some point, permanently relocated to Canada. If a study included both immigrant and Canadian-born older adults, we included it only if at least half of the study sample was born outside Canada, and separate results were available for this group.

A total of 6622 (CINAHL: 1261; Embase: 2223; Cochrane: 312; Medline: 1923; and PsycINFO: 903) records were generated through database searches. Of these, 1453 duplicates were removed and the abstracts of remaining 5169 articles were read for the inclusion criteria. After removing 4304 articles that did not focus on older immigrants, full text of 835 articles was read to determine if they focused on the health of older immigrant women. Twenty articles met our inclusion criteria and were included in the scoping review (see Figure 1).

As per Arksey and O'Malley [12], scoping reviews are undertaken to map the extent, range, and nature of literature, so we did not assess the quality of studies included in the review. We charted the 20 articles in Microsoft Excel 2011 using the following headings: Author/s, Name of Journal, Year of Publication, and Title; Aim of the Study, Focus Area; Ethnicity or Country/Continent of Origin, Age, Sample Size, and Study Setting; Study Method, Study Design, Data Collection, and Data Analysis; and Major Findings (see Table 1).

3. Results

3.1. Characteristics of the Studies Included. Among the 20 articles selected for analysis, seven (35%) were based on data collected for one study that was conducted in seven major cities of Canada: because these articles focused on different aspects of health of older immigrant women in Canada, we included them all. The characteristics reported here, therefore, are for the 14 studies (upon which the 20 articles are based). Their sample sizes ranged from 15 to 88,447. Most studies were based in Ontario (n = 6; 43%), British Columbia (n = 4; 29%), or Alberta (n = 2; 15%). Two were secondary analyses based on large sets of data across multiple provinces. The place of origin of immigrant women was operationalized in different ways across the studies: "country of origin," "country of birth," "continent of birth," or "ethnicity." With the exception of three articles, all (n = 18; 90%) included participants from Mainland China, Hong Kong, Taiwan, and Vietnam. With the exception of one (longitudinal) study, all studies used a cross-sectional design. Most (n = 7; 50%) used mixed methods combining qualitative and quantitative methods, six (n = 6; 43%) used qualitative methods, and one (n = 1; 7%) used a quantitative method. We did not find any articles written in French that met our inclusion criteria.

3.2. Summary of the Studies. We organized the 20 articles into six focus areas: physical health (n = 1; 5%), mental health (n = 3; 15%), abuse (n = 1; 5%), health beliefs/behaviour/practices (n = 8; 40%) and health promotion and chronic disease prevention (n = 5; 25%), and barriers to healthcare access and utilization (n = 3; 15%). One paper addressed both physical and mental health.

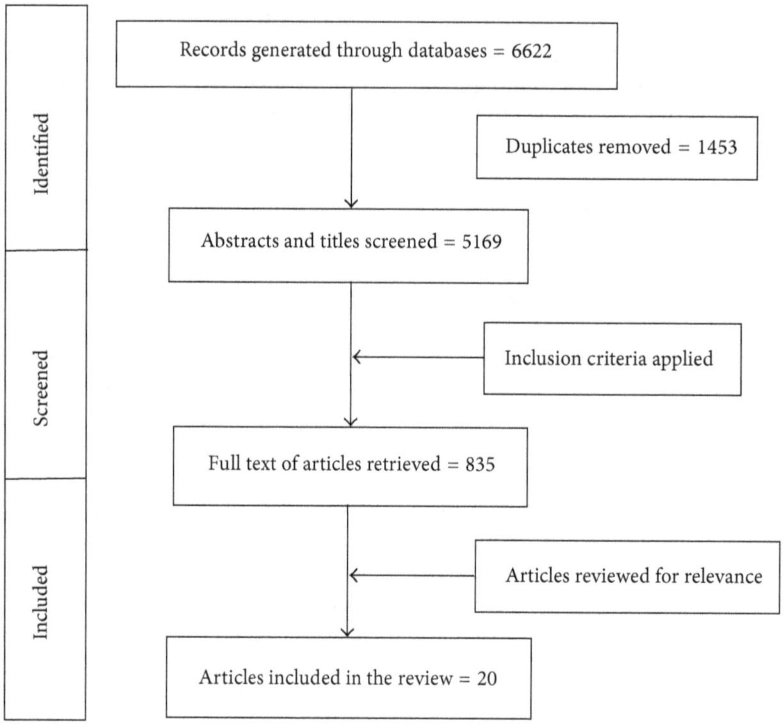

FIGURE 1: Flowchart of literature search and selection.

3.2.1. Physical Health. Chau and Lai [16] investigated the relationship between the size of Chinese communities and the health of older Chinese immigrants in Canada. Older Chinese immigrants residing in communities with a smaller Chinese population reported better physical health than older Chinese immigrants residing in communities with a larger Chinese population. Also, in this particular study, older men tended to score higher than older women did on physical health status scales.

3.2.2. Mental Health. Lai [15] categorized the predictors of depressive symptoms among older Chinese immigrants into three types: physical health factors, circumstantial factors, and psychosocial factors. Physical health factors included general physical health; circumstantial factors included finances, length of residency in Canada, barriers to services, and living arrangement; and psychosocial factors included ethnic identity, life satisfaction, and attitudes toward aging. Lai [15] also reported that older immigrants often encounter additional service barriers, making the transition from their homeland to their life in Canada stressful. Lai [17] later reported that, compared to their male counterparts, Chinese older immigrant women are often more vulnerable, more financially disadvantaged, have fewer resources, and are less healthy physically and mentally and stressed the need for improved support services aimed at older immigrant women. Chau and Lai [16] reported that the size of a Chinese community was a significant predictor of mental health status. As is the case with physical health above, participants residing in cities with a larger Chinese population scored lower on mental health scales. Social support was not a significant predictor of mental health in larger Chinese communities.

3.2.3. Abuse. Lai [18] reported that 4.5% of the study sample ($N = 2{,}272$) had experienced at least one incident of "maltreatment" or "neglect" within the past year: the most common forms of abuse included "being scolded, yelled at, treated impolitely, and ridiculed" (p. 338).

3.2.4. Health Beliefs, Behaviours, and Practices. Lai and Surood [19] reported that the health beliefs of older Chinese adults involve beliefs about "traditional" health practices (such as "Chinese exercise"), traditional Chinese medicine, and preventive diet. MacEntee et al. [20] focused on how acculturation in Canada influenced dental beliefs and behaviours among older Chinese immigrants: they found participants used "western dentistry" in addition to traditional remedies but it was difficult for them to get relevant information about oral health care: the two main barriers to accessing western-based dental care were language and financial costs. Tieu et al. [21] compared beliefs about treatment, etiology, and prognosis about depression among older Chinese immigrants and Canadian-born participants of the same age. They found that older Chinese immigrants would benefit from health education about the symptoms of depression, its etiology, and effective treatments.

Lai et al. [22] reported that participants who identified more strongly with Chinese cultural values and beliefs reported less favourable physical health and more illnesses. Jette and Vertinsky [23] explored how older Chinese immigrant women understood and took up western biomedical beliefs about health and physical activity. They found that the health practices of participants were not influenced by the western narratives of health, rather strongly tied to cultural beliefs. Green et al. [24] assessed the use of vitamin D

Table 1: Summary of charted data.

Author information	Sample information	Research design	Focus area
Lai (2004) [15]	*Ethnicity or country/continent of birth/origin*: Mainland China *Age*: 65+ years *Sample size*: 444 *Location*: Victoria, Vancouver, Calgary, Edmonton, Winnipeg, Toronto, and Montreal	*Method*: mixed *Design*: cross-sectional *Collection*: face-to-face interview *Analysis*: bivariate association using Mann-Whitney test, Kruskal-Wallis test, and Spearman's correlation test	Mental health
Chau and Lai (2011) [16]	*Ethnicity or country/continent of birth/origin*: Mainland China *Age*: 55+ years *Sample size*: 2,272 *Location*: Victoria, Vancouver, Calgary, Edmonton, Winnipeg, Toronto, and Montreal	*Method*: mixed *Design*: cross-sectional *Collection*: face-to-face interview *Analysis*: hierarchical multiple regression analysis	Physical and mental health
Lai (2011a) [17]	*Ethnicity or country/continent of birth/origin*: China *Age*: 65+ years *Sample size*: 151 *Location*: Calgary	*Method*: mixed *Design*: cross-sectional *Collection*: telephone survey *Analysis*: multiple regression analysis	Mental health
Lai (2011b) [18]	*Ethnicity or country/continent of birth/origin*: Mainland China, Hong Kong, Taiwan, Vietnam, and other Southeast Asian countries *Age*: 55+ years *Sample size*: 2,272 *Location*: Victoria, Vancouver, Calgary, Edmonton, Winnipeg, Toronto, and Montreal	*Method*: mixed *Design*: cross-sectional *Collection*: face-to-face interview *Analysis*: hierarchical logistic regression analysis	Abuse
Lai and Surood (2009) [19]	*Ethnicity or country/continent of birth/origin*: Mainland China, Hong Kong, Taiwan, Vietnam, and other Southeast Asian countries *Age*: 55+ years *Sample size*: 2,272 *Location*: Victoria, Vancouver, Calgary, Edmonton, Winnipeg, Toronto, and Montreal	*Method*: mixed *Design*: cross-sectional *Collection*: face-to-face interview *Analysis*: multiple stepwise regression analysis	Health beliefs
MacEntee et al. (2012) [20]	*Ethnicity or country/continent of birth/origin*: China, Hong Kong *Age*: 65+ years *Sample size*: 51 *Location*: Vancouver and Melbourne	*Method*: qualitative *Design*: cross-sectional *Collection*: focus groups *Analysis*: thematic analysis	Health beliefs
Tieu et al. (2010) [21]	*Ethnicity or country/continent of birth/origin*: China *Age*: 55–87 years *Sample size*: 53 *Location*: Calgary	*Method*: mixed *Design*: cross-sectional *Collection*: interview *Analysis*: multiple chi-square analyses	Health beliefs
Lai et al. (2007) [22]	*Ethnicity or country/continent of birth/origin*: Mainland China, Hong Kong, Taiwan, Vietnam, and other Southeast Asian countries. *Age*: 55+ years *Sample size*: 2,272 *Location*: Victoria, Vancouver, Calgary, Edmonton, Winnipeg, Toronto, and Montreal	*Method*: mixed *Design*: cross-sectional *Collection*: face-to-face interview *Analysis*: hierarchical multiple regression using stepwise method	Health beliefs

Table 1: Continued.

Author information	Sample information	Research design	Focus area
Jette and Vertinsky (2011) [23]	*Ethnicity or country/continent of birth/origin*: China *Age*: 65+ *Sample size*: 15 *Location*: Vancouver	*Method*: qualitative *Design*: cross-sectional *Collection*: in-depth semistructured interviews *Analysis*: thematic analysis	Health behaviour
Green et al. (2010) [24]	*Ethnicity or country/continent of birth/origin*: European and Asian *Age*: 50+ years *Sample size*: 1,996 *Location*: British Columbia	*Method*: mixed *Design*: cross-sectional *Collection*: phone-administered survey *Analysis*: multivariate logistic regression	Health behaviour
Johnson and Garcia (2003) [25]	*Ethnicity or country/continent of birth/origin*: Cambodian, Latin-American, Vietnamese, and Polish *Age*: mean age = 68 ± 6 years *Sample size*: 54 *Location*: London, Ontario	*Method*: qualitative *Design*: cross-sectional *Collection*: questionnaire and questionnaire-guided interviews *Analysis*: descriptive analysis using SPSS	Health behaviour
Fornazzari et al. (2009) [26]	*Ethnicity or country/continent of birth/origin*: Latin America *Age*: 55+ years *Sample size*: 125 *Location*: Greater Toronto Area	*Method*: mixed *Design*: cross-sectional *Collection*: questionnaires and scales *Analysis*: descriptive analysis using SPSS	Health beliefs
Sun et al. (2010) [27]	*Ethnicity or country/continent of birth/origin*: Asia *Age*: 50–69 years *Sample size*: 508 *Location*: Canada	*Method*: mixed *Design*: cross-sectional *Collection*: data from the Canadian Community Health Survey cycle 2.1 (2003) *Analysis*: multivariate logistic regression analyses	Health promotion and chronic disease prevention
Todd et al. (2011) [28]	*Ethnicity or country/continent of birth/origin*: China *Age*: 50+ years (mean 63.61) *Sample size*: 103 *Location*: Ontario	*Method*: mixed *Design*: cross-sectional *Collection*: interviews *Analysis*: Fisher's exact tests and independent sample t tests, multivariate logistic regression	Health promotion and chronic disease prevention
Donnelly (2006) [29]	*Ethnicity or country/continent of birth/origin*: Vietnam *Age*: 49–78 years *Sample size*: 15 *Location*: Western Canadian city	*Method*: qualitative *Design*: cross-sectional *Collection*: interviews; semistructured questionnaire using open-ended questions *Analysis*: qualitative data/thematic analysis	Health promotion and chronic disease prevention
Lofters et al. (2010) [30]	*Ethnicity or country/continent of birth/origin*: East Asia and Pacific, Eastern Europe and Central Asia, Latin America and Caribbean, Middle East and North Africa, South Asia, Sub-Saharan Africa, USA, Australia and New Zealand, and Western Europe *Age*: 50–66 years (mean 56.2) *Sample size*: 88,447 *Location*: Ontario	*Method*: quantitative *Design*: population-based cohort study *Collection*: Landed Immigrant Data System *Analysis*: multivariate Poisson regression	Health promotion and chronic disease prevention
Choudhry et al. (2002) [31]	*Ethnicity or country/continent of birth/origin*: South Asian *Age*: 58 and 68 years and 40 and 60 years *Sample size*: 13 *Location*: in and around Toronto	*Method*: qualitative *Design*: cross-sectional *Collection*: focus group discussions *Analysis*: reflexive and dialectical critique	Health promotion and chronic disease prevention

Table 1: Continued.

Author information	Sample information	Research design	Focus area
Lai and Chau (2007) [32]	*Ethnicity or country/continent of birth/origin*: Mainland China, Hong Kong, Taiwan, Vietnam, and other Southeast Asian countries. *Age*: 55+ years *Sample size*: 2,272 *Location*: Victoria, Vancouver, Calgary, Edmonton, Winnipeg, Toronto, and Montreal	*Method*: mixed *Design*: cross-sectional *Collection*: face-to-face interview *Analysis*: multiple regression analysis	Healthcare access
Lai and Kalyniak (2005) [33]	*Ethnicity or country/continent of birth/origin*: Mainland China, Hong Kong, Taiwan, Vietnam, and other Southeast Asian countries. *Age*: 55+ years *Sample size*: 2,272 *Location*: Victoria, Vancouver, Calgary, Edmonton, Winnipeg, Toronto, and Montreal	*Method*: mixed *Design*: cross-sectional *Collection*: face-to-face interview *Analysis*: hierarchical logistic regression analysis	Healthcare utilization
Ballantyne et al. (2011) [34]	*Ethnicity or country/continent of birth/origin*: China, Hong Kong, Vietnam, and Portugal *Age*: 65+ years *Sample size*: 30 *Location*: Toronto	*Method*: qualitative *Design*: cross-sectional *Collection*: interview *Analysis*: inductive content analysis	Healthcare service utilization

supplements among older adults and found that 60% of older British Columbians, including those of "Asian ethnic origin," were using a vitamin D supplement. They also found that older women were more likely than older men to take a supplement containing vitamin D. Having a healthcare practitioner recommend a vitamin D supplement doubled the likelihood of supplement use among older immigrants, demonstrating the importance of healthcare practitioners in influencing positive health behaviours. Johnson and Garcia [25] collected dietary and physical activity profiles and explored the factors that influenced these profiles. They found that older immigrants are at a high level of nutritional risk and identified contributing factors, such as inadequate dietary consumption, tooth and mouth problems, the presence of chronic conditions that require dietary modifications, multiple medications, eating alone, and limited financial resources. Fornazzari et al. [26] reported low levels of knowledge about Alzheimer's disease among a sample of older Latin-American immigrants resulting in both normalization (as a "normal part of aging") and stigmatization (e.g., belief that it is contagious) that may act as a barrier to timely access to health care services.

3.2.5. Health Promotion and Chronic Disease Prevention. Sun et al. [27] reported lower rates of mammography screening among older Asian immigrant women in Canada as compared to Canadian-born women. They found that language differences were a key barrier to mammography screening. Todd et al. [28] explored the predictors of colon and breast cancer screening among older Chinese immigrant women and found that physician recommendation, self-efficacy, and adequate English-language proficiency affected the likelihood of cancer screening. Donnelly [29] explored the processes by which older Vietnamese immigrant women decided to engage in regular breast and cervical cancer screening: key findings were that decision-making should be shared by the patient and the physician, and outreach materials should be provided in a language that is understood by and accessible to this population. Lofters et al. [30] compared the prevalence of cervical cancer screening among older immigrant women from various countries and among Canadian-born women and found that screening rates were much lower among older women from South Asia than among Canadian-born women. Their findings suggested that income and cultural differences contributed significantly to the differences in screening rates between the two groups of women. Choudhry et al. [31] focused on health promotion among South Asian immigrant women and reported that the participants found it important to "maintain culture and tradition," placed family needs before themselves, and survived by "being strong."

3.2.6. Barriers to Healthcare Access and Utilization. Lai and Chau [32] reported that older Chinese immigrants find accessing health services difficult due to communication barriers such as language differences, lack of cultural competence among service providers, and logistical problems in the service delivery system. Lai and Kalyniak's [33] study of predictors related to accessing annual physical examinations among older Chinese immigrants revealed that, in addition to lack of knowledge about healthcare coverage and service availability, the low rates of accessing healthcare could be related to a lack of understanding about the importance and benefits of preventive annual physical examinations.

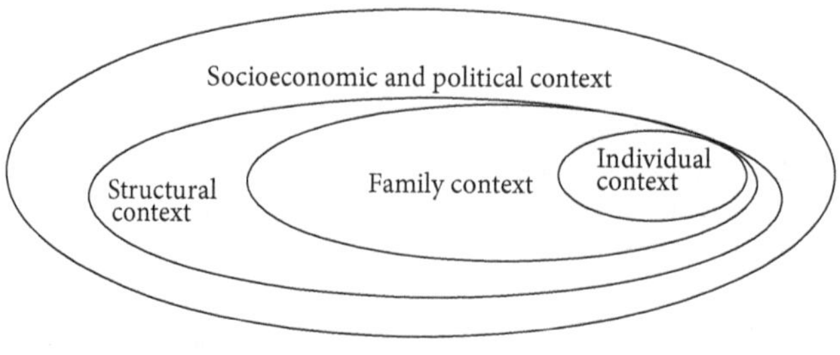

FIGURE 2: Social determinants of health.

Ballantyne et al. [34] investigated medication use among a diverse group of older immigrants and found that older immigrants from China, Hong Kong, Vietnam, and Portugal often avoided discussing their self-care and alternative healthcare practices with their physicians; they also found that the participants often disagreed with the assessment and the recommended treatment and sought out and tried alternative treatments.

4. Discussion

This scoping review summarizes the current literature on the health status of older immigrant women in Canada and the multiple and intersecting factors that affect this population's health. The review makes a significant contribution to the health science literature as it collates the relevant research on the topic.

Many of the studies used narrow recruitment strategies (e.g., telephone surveys) and small samples. Most also focused on one ethnic group and did not compare the results with other immigrant groups or individuals born in Canada. Other limitations of the original studies included potential loss of cultural nuances during translation and interpretation of data; lack of culturally and linguistically relevant data collection instruments; and lack of information about premigration health statuses.

In spite of these limitations, these studies revealed that older immigrant women experience health disadvantages due to intersecting factors such as social isolation, poverty, gender- and generational-specific roles, and other factors linked to the social determinants of health. The World Health Organization defines the Social Determinants of Health as the conditions in which people are born, grow, live, work, and age, including the health system [35]. The social determinants of health are a key element of Canada's framework for improving the health of its population [36].

The social determinants of health can be depicted using three circles to show how each determinant is contextually related to the others [37]. The familial and biologic context is at the centre of Figure 2, reflecting the social determinants of genetic and biological endowment, health practices and coping skills, and healthy child development. The structural context at the next level reflects socially created categories of "identity," which affect individual and group status and, in turn, suboptimal versus optimal health. The socioeconomic and political context, depicted at the outermost level, refers to the structuring of communities and the availability of community-specific resources needed to support health. The three levels are interdependent, but the social determinants of health related to the socioeconomic and political context have the strongest influence on the health and wellbeing of individuals [37]. As is the case with all Canadians, the health priorities and experiences of older immigrant women in Canada are inherently linked to the social determinants of health. Our scoping review has identified six social determinants that strongly affect the health of older immigrant women: physical environment, social environment, economic conditions, cultural beliefs, gendered norms, and the healthcare service delivery system.

4.1. Socioeconomic and Political Context. Physical environment is an important determinant of health. Within the built environment, factors related to housing, the design of communities, and transportation systems can significantly influence the physical and psychological wellbeing of older immigrants [36]. Lack of or limited transportation is known to be a significant barrier for older immigrant women, in particular, in terms of access to health services [20] as well as access to supermarkets and/or "ethnic food stores" [25]. Weather has also been identified as a barrier to physical activity among older immigrant women [25].

Support from families, friends, and communities is associated with better health [36]. Lai and Kalyniak [33] identified social support as a significant enabling factor in gaining adequate access to services. Perceived social support was also associated with positive mental health outcomes in older Hispanic immigrants living in the United States [38]. Further, the size of ethnic communities also affects health and wellbeing. For example, Chau and Lai [16] found that older Chinese immigrants living in larger ethnic communities in Canadian cities reported poorer health status as compared with those living in smaller ethnic communities. They gave several possible explanations for this observation. The first involves segregation of the older Chinese immigrants from individuals of other ethnicities: the large Chinese population in major cities may mean they are unlikely to be integrated into "mainstream" Canadian society, resulting in increased "social distance" from the Canadian-born counterparts and a subsequent decline in health. Members in smaller ethnic communities tend to have stronger social bonds that lead to psychological wellbeing. Also, because smaller communities pose less "less of a threat" to the dominant group, members of smaller ethnic communities may be perceived and treated more positively. Finally, members of smaller ethnic communities may be more resilient in dealing with negative experiences, resulting in better health and functioning.

Lai and Chau [32] found that older Chinese immigrants reported difficulties in accessing services because of lack of knowledge about existing health services, communication barriers, lack of cultural competence on the part of service providers, and administrative problems in the service delivery system. Language was a significant barrier to effective communication with a physician and mammogram use among older Asian immigrant women [32]. Sun et al. [27] reported that older Asian immigrant women who spoke one of the official languages were almost three times more likely to have ever had a screening mammogram. Similarly, studies based in the United States [39] have found language as a significant barrier to access to healthcare services. Publicly insured healthcare and drug benefits reportedly increase the willingness of older immigrant women to regularly consult or attend appointments with a physician and to use "western medicines" [34]. However, more research is needed to clarify the factors affecting the health of older immigrant women, especially their access to and use of healthcare services

4.2. Structural Context. Our findings highlight the negative impact of socioeconomic barriers on health care utilization. Similar findings have been reported in other studies based in the United States [40, 41]. Lai [17] found that being financially stable is important to the physical and mental health of older immigrants: older immigrant women are particularly vulnerable because they have access to fewer resources. In a study of cervical cancer screening use among urban immigrants, older South Asian immigrant women with lower incomes had lower rates of screening [30]. Financial constraints have also been identified as a major barrier to healthy eating practices among older immigrants [25].

The health choices of older immigrants are influenced by their cultural beliefs and values. For example, older Chinese immigrants reportedly believed that mental health problems can be addressed without professional help, which may be one reason for their underutilization of mental health services compared with their non-Chinese counterparts [22]. Lai et al. [22] also reported that older Chinese immigrants who identify more strongly with "traditional" Chinese cultural values and beliefs have less favourable health outcomes in the postmigration context and provided two possible explanations for this finding. First, those with stronger cultural values and beliefs may find it more difficult to adapt to Canadian values and beliefs about health, health practices, and service access. Second, older immigrants often face service barriers, such as language difficulties during encounters with healthcare practitioners. Culture also appears to play a key role in neglect and abuse: Lai and Surood [19] reported that older Chinese immigrants who were more "traditional" were more likely to experience neglect or abuse. But these findings need careful examination in the context of marginalization, stigmatization, loss or devaluation of language and culture, and lack of access to culturally appropriate and safe healthcare and services [37, 42, 43].

Gender refers to the various socially determined roles, attitudes, behaviours, values, relative power, and influence that society ascribes to women and men on a differential basis [36]. Many health issues can be ascribed to gender-based social status or roles [36]. For instance, a literature review on older Asian immigrants in North America found that depression was more prevalent among older Asian women than older Asian men [43]. The intersection of gender with other social identities had a significant effect on the health outcomes. For example, being older, female, single, and poor were all associated with negative influences on health [22]. Older women's access to health services may be related to factors such as the family's financial situation and employment concerns [29]. Often, making time for themselves at the cost of their family's needs is not an option for older immigrant women [31].

4.3. Social Determinants of Health Not Addressed in the Literature. One area of focus absent from the existing body of health research is how employment and working conditions affect the health of older immigrant women. The recent removal of the mandatory retirement age and anecdotal evidence that older women are remaining in the workforce longer indicate the importance of assessing how work and work environments influence the health of older immigrant women. We also did not find studies that assessed literacy and education as a determinant of older immigrant women's health or those that linked child development and the childhood environment with the health statuses of older immigrant women in Canada. No studies addressed genetic predispositions and health statuses of older immigrant women in Canada.

5. Strengths and Limitations of This Review

Scoping reviews are, particularly, useful for topics that have not been reviewed comprehensively before [12], as is the case of health of older immigrant women in Canada. Our review focused on social determinants of health and mirrors the current political trends that guide many health programs in Canada. The factors that shape older immigrant women's health are of importance to key stakeholders around the globe. Thus, our findings can inform practice and policy changes in this area. The findings can also inform future research on the topic.

Our review has several limitations. We excluded grey literature, which can include important research conducted by community organizations. Our literature search also did not include social science databases and thus potentially miss some relevant articles. We also did not search the reference lists of the articles included in the review.

Most of the studies included in our review included immigrants from (South, East, and Southeast) Asia, in general, and Chinese immigrants, in particular. However, the Chinese are the second-largest racialized immigrant group, making up 21% of the racialized population and 4% of the total Canadian population [44], and the findings help to clarify the health issues faced by the (diverse groups of) Asian immigrants in the country. Also, Asians constitute close to 50% of immigrants to most English-speaking countries [45],

Table 2: Key implications from selected studies.

List of studies	Key implications
Lai (2004) [15]	Adequate community support services and networks
Chau and Lai (2011) [16]	Further research to examine the residual confounding effects of the socioeconomic and political environment related to racism and various forms of discrimination in large urban centres
Lai (2011a) [17]	Further research on the influence of cross-cultural differences on health
Lai (2011b) [18]	Community education
Lai and Surood (2009) [19]	Longitudinal studies to clarify the effects of aging and acculturation on health values and beliefs
Tieu et al. (2010) [21]	Mental health education integrated into supports and services
Lai et al. (2007) [22]	Service delivery with attention to individuals' cultural health practices, using an approach that is respectful and nonjudgmental
Johnson and Garcia (2003) [23]	More research about adequate dietary intake and regular physical activity of older immigrants
Fornazzari et al. (2009) [26]	Longitudinal studies about health promotion initiatives
Sun et al. (2010) [27]	Culturally and linguistically appropriate education programs about breast cancer risk and mammography screening and the role of the physician in influencing older immigrant women's mammography screening behaviours
Donnelly (2006) [29]	Research about the influence of culture, social, political, historical, and economic background on cancer screening
Lofters et al. (2010) [30]	Research about cultural barriers to cancer screening
Lai and Chau (2007) [32]	Local health agencies and community health practitioners working more closely to design culturally appropriate methods for health information and promotion activities
Lai and Kalyniak (2005) [33]	Family physicians' proactive engagement in health promotion and local health regions and with community health practitioners

thus making our findings possibly transferable beyond the Canadian context to other countries with similar rates of Asian immigrants.

6. Implications

6.1. Implications for Research. There is an urgent need for more research on various aspects of older immigrant women's health (see Table 2). Studies involving cross-cultural groups would help reveal the degree to which findings are unique to older immigrant women from a specific ethnocultural group or common across immigrant communities. Research in different regions of Canada and different countries of the world would help clarify how geographic locations and healthcare contexts in different regions may affect older immigrant women's health and access to care and services. Studies with a longitudinal design would help delineate and track health changes, the aging process, and sociocultural changes among older immigrant women and their access to services over time. Other methodological issues to consider in future research include more emphasis on comparative research, larger sample sizes, inclusion of older immigrants from different immigration categories (such as refugee, precarious status and family sponsored), and more comprehensive recruitment strategies. An intersectionality approach [46] to examine the interactions of migration, gender, race, ethnicity, and other dimensions of social identity with health could also help further address the knowledge gap.

6.2. Implications for Practice. Overall, our findings suggest that the Canadian healthcare system fails to respond to the health and illness concerns of older immigrant women (see Table 2). First, it lacks holistic and supportive programs that could help older immigrant women cope with postmigration and (re)settlement challenges and achieve a sense of health and wellbeing. Second, services must incorporate community values and strengths, recognize social inequities, and implement new models of collaborative and integrated care. The healthcare and social service sectors need to work together to address the health needs of older immigrant women. There is a need for innovative community outreach strategies that engage key community leaders, to help clarify the barriers in accessing healthcare services. Healthcare practitioners need ongoing training to develop their cross-cultural communication and counselling skills. It is also important to strengthen the curricula of health professions to ensure that graduates in practical disciplines such as nursing are well equipped with the cross-cultural communication skills required for working with culturally diverse older immigrants. Also, with an increasingly aging population, demand for workers to provide care for the elderly population will increase. However, increasing the supply of healthcare providers alone is not a solution; there has to be a key focus on preventive healthcare.

6.3. Implications for Policy. Policy and systematic changes are needed to overcome many health and social challenges faced by older immigrant women (see Table 3). When

TABLE 3: Overview of the policy recommendations offered by selected studies.

List of studies	Key implications
Lai (2004) [15]	*Policy focus*: income security among Chinese immigrants (i) 17.3% of the older Chinese from Mainland China had an inadequate monthly income (<$500/mth) that, in turn, negatively affected all aspects of their health. (ii) Current sponsorship regulation restricts access to government pension benefits within the first ten years after their arrival in Canada. *Recommendation*: policies have to be instituted to help older immigrants access and/or maintain an adequate level of financial stability to protect society from the probable social and fiscal cost of physical and mental health problems that are a direct result of poverty.
Chau and Lai (2011) [16]	*Policy focus*: social support and networks (i) The presence of a larger ethnic community size does not necessarily enhance individual health and wellbeing. (ii) Older immigrants from ethnically diverse populations cannot rely solely on their immediate and community social networks for support to meet their health and wellbeing needs. *Recommendation*: the development of formal social support networks that can attend in culturally safe ways to the needs of ethnically diverse groups is essential to the health and wellbeing of older immigrant women.
Lai (2011a) [17]	*Policy focus*: income security among older Chinese immigrants *Recommendation*: there is a need for policies that will extend income security benefits to realistically account for the nutritional and rent/mortgage supplement needs of older immigrant women.
Lai (2011b) [18]	*Policy focus*: abuse of older immigrants Length of residency in Canada is a significant correlate of neglect and abuse, with long-term immigrants more likely to experience greater levels of abuse and neglect. *Recommendation*: practice policies should evolve to extend screening for abuse and neglect among older immigrant women. There is a need for policies that will support the development of shelters for older immigrant women who may be exposed to various forms of family and even community violence.
MacEntee et al. (2012) [20]	*Policy focus*: income security and dental health *Recommendation*: there is a need for policies that will increase access to routine and emergency dental care particularly among older immigrant women.
Lai et al. (2007) [22]	*Policy focus*: income security *Recommendation*: there is a need for policies that strategically focus on enhancing the health of older immigrant women who are unmarried and who are living in poverty.
Sun et al. (2010) [27]	*Policy focus*: health promotion and illness prevention *Recommendation*: practice and resource distribution policies that target breast cancer prevention need to address culturally safe ways to recruit and treat Asian immigrant women.
Lofters et al. (2010) [30]	*Policy focus*: health promotion and illness prevention *Recommendation*: practice and resource distribution policies that target cervical cancer screening need to address culturally safe ways to recruit and treat older immigrant women living in the lowest-income neighborhoods where service may be absent or where acculturation is likely to affect service uptake.
Lai and Chau (2007) [32]	*Policy focus*: health service access and effectiveness *Recommendation*: enduring and productive changes to improve racialized communities' experience with the healthcare system require the development of equitable and culturally competent systems that respect the rights of culturally diverse populations. Policies that attend to structural changes are needed to ensure that older immigrants are served in a way that prioritizes cultural safety social equity versus equality.

policy recommendations were made, most articles referred to income security as a way to ensure the health of older immigrant women. A number of articles recommended policy changes that would allow for adequate access to a monthly income, rental/mortgage supplements, and extended health benefits, such as dental care. Some referred to the need for resource distribution policies to target the development of formal social support networks, because being surrounded by a large immigrant community does not always translate to social connectedness. One recommendation that was common to several articles was to promote social inclusion of older immigrant women to encourage their physical and social involvement in community life. Addressing abuse of older immigrant women should also be a key policy focus which must address the larger socioeconomic and cultural contexts that contribute to the vulnerability of older immigrant women [47]. Public policies, programs, and services for older immigrant women should extend beyond the health sector and involve collaboration with other sectors, and approaches should be multipronged to incorporate education, awareness-raising, and community-based initiatives.

7. Conclusion

The socioeconomic and political context in which older immigrant women live, work, and grow old has significant implications for their health and wellbeing. This scoping review suggests that older immigrant women, when compared with Canadian-born women, are more vulnerable to poor health, more financially disadvantaged, and face a greater number of barriers when accessing the services needed to maintain and/or promote their health. The findings of this review suggest that Canada's health service system is ill equipped to address the health and illness concerns of this population. Specifically, our findings suggest the need to develop healthcare service delivery approaches that account for the cultural, generational, and gender-based norms of this population. Additionally, improving older immigrant women's health will require innovative community outreach strategies that engage older immigrant women, key community leaders, family members, and other stakeholders across sectors to address barriers to social inclusion, income security, stable housing, healthy relationships, and resources to access health care which will lead to individual transformation, community development, and policy change.

Conflict of Interests

The authors declare that there is no conflict of interests regarding the publication of this paper.

References

[1] Department of Economic and Social Affairs and Population Division, *World Population Ageing 2013, United Nations*, Department of Economic and Social Affairs, Population Division, 2013, http://www.un.org/en/development/desa/population/publications/pdf/ageing/WorldPopulationAgeing2013.pdf.

[2] A. M. Warnes, K. Friedrich, L. Kellaher, and S. Torres, "The diversity and welfare of older migrants in Europe," *Ageing and Society*, vol. 24, no. 3, pp. 307–326, 2004.

[3] United Nations, *World Migration in Figures*, 2013, http://www.oecd.org/els/mig/World-Migration-in-Figures.pdf.

[4] C. B. Tannenbaum, L. Nasmith, and N. Mayo, "Understanding older women's health care concerns: a qualitative study," *Journal of Women & Aging*, vol. 15, no. 1, pp. 3–16, 2003.

[5] E. M. T. Gee, K. M. Kobayashi, and S. G. Prus, "Examining the healthy immigrant effect in mid-to later life: findings from the Canadian Community Health Survey," *Canadian Journal on Aging*, vol. 23, no. 5, pp. 55–63, 2004.

[6] Statistics Canada, *Canadians in Context—AgingPopulation*, Statistics Canada, Ottawa, Canada, 2011, http://well-being.esdc.gc.ca/misme-iowb/.3ndic.1t.4r@-eng.jsp?iid=33.

[7] J. T. McDonald and S. Kennedy, "Insights into the 'healthy immigrant effect': health status and health service use of immigrants to Canada," *Social Science and Medicine*, vol. 59, no. 8, pp. 1613–1627, 2004.

[8] N. Biddle, S. Kennedy, and J. T. Mcdonald, "Health assimilation patterns amongst Australian Immigrants," *Economic Record*, vol. 83, no. 260, pp. 16–30, 2007.

[9] S. Kennedy, J. T. McDonald, and N. Biddle, "The healthy immigrant effect and immigrant selection: evidence from four countries," Social and Economic Dimensions of an Aging Population Research Papers 164, McMaster University, 2006.

[10] E. H. Stephen, K. Foote, G. E. Hendershot, and C. A. Schoenborn, "Health of the foreign-born population: United States, 1989-90," *Advance Data*, no. 241, pp. 1–12, 1994.

[11] E. Ng, R. Wilkins, F. Gendron, and J. M. Berthelot, "Dynamics of immigrants' health in Canada: evidence from the National Population Health Survey," Healthy Today, Healthy Tomorrow? Findings from the National Population Health Survey, Statistics Canada, Ottawa, Canada, 2005.

[12] H. Arksey and L. O'Malley, "Scoping studies: towards a methodological framework," *International Journal of Social Research Methodology*, vol. 8, no. 1, pp. 19–32, 2005.

[13] WHO, *Definition of Older or Elderly Person*, World Health Organization, Geneva, Switzerland, 2011, http://www.who.int/healthinfo/survey/ageingdefnolder/en/index.html.

[14] C. Spencer and G. Gutman, *Sharpening Canada's focus, Developing an Empirical Profile of Abuse and Neglect Among Older Women and Men in the Community*, Human Resources and Social Development, Ottawa, Canada, 2008.

[15] D. Lai, "Depression among elderly Chinese-Canadian immigrants from Mainland China," *Chinese Medical Journal*, vol. 117, no. 5, pp. 677–683, 2004.

[16] S. Chau and D. W. L. Lai, "The size of an ethno-cultural community as a social determinant of health for Chinese seniors," *Journal of Immigrant and Minority Health*, vol. 13, no. 6, pp. 1090–1098, 2011.

[17] D. W. L. Lai, "Perceived impact of economic downturn on worry experienced by elderly Chinese immigrants in Canada," *Journal of Family and Economic Issues*, vol. 32, no. 3, pp. 521–531, 2011.

[18] D. W. L. Lai, "Abuse and neglect experienced by aging Chinese in Canada," *Journal of Elder Abuse & Neglect*, vol. 23, no. 4, pp. 326–347, 2011.

[19] D. W. L. Lai and S. Surood, "Chinese health beliefs of older Chinese in Canada," *Journal of Aging and Health*, vol. 21, no. 1, pp. 38–62, 2009.

[20] M. I. MacEntee, R. Mariño, S. Wong et al., "Discussions on oral health care among elderly Chinese immigrants in Melbourne and Vancouver," *Gerodontology*, vol. 29, no. 2, pp. e822–e832, 2012.

[21] Y. Tieu, C. Konnert, and J. Wang, "Depression literacy among older Chinese immigrants in Canada: a comparison with a population-based survey," *International Psychogeriatrics*, vol. 22, no. 8, pp. 1318–1326, 2010.

[22] D. W. L. Lai, K. T. Ka, N. Chappell, D. C. Y. Lai, and S. B. Y. Chau, "Relationships between culture and health status: a multi-site study of the older Chinese in Canada," *Canadian Journal on Aging*, vol. 26, no. 3, pp. 171–183, 2007.

[23] S. Jette and P. Vertinsky, "'Exercise is medicine': understanding the exercise beliefs and practices of older Chinese women immigrants in British Columbia, Canada," *Journal of Aging Studies*, vol. 25, no. 3, pp. 272–284, 2011.

[24] T. J. Green, S. I. Barr, and G. E. Chapman, "The majority of older British Columbians take vitamin D-containing supplements," *Canadian Journal of Public Health*, vol. 101, no. 3, pp. 246–250, 2010.

[25] C. S. Johnson and A. C. Garcia, "Dietary and activity profiles of selected immigrant older adults in Canada," *Journal of Nutrition For the Elderly*, vol. 23, no. 1, pp. 23–39, 2003.

[26] L. Fornazzari, C. Fischer, T. Hansen, and L. Ringer, "Knowledge of Alzheimer's disease and subjective memory impairment in Latin American seniors in the Greater Toronto Area," *International Psychogeriatrics*, vol. 21, no. 5, pp. 966–969, 2009.

[27] Z. Sun, H. Xiong, A. Kearney et al., "Breast cancer screening among Asian immigrant women in Canada," *Cancer Epidemiology*, vol. 34, no. 1, pp. 73–78, 2010.

[28] L. Todd, E. Harvey, and L. Hoffman-Goetz, "Predicting breast and colon cancer screening among English-as-a-second-language older Chinese immigrant women to Canada," *Journal of Cancer Education*, vol. 26, no. 1, pp. 161–169, 2011.

[29] T. T. Donnelly, "The health-care practices of Vietnamese-Canadian women: cultural influences on breast and cervical cancer screening," *Canadian Journal of Nursing Research*, vol. 38, no. 1, pp. 82–101, 2006.

[30] A. K. Lofters, S. W. Hwang, R. Moineddin, and R. H. Glazier, "Cervical cancer screening among urban immigrants by region of origin: a population-based cohort study," *Preventive Medicine*, vol. 51, no. 6, pp. 509–516, 2010.

[31] U. K. Choudhry, S. Jandu, J. Mahal, R. Singh, H. Sohi-Pabla, and B. Mutta, "Health promotion and participatory action research with South Asian women," *Journal of Nursing Scholarship*, vol. 34, no. 1, pp. 75–81, 2002.

[32] D. W. L. Lai and S. B. Chau, "Effects of service barriers on health status of older Chinese immigrants in Canada," *Social Work*, vol. 52, no. 3, pp. 261–269, 2007.

[33] D. W. L. Lai and S. Kalyniak, "Use of annual physical examinations by aging Chinese Canadians," *Journal of Aging and Health*, vol. 17, no. 5, pp. 573–591, 2005.

[34] P. J. Ballantyne, R. M. Mirza, Z. Austin, H. S. Boon, and J. E. Fisher, "Becoming old as a 'pharmaceutical person': negotiation of health and medicines among ethnoculturally diverse older adults," *Canadian Journal on Aging*, vol. 30, no. 2, pp. 169–184, 2011.

[35] Commission on Social Determinants of Health, *Closing the Gap in a Generation: Health Equity through Action on the Social Determinants of Health*, World Health Organization, 2008, http://www.who.int/social_determinants/en/.

[36] Public Health Agency of Canada, "What makes Canadians healthy or unhealthy?" 2011, http://www.phac-aspc.gc.ca/ph-sp/determinants/determinants-eng.php.

[37] K. Edmunds and J. A. Samuels-Dennis, "Immigrant Canadians," in *Fundamentals: Perspectives on the Art and Science of Canadian Nursing*, D. Gregory, C. Seniuk, L. Patrick, and T. Stephen, Eds., Lippincott Williams & Wilkins, Toronto, Canada, 2014.

[38] S. C. Brown, C. A. Mason, A. R. Spokane, M. C. Cruza-Guet, B. Lopez, and J. Szapocznik, "The relationship of neighborhood climate to perceived social support and mental health in older hispanic immigrants in Miami, Florida," *Journal of Aging and Health*, vol. 21, no. 3, pp. 431–459, 2009.

[39] G. Flores, "Language barriers to health care in the United States," *The New England Journal of Medicine*, vol. 355, no. 3, pp. 229–231, 2006.

[40] F. M. Gany, A. P. Herrera, M. Avallone, and J. Changrani, "Attitudes, knowledge, and health-seeking behaviors of five immigrant minority communities in the prevention and screening of cancer: a focus group approach," *Ethnicity and Health*, vol. 11, no. 1, pp. 19–39, 2006.

[41] A. S. O'Malley, J. Mandelblatt, K. Gold, K. A. Cagney, and J. Kerner, "Continuity of care and the use of breast and cervical cancer screening services in a multiethnic community," *Archives of Internal Medicine*, vol. 157, no. 13, pp. 1462–1470, 1997.

[42] S. Guruge, P. Kanthasamy, J. Jokarasa et al., "Older women speak about abuse & neglect in the post-migration context," *Women's Health and Urban Life*, vol. 9, no. 2, pp. 15–41, 2010.

[43] B. C. H. Kuo, V. Chong, and J. Joseph, "Depression and its psychosocial correlates among older Asian immigrants in North America: a critical review of two decades' research," *Journal of Aging and Health*, vol. 20, no. 6, pp. 615–652, 2008.

[44] Statistics Canada, *Immigration and Ethnocultural Diversity in Canada*, 2011, http://www12.statcan.gc.ca/nhs-enm/2011/as-sa/99-010-x/99-010-x2011001-eng.cfm.

[45] G. Hugo, "The new international migration in Asia: challenges for population research," *Asian Population Studies*, vol. 1, no. 1, pp. 93–120, 2005.

[46] S. Guruge and N. Khanlou, "Intersectionalities of influence: researching the health of immigrant and refugee women," *Canadian Journal of Nursing Research*, vol. 36, no. 3, pp. 32–47, 2004.

[47] A. Matsuoka, S. Guruge, S. Koehn, M. Beaulieu, and J. Ploeg, "Moving forward: prevention of abuse of older women in the post-migration context in Canada," *Canadian Review of Social Policy*, vol. 2, no. 68-69, pp. 107–120, 2012.

14

Geospatial Relationships between Awareness and Utilization of Community Exercise Resources and Physical Activity Levels in Older Adults

Christopher J. Dondzila,[1] Ann M. Swartz,[2,3] Kevin G. Keenan,[2,3] Amy E. Harley,[4] Razia Azen,[5] and Scott J. Strath[2,3]

[1] *Department of Health, Exercise, and Sport Science, The Citadel, Deas Hall, Room 113, 171 Moultrie Street, Charleston, SC 29409, USA*
[2] *Department of Kinesiology, The University of Wisconsin-Milwaukee, Enderis Hall, 2400 East Hartford, Milwaukee, WI 53201, USA*
[3] *Center for Aging and Translational Research, The University of Wisconsin-Milwaukee, NWQ-B, Room 1427, Milwaukee, WI, USA*
[4] *Zilber School of Public Health, The University of Wisconsin-Milwaukee, Zilber School of Public Health Building, Room 409, 1240 North 10th Street, Milwaukee, WI 53205, USA*
[5] *Department of Educational Psychology, The University of Wisconsin-Milwaukee, Enderis Hall, Room 769, 2400 East Hartford, Milwaukee, WI 53201, USA*

Correspondence should be addressed to Christopher J. Dondzila; cdondzil@citadel.edu

Academic Editor: Barbara Shukitt-Hale

Introduction. It is unclear if community-based fitness resources (CBFR) translate to heightened activity levels within neighboring areas. The purpose of this study was to determine whether awareness and utilization of fitness resources and physical activity differed depending on residential distance from CBFR. *Methods*. Four hundred and seventeen older adults (72.9 ± 7.7 years) were randomly recruited from three spatial tiers (≤1.6, >1.6 to ≤3.2, and >3.2 to 8.0 km) surrounding seven senior centers, which housed CBFR. Participants completed questionnaires on health history, CBFR, and physical activity, gathering data on CBFR awareness, utilization, and barriers, overall levels, and predictors to engagement in moderate to vigorous physical activity (MVPA). *Results*. Across spatial tiers, there were no differences in positive awareness rates of CBFR or CBFR utilization. Engagement in MVPA differed across spatial tiers ($P < 0.001$), with the >3.2 to 8.0 km radius having the highest mean energy expenditure. Across all sites, age and income level ($P < 0.05$) were significant predictors of low and high amounts of MVPA, respectively, and current health status and lack of interest represented barriers to CBFR utilization ($P < 0.05$). *Conclusion*. Closer proximity to CBFR did not impact awareness or utilization rates and had an inverse relationship with physical activity.

1. Introduction

Older adults (65+ years) are among the most rapidly growing segments in the United States population, and projections predict this trend to continue into the future [1, 2]. Despite modern advancements in medicine and technology, there are continual health concerns in the older adult population. The prevalence of chronic conditions, such as diabetes, osteoporosis, hypertension, hyperlipidemia, obesity, and cancer, remains high, having a detrimental effect on an older adult's overall health and quality of life and placing excessive economic strain on our nation's health care system [3, 4]. Accordingly, there is an increased emphasis on exploring the effectiveness of preventative efforts to ameliorate the burden of such adverse health outcomes in older adults.

Regular physical activity and exercise have long been promoted as a means to treat and prevent a multitude of health conditions [5], yet the number of older adults who are regularly active is staggeringly low. Based on objective physical activity assessments, it is estimated that only 3.5–10% of older adults are meeting physical activity recommendations [6, 7]. Furthermore, the amount of physical activity performed across the older adult years steadily decreases as sedentary behaviors begin to dominate everyday life [8, 9].

There is a complex interaction of factors that influence habitual physical activity engagement. A key barrier to physical activity for the older adult population is access to resources that promote regular physical activity and exercise [10–12]. Community-based fitness resources (CBFR) can provide older adults a wealth of opportunities to promote increases in physical activity levels, such as removing/minimizing barriers to physical activity, including the availability, supervision, and instruction on use of exercise equipment, and developing a supportive network of peers. Such factors have been shown to be critical in influencing physical activity levels in older adults [13]. Proximity to CBFR is likely to be important, as it further reduces a potential transportation barrier [10–13] and may also result in a greater awareness of programming opportunities and their associated benefits.

Senior centers offer an excellent conduit in which to promote CBFR and could serve as an organizational mediator to physical activity behavior in older adults. To date, it remains unclear whether proximity to senior centers with CBFR has an impact on awareness and utilization of resources and ultimately overall physical activity levels of older adults. Thus, the purpose of the current study was to assess awareness and utilization of CBFR, based on residential spatial tiers of increasing distance from said resources. It was hypothesized that individuals living in closer proximity to CBFR would have greater awareness, utilization rate, and overall higher physical activity levels, compared to those residing further away from CBFR.

2. Methods

2.1. Study Design. This cross-sectional study involved gathering a series of information regarding awareness and utilization of CBFR and current physical activity levels, based on proximity to the facilities. Participation consisted of the completion of a series of questionnaires mailed to participants, which included a health history questionnaire, a community-based resources questionnaire, and the CHAMPS physical activity questionnaire. In addition to the questionnaires, a cover letter was enclosed to orient the participant on completing the forms, as well as a preaddressed, stamped envelope for the questionnaires to be returned to the investigative team.

The surrounding areas of seven local senior centers with CBFR throughout a large metropolitan area were included in the current study. Extensive calling lists of those aged ≥60 years were compiled to recruit potential participants. These lists were designated to include all older adults residing within 5 miles of targeted senior centers, obtained through marketing companies. Calling lists were then segmented by geographic information systems software into those who resided ≤1.6, >1.6 to ≤3.2, and >3.2 to 8.0 km from targeted senior centers. Within the stratified calling lists, a random sample of potential participants was contacted via telephone to inquire if they would be interested in participating in this study. Upon receiving verbal consent to participate, as approved by the University's Institutional Review Board, all documents were sent out in the mail. All data collection was conducted within a single season, thus reducing the confounding of seasonality on responses.

2.2. Participants. Inclusion criteria for participating in the study consisted of being between 60 and 90 years and willingness to complete and return all questionnaires. By nature of the study design, all participants contacted were previously stratified to be residing within 8.0 km of a targeted senior center.

2.3. Study Measures

2.3.1. Community-Based Fitness Resource Questionnaire. An 11-point questionnaire was developed by the investigators to amass descriptive data pertaining to CBFR awareness, utilization, transportation, and barriers to utilization.

Community-Based Fitness Resource Awareness. To assess awareness of CBFR, participants checked a box either "yes" or "no" to the following question: "Are you aware of any exercise/fitness programs or classes at your local senior center?"

Community-Based Fitness Resource Utilization. To assess utilization of CBFR, participants checked a box either "yes" or "no" to the following question: "Do you currently attend or participate in any of the exercise/fitness programs or classes at your local senior center?"

Barriers to Community-Based Fitness Resource Utilization. Additionally, participants were given the opportunity to identify what barriers pertaining to CBFR use were applicable to them from the following question: "What barriers prevent you from attending and participating in any exercise/fitness programs or classes at your local senior center more often/if at all?" A list of common barriers was provided, including knowledge of services, time, transportation, work/other commitments, health, lack of interest, and distance from resources, prompting participants to check a box adjacent to each applicable barrier that contributed to limiting their engagement. There was no limit to how many barriers could be marked as influencing CBFR utilization.

2.3.2. Physical Activity Assessment. The CHAMPS physical activity questionnaire was used to collect information on physical activity engagement, targeting frequency (days/week) and weekly duration spent engaging in various exercise behaviors, everyday activities, and leisure-time activities common to older adults. For the current study, the outcome measurement from the CHAMPS questionnaire was weekly caloric expenditure in moderate to vigorous intensity activities, using adapted MET values for older adults [14]. Calculating energy expenditure from the CHAMPS questionnaire requires calculating weekly duration engaged in each activity, which has been shown to have acceptable measures of reliability, with r values ranging from 0.67 to 0.76

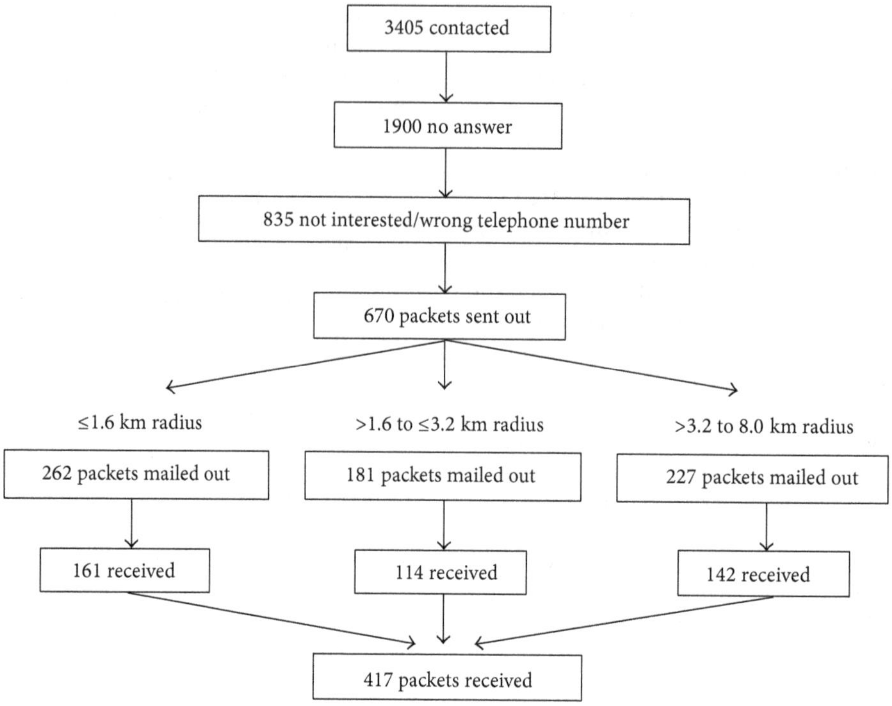

FIGURE 1: Participant flow diagram.

[14, 15]. The CHAMPS questionnaire has also been shown to appropriately demarcate varying physical activity levels with a level of precision similar to more intensive physical activity interviewing assessments ($F_{2,246} = 20.85$, $P < 0.001$), providing evidence for the CHAMPS questionnaire to be a valid physical activity assessment tool [14].

2.4. Data and Statistical Analysis. Descriptive statistics are expressed as mean ± standard deviation. Chi-square tests were performed to examine if awareness and utilization rates of CBFR differed across spatial tiers. Results were calculated as the overall percentage of those who responded "yes" to the inquiries on awareness and utilization over the total sample. Kruskal-Wallis tests were performed to examine if engagement in moderate to vigorous physical activity (MVPA) differed across spatial tiers. Multinomial logistic regression analyses were performed to identify which mediators to physical activity (age, gender, income, car ownership, and CBFR utilization) were significant predictors to overall activity levels, represented by caloric expenditure. The dependent physical activity categories included sedentary (0 kcals/wk; referent category), low levels of physical activity (>0–6710 kcals/wk), and high levels of physical activity (>6710 kcals/wk). The cut point used to delineate low and high physical activity levels was based on the median energy expenditure values among all nonsedentary (>0 kcals/wk) participants in the current sample. Binary logistic regression analyses were performed to identify which barriers significantly inhibited CBFR utilization, including knowledge of services, time, transportation, work/other commitments, health, lack of interest, and distance from resources. All statistical analyses were performed utilizing SPSS 19.0 for Windows (Chicago, IL).

3. Results

3.1. Participant Characteristics. A total of 3405 participants were contacted for participation in this study. Figure 1 depicts the recruitment flow, leading to the final sample of 417 older adults. Of the final sample, 161 were included in the ≤1.6 km radius group, 114 in the >1.6 to ≤3.2 km radius, and 142 in the >3.2 to 8.0 km radius. The successful return rates of complete questionnaires for the aforementioned spatial tiers were 61.5%, 63.0%, and 62.6%, respectively.

Participant demographics are listed in Table 1. There was an even distribution of female (n = 208) and male (n = 206) respondents, and participants were primarily Caucasian, had at least a high school education, and owned a car. No clear trend was discernable between education and income levels with car ownership across spatial tiers, although little variation was evident among these variables to allow such a distinction to be made. Body mass index (BMI) for all participants averaged just below the threshold (30 kg/m^2) to define obesity [16].

3.2. Community-Based Fitness Resource Awareness and Utilization. The responses for awareness and utilization of CBFR are reported in Figure 2. Among all respondents in the ≤1.6 km, >1.6 to ≤3.2 km, and the >3.2 to 8.0 km radii, 48.4%, 50.0%, and 44.4% were aware of CBFR, respectively. Respondents' overall utilization rates of CBFR, however, were extremely low (2.9%), with no differences across the spatial

TABLE 1: Participant demographics (mean ± SD).

	All (N = 417)	≤1.6 km radius (n = 161)	>1.6 to ≤3.2 km radius (n = 114)	>3.2 to 8.0 km radius (n = 142)
Age (yrs, n = 414)	72.9 ± 7.7	73.4 ± 7.9	72.5 ± 7.7	72.6 ± 7.6
Height (m, n = 381)	1.7 ± 0.1	1.7 ± 0.1	1.7 ± 0.1	1.7 ± 0.1
Weight (kg, n = 385)	82.9 ± 20.0	83.9 ± 21.3	81.9 ± 19.5	82.6 ± 19.0
Body mass index (kg/m^2, n = 373)	29.3 ± 6.6	29.7 ± 6.6	29.2 ± 6.0	29.0 ± 7.1
Gender (%, n = 414)	50.2	50.9	56.8	44.4
Ethnicity (%, n = 412)	82.3	81.3	80.2	87.9
Education (%, n = 409)	96.3	96.2	98.2	94.9
Income (%, n = 376)				
<$5,000	1.7	1.9	2.6	0.7
$5000–$14999	11.3	13.7	10.5	9.2
$15000–$24999	18.9	19.9	17.5	19.0
$25000–$34999	19.2	18.0	20.2	19.7
$35000–$49999	15.1	16.1	14.0	14.8
>$50000	24.0	19.9	24.6	28.2
Car (n = 417)	85.0	84.5	86.8	83.8

Note. Gender: percentage of female participants. Ethnicity: percentage of Caucasian participants. Education: percentage of those with at least a high school education. Car ownership reflects the percentage of participants that own a car.

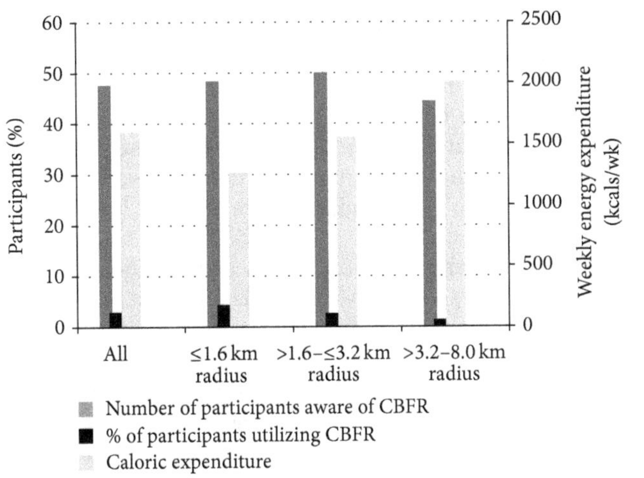

FIGURE 2: Awareness and utilization of community-based fitness resources (CBFR) compared to weekly energy expenditure (mean ± SE).

tiers (χ^2 = 2.37, df = 2, P = 0.306). Among those residing in the ≤1.6 km, >1.6 to ≤3.2 km, and the >3.2 to 8.0 km radii, only 4.3%, 2.6%, and 1.4% of participants responded positively to utilizing CBFR, thus exhibiting a weak trend of decreased utilization with increasing distance from CBFR.

3.3. Barriers to Community-Based Fitness Resources. Among the barriers listed that had a negative influence on CBFR utilization, lack of interest in CBFR was the most frequently cited barrier (51.6% of participants), followed by time (18.2%), work (16.1%), health (14.1%), transportation (9.1%), and distance (2.9%). Including all participants across all spatial tiers, only health (β = 1.408, P = 0.004) and lack of interest (β = −2.302, P = 0.002) were significant predictors of individuals not utilizing CBFR. Specific to spatial tiers, the only significant barriers were transportation (β = 5.47, P = 0.002) in the >1.6 to ≤3.2 km radius and health (β = 2.27, P < 0.05) in the >3.2 to 8.0 km radius.

3.4. Physical Activity Engagement. The average energy expenditure in MVPA for all participants across all sites was 1601 ± 2293 kcals/wk (n = 378), represented in Figure 2. Engagement in MVPA differed across spatial tiers (χ^2 = 15.74, df = 2, P = 0.000), with mean caloric expenditures rising in conjunction with increasing distance from CBFR: from 1263 ± 2177 kcals/wk (n = 146) to 1555 ± 1793 kcals/wk (n = 101) to 2013 ± 2680 kcals/wk (n = 131), respectively. Overall, 27.8% reported an energy expenditure of 0 kcals/wk (n = 105), 29.1% from >0 to 999 kcals/wk (n = 110), 8.7% from 1000 to 1499 kcals/wk (n = 33), 8.5% from 1500 to 1999 kcals/wk (n = 32), 5.8% from 2000 to 2499 kcals/wk (n = 22), and 20.6% >2500 kcals/wk (n = 78). Including participants from all spatial tiers, the multinomial regression model accounted for 16.7% of variability in MVPA values, with age and income being significant predictors of low (β = −0.04, P < 0.05) and high (β = 0.92, P < 0.05) levels of physical activity, respectively. Specific to spatial tiers, age was a significant predictor of low levels of physical activity within the ≤1.6 km radius (β = −0.062, P < 0.05) and >2–5 mile radius (β = −0.07, P < 0.05). No other independent variables were significant predictors of low or high levels of physical activity.

4. Discussion

National data suggest only a small percentage of older adults are active enough to receive the health benefits of physical activity, raising the susceptibility to poor overall health with increasing age. One approach to promoting physical activity and exercise specific to older adults is through local senior centers, providing an environment conducive to support physical activity and exercise by way of exercise equipment/rooms and supervised fitness classes. Such CBFR aim to reduce the influence of barriers that negatively impact regular physical activity, including lack of access to facilities, guidance, and social support. Still, other factors remain potentially unresolved by CBFR that contribute to their utilization (or lack thereof). Mainly, the influence of the availability of transportation and lack of time constraints remain unaffected and are heavily governed by one's residence distance from such resources. However, it is unclear how awareness and utilization of CBFR are thus impacted by distance from centers promoting and providing resources for active lifestyles. The main findings of this study show that, among spatial tiers of increasing distance surrounding CBFR, there were no statistical differences in awareness or utilization of CBFR. Moreover, despite approximately one-half of participants being currently aware of CBFR, utilization rates were less than 5% among those surveyed. Additionally, respondents reported greater physical activity levels the further one resided from CBFR.

An estimated 25% of older adults report utilizing senior centers [17], providing a promising setting for physical activity promotion efforts. Despite this, the results of the current study suggest that CBFR have a negligible impact on physical activity. There was a substantial decline in the number of individuals who used CBFR, relative to those who were aware of the resources (only 3% utilized CBFR, out of approximately 50% who were aware). Similar awareness-to-active engagement statistics are also available at the national level, were one to consider that an estimated 36% of US adults are aware of physical activity recommendations, with only 10% meeting such benchmarks [18, 19]. There is evidence to suggest that increasing the density of community resources positively relates to physical activity levels [20], specifically with increasing overall exercise frequency [21]. Therefore, implementing such resources is a first step in promoting exercise in older adults, given the noted positive relationships between the presence of fitness resources within the community and physical activity levels [22]. Still, awareness of the benefits of exercise towards health is a critical determinant of exercise adoption and adherence [23]. Given that 50% of the current study population was aware of CBFR, it is plausible that many did not favorably view CBFR or were possibly not aware of specific opportunities within community centers to tailor physical activity and exercise to their preferences.

Provided the disconnect between awareness of CBFR and the use of these available resources, other factors pertaining to facility use are likely more influential. Barriers, both personal and environmental, represent factors that inhibit CBFR utilization. Among barriers measured in the current study across all spatial tiers, health and interest were the only significant predictors of not utilizing CBFR, although interest was the most commonly reported barrier. Health, in the context of reporting multiple chronic conditions, has been shown to decrease the amount of adults meeting physical activity guidelines by up to 30% [24]. In the current study, 34% reported multiple chronic conditions, suggesting that this sample population may have been in poor health overall, which resulted in low CBFR utilization rates. Although health status has been noted as a critical barrier [23], it has also been viewed as a powerful physical activity motivator among older adults [25]. Accordingly, this sample population also represents the massive potential benefit to promote health as a theme to increase interest in CBFR. Educational components have been shown to have positive relationships with physical activity and health [26]. Thus, intervening and educating on health is a logical first step towards bolstering interest rates, targeting both barriers reported for not utilizing CBFR.

Among other barriers, only transportation and health were significant barriers in the >1.6 to ≤3.2 km and >3.2 to 8.0 km radii, respectively. Approximately 10% of the sample population reported difficulties with transportation to CBFR. The term "transportation" is one of the most influential barriers to physical activity in older adults [27–29] and includes multiple contexts, spanning financial, health, distance, time, and built environment factors [30, 31]. Among factors related to transportation that require extended time and/or monetary investments and thus are less feasible to modify in the short term, are environmental aesthetics, safety, and walkability (sidewalks, traffic lights) [32]. Conversely, factors more easily modified are often specific to each individual. Given that both health and transportation were significant barriers in the current study, there is more evidence to suggest a poor level of health in the population that would inhibit transportation to CBFR and, therefore, result in low levels of utilization.

Based on current physical activity recommendations, the current sample population can be classified as, on average, sufficiently active with an average energy expenditure exceeding 1500 kcals/wk, assuming 100 kcals per 10 minutes of moderate intensity activity. Although this is higher compared to other reported activity levels in older adults, there were large variations in energy expenditure, from sedentary to extremely active. Only 132 participants (35.0%) reported actually engaging in over 1500 kcals/wk, providing evidence that bolsters the potential for CBFR to increase physical activity among those insufficiently active. In particular, such resources have been shown to be linked to increased participation in more intense, exercise-type behaviors [33], which is increasingly important, given the combination of low utilization rates of such resources and overall inactivity of the sample population (two-thirds not meeting recommended activity levels). Despite low utilization rates of CBFR, there was a marginal trend of increased utilization of exercise bikes, aerobic machines, and strength training equipment (in general) with increased distance from CBFR. Coupled with the observation that overall physical activity increased the further one resided from CBFR, this evidence reinforces the potential of CBFR to increase overall physical activity levels via exercise equipment should utilization rates increase.

This study is not without limitations. By design, the study was cross-sectional, so one is not able to glean causation between awareness and use of CBFR and overall physical activity levels. However, there is benefit to the random sampling of participants from surrounding neighborhoods, providing a large and diverse population to draw conclusions from. Another limitation is that physical activity data were obtained from subjective methodologies, specifically pertaining to the risk of participant bias based on expectant outcomes and recall error [34]. Considering such weaknesses, though, self-report questionnaires have been shown to accurately rank individuals across varying levels of physical activity [35].

5. Conclusions

Overall, closer proximity to CBFR did not impact awareness or utilization rates of such resources, while physical activity levels marginally increased the further one resided from CBFR. Future work in objectively assessing physical activity while utilizing CBFR is warranted to explore the utility of such resources to promote meaningful increases in energy expenditure in older adults, while investigating strategies to increase awareness and utilization of such resources.

Conflict of Interests

The authors declare that there is no conflict of interests regarding the publication of this paper.

Authors' Contribution

Christopher J. Dondzila and Scott J. Strath conceptualized the study. Christopher J. Dondzila collected the data, performed data analysis, and drafted the paper. Christopher J. Dondzila, Ann M. Swartz, Kevin G. Keenan, Amy E. Harley, Razia Azen, and Scott J. Strath all substantially edited and revised the draft prior to submission.

Acknowledgment

The authors acknowledge Kristi Farmer for efforts in assisting with participant recruitment. This study was partially funded by grants received from the University of Wisconsin-Milwaukee Research Growth Initiative and the College of Health Sciences Doctoral Student award.

References

[1] "United States Department of Health and Human Services: A profile of older Americans," 2011, http://www.aoa.gov/Aging_Statistics/Profile/2011/docs/2011profile.pdf.

[2] L. Ferrucci, F. Giallauria, and J. M. Guralnik, "Epidemiology of Aging," *Radiologic Clinics of North America*, vol. 46, no. 4, pp. 643–652, 2008.

[3] T. Lehnert, D. Heider, H. Leicht et al., "Review: health care utilization and costs of elderly persons with multiple chronic conditions," *Medical Care Research and Review*, vol. 68, no. 4, pp. 387–420, 2011.

[4] J. H. Thrall, "Prevalence and costs of chronic disease in a health care system structured for treatment of acute illness," *Radiology*, vol. 235, no. 1, pp. 9–12, 2005.

[5] M. E. Nelson, W. J. Rejeski, S. N. Blair et al., "Physical activity and public health in older adults: recommendation from the American College of Sports Medicine and the American Heart Association," *Circulation*, vol. 116, no. 9, pp. 1094–1105, 2007.

[6] J. M. Tucker, G. J. Welk, and N. K. Beyler, "Physical activity in U.S. adults: compliance with the physical activity guidelines for Americans," *The American Journal of Preventive Medicine*, vol. 40, no. 4, pp. 454–461, 2011.

[7] R. P. Troiano, D. Berrigan, K. W. Dodd, L. C. Mâsse, T. Tilert, and M. Mcdowell, "Physical activity in the United States measured by accelerometer," *Medicine and Science in Sports and Exercise*, vol. 40, no. 1, pp. 181–188, 2008.

[8] R. A. Winett, D. M. Williams, and B. M. Davy, "Initiating and maintaining resistance training in older adults: a social cognitive theory-based approach," *British Journal of Sports Medicine*, vol. 43, no. 2, pp. 114–119, 2009.

[9] B. H. Hansen, E. Kolle, S. M. Dyrstad, I. Holme, and S. A. Anderssen, "Accelerometer-determined physical activity in adults and older people," *Medicine and Science in Sports and Exercise*, vol. 44, no. 2, pp. 266–272, 2012.

[10] M. L. Booth, N. Owen, A. Bauman, O. Clavisi, and E. Leslie, "Social-cognitive and perceived environment influences associated with physical activity in older Australians," *Preventive Medicine*, vol. 31, no. 1, pp. 15–22, 2000.

[11] S. L. Huston, K. R. Evenson, P. Bors, and Z. Gizlice, "Neighborhood environment, access to places for activity, and leisure-time physical activity in a diverse North Carolina population," *The American Journal of Health Promotion*, vol. 18, no. 1, pp. 58–69, 2003.

[12] C. L. Addy, D. K. Wilson, K. A. Kirtland, B. E. Ainsworth, P. Sharpe, and D. Kimsey, "Associations of perceived social and physical environmental supports with physical activity and walking behavior," *The American Journal of Public Health*, vol. 94, no. 3, pp. 440–443, 2004.

[13] A. E. Mathews, S. B. Laditka, J. N. Laditka et al., "Older adults' perceived physical activity enablers and barriers: a multicultural perspective," *Journal of Aging and Physical Activity*, vol. 18, no. 2, pp. 119–140, 2010.

[14] A. L. Stewart, K. M. Mills, A. C. King, W. L. Haskell, D. Gillis, and P. L. Ritter, "CHAMPS physical activity questionnaire for older adults: outcomes for interventions," *Medicine and Science in Sports and Exercise*, vol. 33, no. 7, pp. 1126–1141, 2001.

[15] N. D. Harada, V. Chiu, A. C. King, and A. L. Stewart, "An evaluation of three self-report physical activity instruments for older adults," *Medicine and Science in Sports and Exercise*, vol. 33, no. 6, pp. 962–970, 2001.

[16] World Health Organization, "Obesity: preventing and managing the global epidemic," WHO Technical Report Series 894, World Health Organization, Geneva, Switzerland, 2000.

[17] J. I. Wallace, D. M. Buchner, L. Grothaus et al., "Implementation and effectiveness of a community-based health promotion program for older adults," *Journals of Gerontology Series A: Biological Sciences and Medical Sciences*, vol. 53, no. 4, pp. M301–M306, 1998.

[18] M. A. Cunningham, D. D. Carroll, S. A. Carolson, and J. E. Fulton, "Awareness and knowledge of the 2008 Physical Activity Guidelines for Americans," *Journal of Physical Activity & Health*, vol. 11, no. 4, pp. 693–698, 2014.

[19] J. M. Tucker, G. J. Welk, and N. K. Beyler, "Physical activity in U.S. adults: compliance with the physical activity guidelines for Americans," *American Journal of Preventive Medicine*, vol. 40, no. 4, pp. 454–461, 2011.

[20] U. Eriksson, D. Arvidsson, and K. Sundquist, "Availability of exercise facilities and physical activity in 2,037 adults: cross-sectional results from the Swedish neighborhood and physical activity (SNAP) study," *BMC Public Health*, vol. 12, article 607, 2012.

[21] J. F. Sallis, M. F. Hovell, C. R. Hofstetter et al., "Distance between homes and exercise facilities related to frequency of exercise among San Diego residents," *Public Health Reports*, vol. 105, no. 2, pp. 179–185, 1990.

[22] J. A. Carlson, J. F. Sallis, T. L. Conway et al., "Interactions between psychosocial and built environment factors in explaining older adults' physical activity," *Preventive Medicine*, vol. 54, no. 1, pp. 68–73, 2012.

[23] K. A. Schutzer and B. S. Graves, "Barriers and motivations to exercise in older adults," *Preventive Medicine*, vol. 39, no. 5, pp. 1056–1061, 2004.

[24] W.-C. Lee and M. G. Ory, "The engagement in physical activity for middle-aged and older adults with multiple chronic conditions: findings from a community health assessment," *Journal of Aging Research*, vol. 2013, Article ID 152868, 8 pages, 2013.

[25] E. Costello, M. Kafchinski, J. Vrazel, and P. Sullivan, "Motivators, barriers, and beliefs regarding physical activity in an older adult population," *Journal of Geriatric Physical Therapy*, vol. 34, no. 3, pp. 138–147, 2011.

[26] S. Wunderlich, C. McKinnon, J. Piemonte, and Z. N. Ahmad, "Measuring the impact of nutrition education and physical activity on older adults participating in government sponsored programs," *Journal of Nutrition for the Elderly*, vol. 28, no. 3, pp. 255–271, 2009.

[27] A. Patel, G. S. Kolt, J. W. L. Keogh, and G. M. Schofield, "The green prescription and older adults: what do general practitioners see as barriers?" *Journal of Primary Health Care*, vol. 4, no. 4, pp. 320–327, 2012.

[28] S. Wilcox, L. Oberrecht, M. Bopp, S. K. Kammermann, and C. T. McElmurray, "A qualitative study of exercise in older African American and white women in Rural South Carolina: perceptions, barriers, and motivations," *Journal of Women and Aging*, vol. 17, no. 1-2, pp. 37–53, 2005.

[29] S. Lachenmayr and G. Mackenzie, "Building a foundation for systems change: increasing access to physical activity programs for older adults.," *Health promotion practice*, vol. 5, no. 4, pp. 451–458, 2004.

[30] J. H. Rimmer, E. Wang, and D. Smith, "Barriers associated with exercise and community access for individuals with stroke," *Journal of Rehabilitation Research and Development*, vol. 45, no. 2, pp. 315–322, 2008.

[31] D. E. Rosenberg, D. L. Huang, S. D. Simonovich, and B. Belza, "Outdoor built environment barriers and facilitators to activity among midlife and older adults with mobility disabilities," *Gerontologist*, vol. 53, no. 2, pp. 268–279, 2013.

[32] J. A. Carlson, J. F. Sallis, T. L. Conway et al., "Interactions between psychosocial and built environment factors in explaining older adults'physical activity," *Preventive Medicine*, vol. 54, no. 1, pp. 68–73, 2012.

[33] M. L. Pollock, J. F. Carroll, J. E. Graves et al., "Injuries and adherence to walk/jog and resistance training programs in the elderly," *Medicine and Science in Sports and Exercise*, vol. 23, no. 10, pp. 1194–1200, 1991.

[34] S. A. Prince, K. B. Adamo, M. E. Hamel, J. Hardt, S. Connor Gorber, and M. Tremblay, "A comparison of direct versus self-report measures for assessing physical activity in adults: a systematic review," *International Journal of Behavioral Nutrition and Physical Activity*, vol. 5, article 56, 2008.

[35] S. J. Strath, L. A. Kaminsky, B. E. Ainsworth et al., "Guide to the assessment of physical activity: clinical and research applications: a scientific statement from the American Heart association," *Circulation*, vol. 128, no. 20, pp. 2259–2279, 2013.

15

Functional Fitness and Self-Reported Quality of Life of Older Women Diagnosed with Knee Osteoarthrosis

Paula Andréa Malveira Cavalcante,[1] Márcio Roberto Doro,[1] Frank Shiguemitsu Suzuki,[1,2] Roberta Luksevicius Rica,[1] Andrey Jorge Serra,[2,3] Francisco Luciano Pontes Junior,[4] Alexandre Lopes Evangelista,[1,2] Aylton José Figueira Junior,[1] Julien Steven Baker,[5] and Danilo Sales Bocalini[1]

[1] *Postgraduate Program in Physical Education and Aging Science of São Judas Tadeu University (USJT), São Paulo, SP, Brazil*
[2] *Department of Physical Education, Nove de Julho University (UNINOVE), São Paulo, SP, Brazil*
[3] *Postgraduate Program in Biophotonics Applied to Health Sciences, Nove de Julho University (UNINOVE), São Paulo, SP, Brazil*
[4] *Department of Gerontology of Arts, Science and Humanities School of University of São Paulo, São Paulo, SP, Brazil*
[5] *School of Science and Sport, University of the West of Scotland, Hamilton, Lanarkshire, UK*

Correspondence should be addressed to Danilo Sales Bocalini; bocaliniht@hotmail.com

Academic Editor: David William Molloy

Aim. Utilizing a cross-sectional case control design, the aim of this study was to evaluate the functional fitness and self-reported quality of life differences in older people diagnosed with knee osteoarthrosis (O) who participated in health promotion groups. *Methods.* Ninety older women were distributed into two groups: control without O of the knee (C, $n = 40$) and a group diagnosed with primary and secondary knee O with grade II or higher, with definite osteophytes (OA, $n = 50$). Functional fitness was evaluated by specific tests, and the time spent in physical activity and quality of life was evaluated by the IPAQ and WHOQOL (distributed in four domains: physical: P, psychological: PS, social: S, and environmental: E) domain questionnaires. *Results.* No differences were found between ages of groups (C: 66 ± 7; OA: 67 ± 9; years). The values of the chair stand test (rep) in the OA (13 ± 5) group were different when compared to C group (22 ± 5). For the 6-minute walk test (meters), the values obtained for the C (635 ± 142) were higher ($P < 0.01$) than the OA (297 ± 143) group. The time spent in physical activity (min) was greater ($P < 0.001$) in the control (220 ± 12) group compared to OA (100 ± 10) group. Higher values ($P < 0.001$) in all domains were found in the C (P: 69 ± 16, PS: 72 ± 17, S: 67 ± 15, E: 70 ± 15) group compared to OA (P: 48 ± 7, PS: 43 ± 8, S: 53 ± 13, E: 47 ± 14) group. *Conclusion.* Our data suggests that knee O, in older women, can promote a decline in time spent performing physical activity and functional fitness with decline in quality of life with an increase in sitting time.

1. Introduction

Osteoarthritis (OA) is a chronic, multifactorial disease that leads to progressive functional disability [1] and has been considered one of the most frequent causes of incapacity for work in Brazil [1, 2] and worldwide [3]. Among the joints, knee, hip, hand, foot, and spine [3] are the most common areas for the development of osteoarthritis; however, the knee joint has been the most studied [4].

In histological studies, OA is characterized by focal areas of loss of cartilage in synovial joints by joining capsule thickening and bone hypertrophy with consequent formation of osteophytes and bone sclerosis [3, 5]. Joint pain, tenderness, limitation of movement, crepitus, occasional effusion, and variable degrees of local inflammation are usual signs in the clinical condition of impairment [3, 4]. Around the risk factors, age, female gender, previous joint injury, genetics, and muscle weakness [5] are important factors to pathogenesis;

however, many individuals are affected by lifestyle factors such as obesity and lack of physical activity [3, 5].

In the USA it is estimated that 25% of people aged over 65 years suffer from pain and other disabilities associated with OA [6]. In Brazil, there are no precise data on prevalence; however, Coimbra et al. [1] report that it is the most common rheumatic disease found in women in Brazil among individuals over 65 years [6]. As a result, OA will be an important public health problem in future years in Brazil due to the increase in age of the population [7].

The conservative treatment of knee OA requires analgesic therapy for long periods [8]; however, the pharmacological treatment should always be multifactorial [1]. Physical exercise had been used in conjunction with pharmacological treatments. No pharmacologic strategy alone has been identified as an effective method of therapeutic intervention demonstrating pain relief and increased mobility related to patients with knee OA [1, 4, 5, 9, 10]. Additionally, local physical therapy, rehabilitation, and reduction of mechanical stress on joints may provide improvements in pain symptoms and maintain joint function, which mainly reflects the improvement in the quality of life of people affected by the disease [4].

In older patients, functional fitness is impaired by pain, joint stiffness, and muscle atrophy and bone crepitus [4, 5]. In this context, functional fitness evaluation had been highlighted as a relevant strategy utilized for older people [11] and is an indicative measure that individuals have to decide about their functional capacity and that relates to their day to day living and capacity to perform [6, 12, 13]. Another important disclosure has been to address the quality of life [14]. Additionally, studies [6, 13] have shown significant reductions in self-reported quality of life, including pain increase and physical and psychological stress [13]. Considering these points and to address some of the gaps observed in both the literature and experimental studies, the aim of this study was to evaluate the functional fitness and self-reported quality of life differences in older people. Two groups were evaluated, subjects diagnosed with knee osteoarthrosis and a control group without osteoarthrosis of the knee.

2. Material and Methods

After approval by the Research Ethics Committee of Nove de Julho University (466/2012), ninety older women (over 60 years) participants of health promotion groups (method of collective and interdisciplinary health intervention, consisting of a group process) were recruited from the Regional Community Adult Day Care facilities by Nove de Julho University and distributed into two groups: without osteoarthrosis of knee (control, *n*: 40) and with primary and secondary knee osteoarthrosis (OA, *n*: 50). All participants had medical examinations and completed questionnaires regarding medical history. All protocols used in the study were performed in accordance with the ethical standards of the Helsinki Declaration.

The following exclusion criteria were assigned: chronic knee pain, knee surgery, current or previous participation in regular exercise programs in the past six months, recent hospitalization, cardiorespiratory disease, severe hypertension, metabolic syndrome and liver or kidney disease, cognitive impairment or progressive conditions with debilitating inability to exercise, recent bone fractures, any knee surgery earlier, and any other medical contraindications for training.

Table 1: The radiographic parameters for knee OA diagnosis.

Grade	Criteria
0	Normal
1	Doubtful joint space narrowing, possibly developing osteophytes
2	Definite osteophytes, narrowing missing or questionable joint space
3	Osteophytes moderate, definite narrowing some sclerosis possible joint deformity
4	Large osteophytes marked narrowing sclerosis severe joint deformity established

The OA diagnosis was based on clinical and radiographic parameters, in line with the American College of Rheumatology [15] and individual medical history. The radiographic parameters for knee OA diagnosis were established according to the classification of Kellgren and Lawrence [16], with involvement of the knee on or above grade II, conform described on Table 1.

2.1. Physical Activity Level. Utilizing the interview strategy, the short form International Physical Activity Questionnaire (IPAQ) was used to estimate physical activity levels. The questions were asked of all subjects on the week preceding the physical activity measures. The questions asked explored the frequency and duration of physical activity including walking, moderate and vigorous physical exercise, and sitting time. Individuals were considered active if they participated in physical activity for more than 150 minutes per week and inactive if their participation levels were less than 150 minutes per week.

2.2. Anthropometric Parameters. The anthropometric measures used in this study were similar to those previously reported by our group [14, 17]. Stature was measured to the nearest 0.1 cm using a Cardiomed WCS stadiometer (Curitiba, Brazil). Body mass was measured to the nearest 0.1 kg using a Filizola Personal Line 150 scale (São Paulo, Brazil). Body mass index (BMI) was calculated as follows: BMI = weight/height^2.

2.3. Functional Fitness. Functional fitness evaluation comprised six tests previously reported in the literature to assess physical performance parameters concerning mobility and balance in older adults [12, 14, 17, 18]. The following tests were utilized.

2.3.1. Arm Curl Test. It was used to evaluate upper limb fitness, with the analyzed score as the total number of hand weight curls through the full range of motion.

TABLE 2: Anthropometric parameters.

Parameters	Control	OA	95% of IC	Significance
Age (years)	66 ± 7	67 ± 9	−1.932–4.922	$P > 0.05$
Body mass (kg)	66 ± 7	67 ± 9	−0.631–7.672	$P > 0.05$
Height (cm)	167 ± 0.12	164 ± 0.13	−0.090–0.011	$P > 0.05$
BMI (kg/m^2)	30 ± 5	33 ± 5	0.690–4.920	$P < 0.01$

Values expressed in mean ± SEM of control and osteoarthrosis (OA) groups. BMI: body mass index.

2.3.2. Chair Stand Test. It was used to evaluate lower limb strength, scored by the number of full stand-ups executed correctly within 30 seconds.

2.3.3. Agility. It was evaluated by the 8-foot up-and-go test (TUG), and the score recorded was considered the shortest time to rise from a seated position, walk eight feet, turn back, and return to the seated position.

2.3.4. Sit and Reach Test. It was used to evaluate the lower body flexibility scored by the shortest distance achieved between the extended fingers and the toe when seated with extended leg and heel resting on the floor.

2.3.5. Static Balance. It was assessed by having subjects stand on one leg for a maximum of 30 seconds on each side. The score was measured, allowing only minimal fluctuations of ankle position or obvious toe clawing, without hopping or upper limb movement. The test was stopped after 30 seconds if hopping occurred, the ankle movement was excessive, or the hanged foot touched the floor or contacted the stance leg/foot.

2.3.6. Functional Exercise Capacity. It was measured by 6-minute walk test [6].

2.4. Quality of Life. Quality of life was evaluated by a shortened WHO quality of life questionnaire as outlined previously [14, 17, 19]. The questionnaire comprised 25 questions about several aspects of quality of life, including the following.

2.4.1. Physical Domain. It concerns pain or discomfort, energy or fatigue, sleep, rest, mobility, daily activities, medicine dependency, and job performance.

2.4.2. Psychological Domain. It includes feelings, learning, memory and attention, self-esteem, aspect, spirituality, religiousness, and positive or negative thinking.

2.4.3. Social Domain. It deals with personal relationships, social support, and sexuality.

2.4.4. Environmental Domain. It includes physical security, home environment, financial security, opportunity for information assessment, social or cultural event participation, and activities undertaken during spare time. Each domain was scored from 0 to 100 points, and higher scores represented improvement.

2.5. Statistical Analyses. All statistical analyses were performed using SPSS software (v 12.0; IBM, Armonk, NY, USA). The D'Agostino-Pearson test was applied to Gaussian distribution analysis. Analysis of comparisons between groups over time was performed by Student's t-test or Mann-Whitney test. Statistical significance was established at $P < 0.05$. Data are expressed as mean ± SEM.

3. Results

During functional fitness evaluation phase program, 10 women of OA group dropped out of study due to knee pain during execution of the test. Therefore, fifty women were included on OG group.

The anthropometric parameters are presented in Table 2. The body mass and stature did not differ between groups. However, the BMI of OA group was higher than control group.

Significant differences ($P < 0.01$) were found between time spent in physical activity (control: 220 ± 12 versus OA: 100 ± 10; minutes) and sitting time (control: 1673 ± 532 versus OA: 2675 ± 680; minutes) between groups.

Functional fitness scores are outlined in Figure 1. Statistical differences ($P < 0.01$) were found between groups between the chair stand test (control: 22 ± 5 versus OA: 13 ± 5 rep.), arm curl test (control: 22 ± 6 versus OA: 18 ± 4), sit and reach test (control: 23 ± 4 versus OA: 12 ± 5; cm), TUG (control: 18 ± 6 versus OA: 29 ± 4; sec), 6-minute walk test (control: 635 ± 142 versus OA: 297 ± 143, m), and balance (control: 18 ± 4 versus OA: 11 ± 3; sec).

In all quality of life domains the control (physical: 69 ± 16, psychological: 72 ± 17, environmental: 67 ± 15, and social: 70 ± 15) was higher ($P < 0.001$) than OA (physical: 48 ± 7, psychological: 43 ± 8, environmental: 53 ± 13, and social: 47 ± 14) as shown in Figure 2.

4. Discussion

The main objectives of this study were to identify differences in time spent in physical activity, functional fitness, and quality of life with increase in sitting time in older people diagnosed with knee OA. Previous studies [3, 6] suggested that obesity may be considered a risk factor for the development of OA. Falsarella et al. [6] demonstrated that individuals with a high BMI (above 25 kg/m^2) had an association with

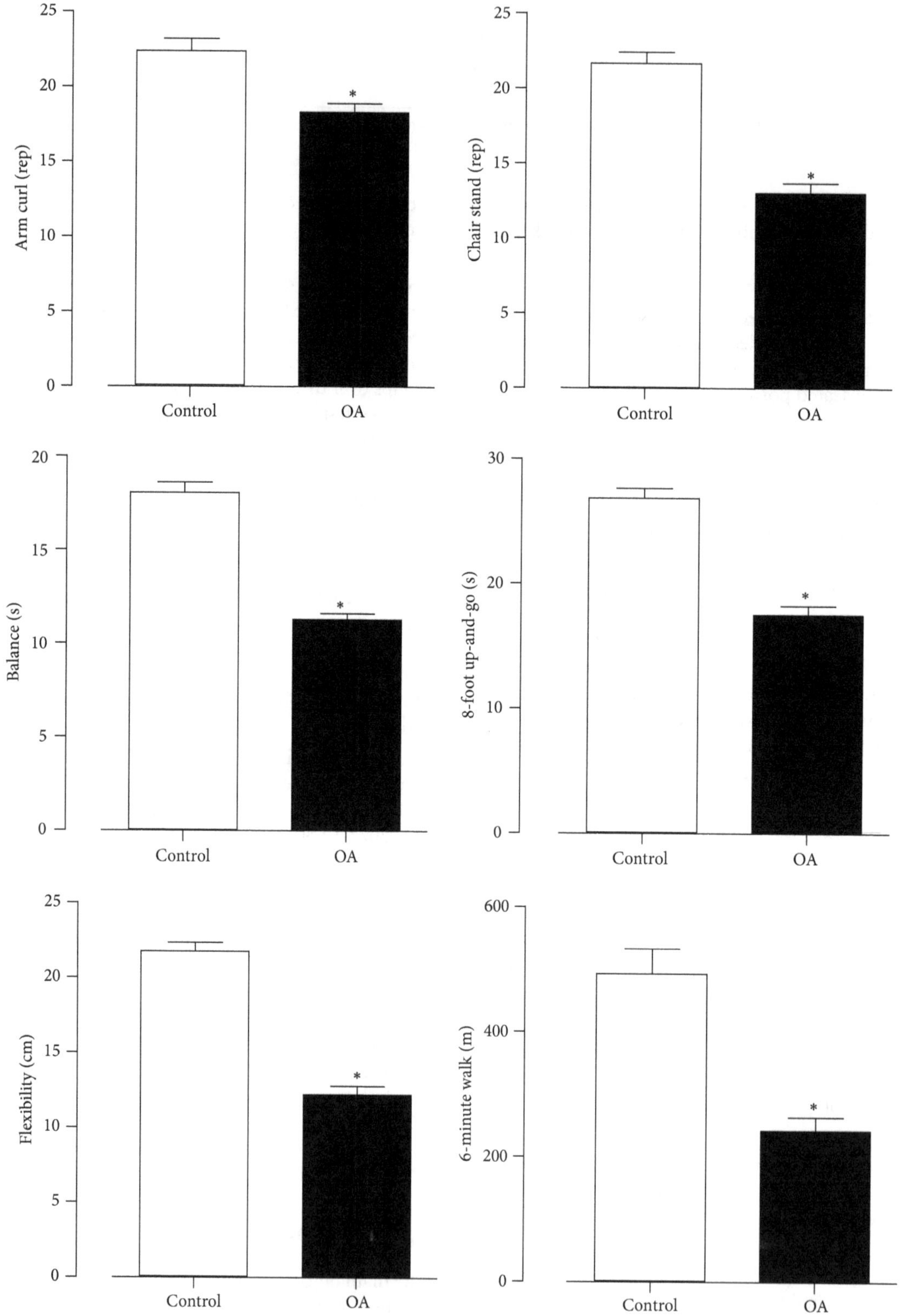

FIGURE 1: Values expressed in ± SEM of functional fitness test of control and osteoarthrosis (OA) groups. $^{*}P < 0.05$.

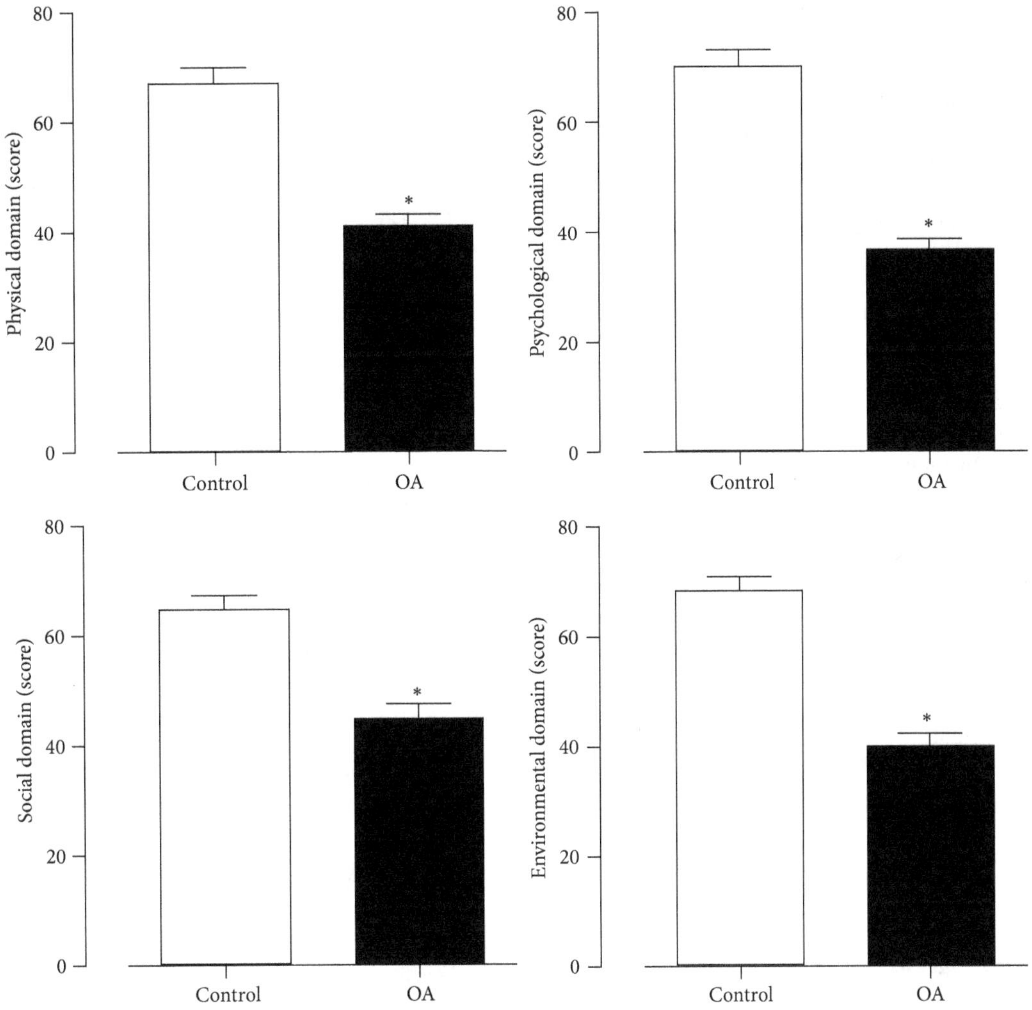

FIGURE 2: Values expressed in ± SEM of quality of life of control and osteoarthrosis (OA) groups. $^*P < 0.05$.

joint symptoms; however, Niu et al. [20] demonstrated that obesity is not related to the progression of knee OA.

The decrease in muscle strength is associated with reduced joint flexibility and impairment of functionality, limiting the realization of occupational activity and compromising the welfare on aging [21]. The strength deficits in OA people, evaluated by electrical stimulation of quadriceps muscle by maximal strength voluntary contraction, varied between 15% and 18% on early disease, 24% in level II, according to Kellgren and Lawrence [16], and 38% in level IV [22]. In our study, we found a deficit of muscular strength of 40% in the lower limb when compared to control group. Additionally, our lower limb values (22 ± 5 repetitions) correspond to the findings of previous studies [17, 23].

However, cause-effect relationships between muscle weakness and OA are complex and have been widely debated [10]. Although the muscular strength probably decreases in people with OA as a secondary result of reduced activity, there is evidence that muscle weakness directly contributes to development and progression of OA [24]. Therefore, it may be possible that muscular weakness of the quadriceps could be responsible for functional impairment, predisposing structural damage to the knee, since this muscle acts as a shock absorber in this joint [25].

Ueno et al. [26] reported that changes in older people's flexibility may compromise functional fitness, reducing some activities of daily living. In this study the greater decline in flexibility in OA group was observed. Additionally, Oliveira et al. [2] suggested that improvement in muscular stretching may reduce stiffness and joint pain and improve physical function in osteoarthritis subjects.

The TUG is the most favorable test developed to assess parameters of physical mobility, translated agility, speed, and dynamic balance [18]. Evidence [11] indicates that the knee receptors have an important role in the control of posture, balance, and locomotion capacity. The changes in these receptors may be responsible for the dysfunction on gait pattern in aging, which may be related to muscle reflexes protectors [27]. Although no neural measurements had been done, we considered that alterations may be associated with performance testing changes in OA group.

In relation to aerobic capacity, Jackson et al. [28] showed a reduction by 1% per year and about 50% of this decline is related to inactive lifestyle and a poor body composition. In OA patients, weight loss can lead to significant improvements in reduction of disability and knee burden [5]. Additionally, aerobic exercises can improve VO_2 peak in this population [5]; however, in the OA group, the time spent in physical activity was lower and sitting time was higher than WHO recommendations. This probably contributed to the poor aerobic fitness levels observed. Similar to our study, Tamegushi et al. [13] demonstrated significant impairment on 6MWT outcome in OA knee patients.

Studies [5, 6, 29] have demonstrated that functional fitness reductions affect significantly self-reported quality of life in the OA older patients. Falsarella et al. [6] indicated that a reduction in joint pain is the most important fact related to this statement; conversely, Alves and Bassitt [29] observed that OA patients have a good quality of life, regardless of functional fitness impairment.

This is a relatively small sample and case control study, with no information about long-term outcomes. Nevertheless, for future public health strategies, this work reinforces the message of the importance of the frequency and regularity of clinical investigation. In addition, there may be some small inaccuracies in estimating maximum aerobic fitness (indirect test). Nevertheless this drawback was common to both the control and OA groups and for all evaluations, thus reducing inaccuracy.

5. Conclusion

The present study suggests that knee osteoarthrosis in older women can promote a decline in time spent performing physical activity, functional fitness, and quality of life with consequent increase in sitting time. Thus, despite inherent limitations, our data reinforce the safety and utility of clinical approach strategies that should be considered to address issues observed in this population.

Conflict of Interests

The authors declare that there is no conflict of interests regarding the publication of this paper.

Acknowledgments

The authors thank CAPES (Coordenação de Aperfeiçoamento de Pessoal de Nível Superior) fellowships addressed to P. A. M. Cavalcante, F. S. Suzuki, and R. L. Rica. The fund providers had no role in decision to publish and preparation of the paper.

References

[1] I. B. Coimbra, E. H. Pastor, J. M. D. A. Greve et al., "Osteoartrite (Artrose): tratamento," *Revista Brasileira de Reumatologia*, vol. 44, no. 6, pp. 450–453, 2004.

[2] A. M. I. Oliveira, M. S. Peccin, K. N. G. da Silva, L. E. P. de Paiva Teixeira, and V. F. M. Trevisani, "Impact of exercise on the functional capacity and pain of patients with knee osteoarthritis: a randomized clinical trial," *Revista Brasileira de Reumatologia*, vol. 52, no. 6, pp. 876–882, 2012.

[3] A. D. Woolf and B. Pfleger, "Burden of major musculoskeletal conditions," *Bulletin of the World Health Organization*, vol. 81, no. 9, pp. 646–656, 2003.

[4] V. S. Duarte, M. L. dos Santos, K. A. Rodrigues, J. B. Ramires, G. P. T. Arêas, and G. F. Borges, "Exercise and osteoarthrosis: a systematic review," *Fisioterapia em Movimento*, vol. 26, no. 1, 2013.

[5] K. L. Bennell and R. S. Hinman, "A review of the clinical evidence for exercise in osteoarthritis of the hip and knee," *Journal of Science and Medicine in Sport*, vol. 14, no. 1, pp. 4–9, 2011.

[6] G. R. Falsarella, I. B. Coimbra, C. C. Barcelos, L. T. L. Costallat, O. M. F. Carvalho, and A. M. V. Coimbra, "Prevalence and factors associated with rheumatic diseases and chronic joint symptoms in the elderly," *Geriatrics and Gerontology International*, vol. 13, no. 4, pp. 1043–1050, 2013.

[7] World HealthOrganization (WHO), *Envelhecimento ativo: uma política de saúde*, Organização Pan-Americana da Saúde, Brasília, Brazil, 2005.

[8] Sociedade Brasileira de Reumatologia e Sociedade Brasileira de Medicina de Família e Comunidade, "Uso dos antiinflamatórios não hormonais na dor crônica em pacientes com Osteoartrite (osteoartrose)," Diretrizes Clínicas na Saúde Suplementar, 2011.

[9] J. Iwamoto, Y. Sato, T. Takeda, and H. Matsumoto, "Effectiveness of exercise for osteoarthritis of the knee: a review of the literature," *World Journal of Orthopaedics*, vol. 2, no. 5, pp. 37–42, 2011.

[10] N. Latham and C.-J. Liu, "Strength training in older adults: the benefits for osteoarthritis," *Clinics in Geriatric Medicine*, vol. 26, no. 3, pp. 445–459, 2010.

[11] M. J. Daley and W. L. Spinks, "Exercise, mobility and aging," *Sports Medicine*, vol. 29, no. 1, pp. 1–12, 2000.

[12] S. M. Matsudo, *Avaliação do Idoso: Física e Funcional*, Midiograf, Londrina, Brazil, 2000.

[13] A. S. Tamegushi, C. S. Trelha, M. S. G. Dellaroza, M. Cabrera, and T. N. Ribeiro, "Functional capacity of elderly with osteoarthritis of knees and hip," *Revista Espaço para a Saúde*, vol. 9, no. 2, pp. 8–16, 2008.

[14] D. S. Bocalini, L. Dos Santos, and A. J. Serra, "Physical exercise improves the functional capacity and quality of life in patients with heart failure," *Clinics*, vol. 63, no. 4, pp. 437–442, 2008.

[15] R. Altman, E. Asch, and D. Bloch, "Development of criteria for the classification and reporting of osteoarthritis. Classification of osteoarthritis of the knee," *Arthritis and Rheumatism*, vol. 29, no. 8, pp. 1039–1049, 1986.

[16] J. H. Kellgren and J. S. Lawrence, "Radiological assessment of osteo-arthrosis," *Annals of the Rheumatic Diseases*, vol. 16, no. 4, pp. 494–501, 1957.

[17] R. L. Rica, R. M. M. Carneiro, A. J. Serra, D. Rodriguez, F. L. Pontes Junior, and D. S. Bocalini, "Effects of water-based exercise in obese older women: impact of short-term follow-up study on anthropometric, functional fitness and quality of life parameters," *Geriatrics and Gerontology International*, vol. 13, no. 1, pp. 209–214, 2013.

[18] R. E. Rikli and C. J. Jones, "Development and validation of a functional fitness test for community-residing older adults,"

Journal of Aging and Physical Activity, vol. 7, no. 2, pp. 129–161, 1999.

[19] M. P. A. Fleck, S. Louzada, M. Xavier et al., "Aplicação da versão em português do instrumento abreviado de avaliação da qualidade de vida 'WHOQOL-bref'," *Revista de Saúde Pública*, vol. 34, no. 2, pp. 178–183, 2000.

[20] J. Niu, Y. Q. Zhang, J. Torner et al., "Is obesity a risk factor for progressive radiographic knee osteoarthritis?" *Arthritis Care and Research*, vol. 61, no. 3, pp. 329–335, 2009.

[21] W. J. Chodzko-Zajko, D. N. Proctor, M. A. Fiatarone Singh et al., "Exercise and physical activity for older adults," *Medicine and Science in Sports and Exercise*, vol. 41, no. 7, pp. 1510–1530, 2009.

[22] S. C. Petterson, P. Barrance, T. Buchanan, S. Binder-Macleod, and L. Snyder-Mackler, "Mechanisms underlying quadriceps weakness in knee osteoarthritis," *Medicine and Science in Sports and Exercise*, vol. 40, no. 3, pp. 422–427, 2008.

[23] D. S. Bocalini, A. J. Serra, N. Murad, and R. F. Levy, "Water- versus land- based exercise effects on physical fitness in older women," *Geriatrics and Gerontology International*, vol. 8, no. 4, pp. 265–271, 2008.

[24] C. Slemenda, K. D. Brandt, D. K. Heilman et al., "Quadriceps weakness and osteoarthritis of the knee," *Annals of Internal Medicine*, vol. 127, no. 2, pp. 97–104, 1997.

[25] G. K. Fitzgerald, S. R. Piva, J. J. Irrgang, F. Bouzubar, and T. W. Starz, "Quadriceps activation failure as a moderator of the relationship between quadriceps strength and physical function in individuals with knee osteoarthritis," *Arthritis Care and Research*, vol. 51, no. 1, pp. 40–48, 2004.

[26] L. M. Ueno, S. S. Okuma, M. L. Miranda, and W. J. Filho, "Análise dos Efeitos Quantitativos e Qualitativos de um Programa de Educação Física sobre a Flexibilidade do Quadril em Indivíduos Com Mais de 60 Anos," *Motriz*, vol. 6, no. 1, pp. 9–16, 2000.

[27] K. D. Brandt, E. L. Radin, P. A. Dieppe, and L. van de Putte, "Yet more evidence that osteoarthritis is not a cartilage disease," *Annals of the Rheumatic Diseases*, vol. 65, no. 10, pp. 1261–1264, 2006.

[28] A. S. Jackson, L. T. Wier, G. W. Ayers, E. F. Beard, J. E. Stuteville, and S. N. Blair, "Changes in aerobic power of women, ages 20–64 yr," *Medicine and Science in Sports and Exercise*, vol. 28, no. 7, pp. 884–891, 1996.

[29] J. C. Alves and D. P. Bassitt, "Qualidade de vida e capacidade funcional de idosas com osteoartrite de joelho," *Einstein*, vol. 11, no. 2, pp. 209–215, 2013.

16

Flexibility Training and Functional Ability in Older Adults

Liza Stathokostas,[1] Robert M. D. Little,[1] A. A. Vandervoort,[2] and Donald H. Paterson[1]

[1] *Canadian Centre for Activity and Aging, School of Kinesiology, The University of Western Ontario, London, 3M Centre 2225, ON, Canada N6A 3K7*
[2] *School of Physical Therapy, Elborn College 1400, The University of Western Ontario, London, ON, Canada N6A 3K7*

Correspondence should be addressed to Liza Stathokostas, lstatho2@uwo.ca

Academic Editor: Wojtek Chodzko-Zajko

Background. As indicated in a recent systematic review relating to Canada's Physical Activity Guidelines for Older Adults, exercise interventions in older adults can maintain or improve functional abilities. Less is known about the role of flexibility in the maintenance or improvement of functional abilities, and there currently does not exist a synthesis of the literature supporting a consensus on flexibility training prescription. *Purpose.* To systematically review the effects of flexibility-specific training interventions on measures of functional outcomes in healthy older adults over the age of 65 years. *Methods.* Five electronic databases were searched for intervention studies involving concepts related to aging, flexibility, functional outcomes, and training interventions. After evaluating the articles for relevance, 22 studies were considered. *Results.* The results suggested that while flexibility-specific interventions may have effects on range of motion (ROM) outcomes, there is conflicting information regarding both the relationship between flexibility interventions and functional outcomes or daily functioning. *Conclusions.* Due to the wide range of intervention protocols, body parts studied, and functional measurements, conclusive recommendations regarding flexibility training for older adults or the validity of flexibility training interventions as supplements to other forms of exercise, or as significant positive influences on functional ability, require further investigation.

1. Introduction

As indicated in a recent systematic review relating to Canada's Physical Activity Guidelines for Older Adults, exercise interventions (comprised of aerobic and strength training) in older adults can maintain or improve functional abilities [1]. Less is known about the role of flexibility in the maintenance or improvement of functional abilities. While joint flexibility may decrease with age, with the potential to affect normal daily function, older adults do maintain the ability to improve flexibility through stretching exercises [1]. The 2009 American College of Sports Medicine (ACSM) position statement "Exercise and Physical Activity for Older Adults" [2] noted there is a lack of studies of the effects of range of motion exercises on flexibility outcomes in older populations and a lack of consensus regarding the prescription of stretching exercises for older adults. Despite the lack of a synthesis of the literature to support the recommendation of the inclusion of a flexibility component to older adult exercise programs, many older adult activity programs place a considerable emphasis on flexibility. Stretching exercises are used extensively in the rehabilitation context wherein injury or disease may have resulted in a restricted range of motion specific to given joints, and the goal is to regain "normal" range of motion [3]. However, the present paper is focused not on stretching exercise for rehabilitation purposes but for the role of flexibility in general exercise prescription for older adults.

In light of the significant benefits of an exercise program for an aging population, it is important to provide evidence-based prescription for older adult exercise programs and highlight areas of research requiring further investigation in order to maximize these benefits. The goal of a flexibility program is to improve range of motion in the major muscle-tendon groups in accordance with individualized goals [4]. For the majority of the aging population, the goals may not be related to athletic performance, but rather performance of functional abilities in activities of daily living. Nevertheless, there is relatively little research on the potential benefits of flexibility-specific training interventions for this population in that context. Despite the lack of research and no "known health benefits" [5], again, there is still a tendency in the literature to mention flexibility training as a presumed "component of fitness" and beneficial adjunct to other forms of exercise. Therefore, the purpose of this systematic review is to investigate the functional outcomes of flexibility specific training in older adults.

2. Methods

2.1. The Literature Search and Inclusion Criteria. A search strategy was developed, where all reasonable expressions of the concepts of aging, flexibility, functional outcomes, and training interventions were considered (see Appendix for a sample search strategy). A comprehensive electronic literature search was conducted on five online databases: PubMed (NCBI; 1950-), Embase (OVID; 1974-), CINAHL (OVID & EBSCO; 1982-), Scopus (1823-), and SportDiscus (EBSCO; 1800-). The literature was searched up to January 2011. The final inclusion criteria for this paper were (1) an original research article, (2) human subjects, (3) an intervention study, (4) flexibility training was an independent intervention or was used as a control, (5) aged population (mean age ≥ 65 years), and (6) the population was healthy but allowing for arthritis, osteoarthritis, and those residing in assisted living (based on age and risk, not diseases or other medical conditions). For this paper, healthy was operationally defined as community-dwelling and assisted living with the health and function and cognitive ability to participate in light physical activity interventions and complete physical function measures. Interventions targeting specific chronic conditions (aside from arthritis and osteoarthritis) were excluded from review. Despite their use in flexibility training, tai chi- and yoga-based studies were excluded from this paper because by nature they include strength components. The electronic search yielded 4037 citations. The citations and applicable electronic versions of the article (where available) were downloaded to an online research management system (RefWorks, Bethesda, MD, USA).

2.2. Screening. Two reviewers independently (RL, LS) evaluated the articles for relevance using standard systematic review methodology leading to further consideration of 22 articles.

Two reviewers independently completed standardized data extraction forms for each level of screening. Three levels of screening were utilized. Level 1 screening was based on article titles, Level 2 was based on the title and abstract, and Level 3 was a full text screening. The articles that progressed through to Level 3 were retrieved electronically or manually via the Canadian interlibrary system and were printed from electronic copy. Any cross-referenced articles from the reference section of Level 3 articles were hand-screened. Disagreements regarding inclusion were resolved through discussion with a third reviewer (DP).

2.3. Data Extraction. Data from the included studies were extracted (Table 1) and organized by the target muscle groups of the flexibility interventions. Two reviewers completed standardized data extraction forms. One reviewer performed the data extraction for each paper assigned to them and the extraction was verified by another reviewer. The reviewers were not blinded to the journal or the author names when extracting information from the articles.

2.4. Level of Evidence. The approach used to establish the level and grade of evidence was consistent with Lau et al. [6] which provide predefined and objective criteria. Thus, the strength of the evidence was assessed for flexibility interventions and functional outcomes in older adults with respect to general recommendations and appropriate dose.

2.5. Quality Assessment. Quality assessment of the included studies was also performed (Table 1). The Downs and Black [7] scale was selected to assess the quality of each study as it is appropriate to evaluate nonrandomized investigations, and it contained the highest number of relevant items for the needs of this paper. However, as not all items were relevant to the various study types included in this paper, a modified version of the checklist was employed for each of RCTs (randomized control trials), and non-RCTs study types. Thus, the quality of each study was also established similar to the method of Gorber et al. [8] to include the most relevant components of the scoring tool. Therefore, a modified version of the Downs and Black checklist was used with the final checklist consisting of 22 items with a maximum score of 24 points for the studies of a RCT design; 22 items for non-RCT designs with a maximum score of 23; experimental single group interventions had a maximum score of 18 from 18 items; experimental single-group and single-session studies were based on 14 items for a maximum score of 14. Higher scores reflected a superior quality of investigation.

2.6. Integration of Findings. Due to the heterogeneity across study populations, methods used, and outcomes assessed, we conducted a narrative synthesis of the results.

3. Results

3.1. Description of Studies. The initial search yielded 4037 articles. Twenty-two articles were ultimately included after meeting Level 3 inclusion criteria (Figure 1). Of the final 22 articles, 18 were from electronic database searching, and 4 were found by hand searching. Quality assessment indicated that the RCT studies ($n = 13$) were of good quality with an average score of 18 out of 24. The non-RCT studies ($n = 6$) had an average score of 14 out 23. An average score of 12 out of 18 was assessed for the experimental single-group studies ($n = 3$). Fourteen articles were conducted in the United States [10–12, 14, 15, 17, 18, 20, 22, 25–29], while the remainder of the studies were from Japan [19], Brazil

TABLE 1: Table-Flexibility training studies examining the relationship between flexibility and functional abilities in older adults.

Publication country/study type	Objective	Population	Methods	Outcomes	Comments and conclusions	Quality
Barrett and Smerdely, 2002 [9]. Australia. RCT (single-blinded, assessor). **Focus** Major muscle groups.	To determine whether a resistance training program could improve strength, mobility, and quality of life of community-dwelling elderly people versus flexibility control group.	$n = 40$. Age: 67 yr. 10 males, 30 females. Experimental $n = 20$. Age: 64 ± 3 yr. 5 male, 15 female. Control $n = 20$ Age: 70 ± 3 yr. 5 male, 15 female. **Inclusion criteria** >60 yr, healthy.	Prepost 10 wks. Both groups attended class 1 hr, twice wk^{-1}, 10 wks. **Intervention** 5 min warm-up including stretching, 8–10 resistance exercises (~45 min) with free weights for both upper and lower limbs, followed by 5 min of stretching. **Control** Stretching of major muscle groups (25 min) light cardiovascular (20 min) and low intensity strengthening (15 min). **Assessment** Isometric strength bilaterally with hand dynamometer: biceps, quads; time to stand and sit 5 times for leg strength. Balance: Functional reach test and step test. Quality of Life: SF36 Health. Survey self-reported. **Analysis** Independent sample t-tests. Gender: Chi-square tests. Bonferroni adjustment.	Progressive resistance training group improved significantly in all physical measurements. Flexibility group improved significantly in sit-to-stand (9.6% from 10.2 to 9.2 s) and step test (23.5% from 17 to 20 steps) only. Progressive resistance training had a greater effect than flexibility training on quadriceps strength, left biceps strength, functional reach test and step test. Neither group improved significantly in any subscale of quality of life.	Progressive high intensity resistance training produces greater strength, balance, and gait improvements than a nonspecific flexibility group.	13/18

TABLE 1: Continued.

Publication country/study type	Objective	Population	Methods	Outcomes	Comments and conclusions	Quality
Klein et al. 2002 [10]. USA. Prospective two-stage intervention. **Focus** Major muscle groups.	To examine the impact of PNF on physical function in an assisted-living population by assessing ROM and isometric strength.	$n = 14$. Age: 87 ± 6.5 yr. Male = 2. Female = 12. **Inclusion criteria** ≥65 yr, no neurological or cognitive impairments, resting BP < 160/100 mmHg, no limiting cardiorespiratory condition or recent surgery Living in assisted-living facility, frail.	Baseline (T1), pretraining (T2, 5 wks), posttraining (T3, 10 wks). **Pre-training** 1 wk^{-1} visit with trainer to increase rapport and interest in participation. **Training program** 40–60 min, 2 wk^{-1}Warm-up, cool down, and flexibility (single set 15–20 min, later 2-3 sets) Flexibility: 8 exercises using passive contract-relax PNF technique (6 s isometric contraction then passive stretch held for 20 s then 20 s rest). Hamstrings, gluteals, shins, calves and back). **Assessments** Isometric strength (dynamometer), flexibility (bubble inclinometer for shoulders, hips, and ankles, sit-and-reach for spine, functional-reach for shoulder). Mobility: get-up-and-go test, 5-sit-to-stand. **Analysis** Listwise repeated measures, univariate ANOVA, paired t-tests, and Bonferroni adjustment	$n = 11$ Statistically significant differences in 6 of 18 variables: sit-to-stand decreased significantly from 9.33 to 7.91 s ($P = 0.42$). No change in balance, get up and go, single leg stand. Ankle-flexion ROM decreased (improved) from 26.25 to 20.27° ($P = 0.009$). Shoulder-flexion ROM increased from 163.8 to 177.6° ($P = 0.016$) No change in hip flexion, hip extension, ankle extension, functional reach, and sit-and-reach. Significant increases in strength for hip extension and ankle flexion/extension. No change in hip flexion, shoulder extension, and shoulder flexion strength	PNF flexibility training can improve ROM, isometric strength, and selected physical-function tasks in assisted-living older adults. Because the training period was short, 10 weeks, the results suggest that continued training might have a greater impact on physical function and the ability to perform routine daily activities.	13/18

Table 1: Continued.

Publication country/study type	Objective	Population	Methods	Outcomes	Comments and conclusions	Quality
Brown et al. 2000 [11]. USA. RCT. **Focus** Major muscle groups.	To examine effects of low-intensity exercise on factors associated with frailty (gait, flexibility, strength, balance, sensation, response time, and coordination) versus flexibility control group.	$n = 87$. Age: 83 ± 4 yr. **Experimental group (exer)** $n = 48$. Male = 20, Female = 28. Age: 83 ±4 yr. **Control group (home)** $n = 39$. Male = 17, female = 22. Age: 83 ±4 yr. **Characteristics** Sedentary, over 78 yrs, living independently but with difficulty. **Inclusion criteria** Medical screening, physical performance test (PPT) for frailty: 17 < score < 32.	Pre-post 3 mo **Intervention** **exer** 22 low intensity strength and flexibility exercise for upper and lower body 3x/week for total of 36 sessions (∼3 mo) **HOME** 9 upper and lower body flexibility exercises. Conducted at home (self-report), option to participate on site 1 wk^{-1}. **Assessments** *Strength:* physical performance test, isokinetic dynamometer (knee flexors/extensors, ankle flexors/extensors), and hand-held dynamometer (upper extremities) *ROM*: goniometry (shoulders, hips, knees, ankles, and trunk). *Balance:* static (Romberg test), dynamic (balance bean, obstacle course, and gait speed), and weight-shift (Berg balance test). *Gait:* pressure-sensitive foot switches. *Coordination:* Purdue peg board. *Speed of response:* red light to green light, stepping on brake and gas pedals. *Sensation:* Semmes-Weinstein monofilaments. **Analysis** 2 × 2 ANOVA; paired *t*-tests for EXER group only	**Physical performance test** Significant improvements in PPT scores from 29 ± 4 to 31 ± 4; unchanged in control group); improvements were in chair rise, putting on/taking off coat, picking up penny, and Romberg test. **Strength** Significant increases in knee flexor and extensor strength (9% change versus−1% in control) and shoulder abductors. **Range of motion** Flexibility increased in all measurements and in both groups. **Balance** Significant improvements in EXER group for obstacle course, full-tandem of Romberg, Berg balance test, and one-limb standing time. No significant changes in control group **Gait** Significant change in preferred walking cadence in EXER group. **Coordination** Difference between groups was "*almost* significant." **Response time** Unchanged in both groups. **Sensation** No apparent differences.	The control group lost a small amount of strength and balance in just 3 months, even though flexibility improved. These results suggest that the more comprehensive the exercise intervention, the greater the likely scope of improvement in frailty.	14/24

Table 1: Continued.

Publication country/study type	Objective	Population	Methods	Outcomes	Comments and conclusions	Quality
King et al. 2000 [12]. USA. RCT. **Focus** Major muscle groups.	To evaluate the effects of two different community-based physical activity regimens—on one year physical performance outcomes, perceived functioning and well-being in a sample of community-dwelling, sedentary women and men.	$n = 103$ Age: 70 ± 4 yr Males = 36, females = 67 **Inclusion criteria** >65 yrs, absence of cardiovascular disease or stroke, regularly active no more than 2x/week during the preceding 6 mo, free of musculoskeletal problems that would prevent participation in moderate levels of physical activity.	Pre-post 12 month, 6 month interim assessment 2 exercise classes/week and home exercise at least 2 wk^{-1}. Classes one hour, home exercise built up to 40 min sessions. **Experimental group** (fit and firm) Progressive moderate-intensity endurance and strengthening exercises. 5–10 min warm-up, 40–45 min aerobic and strength training circuit, 5–10 min cool-down; target heart rate 60–75% HRR. **Control group** (stretch and flex) Stretching and flexibility exercises. 5–10 min warm-up, 40 min stretching section, 5–10 min relaxation exercises. Stretching for neck, shoulders, back, chest, waist, hamstrings, calves, and hands. **Assessments** *Functional capacity/endurance*: Graded treadmill exercise test (GXT). *Strength and flexibility:* upper body strength (lift and reach task), lower body strength (sit to stand), and flexibility (sit and reach w/Accuflex 1 sit and reach box. *Self-rated physical performance:* a self-efficacy questionnaire. *Perceived functioning and well-being:* scales from the Medical Outcomes Study (MOS) incl. physical functioning, bodily pain, emotional well-being,	(values reported separately for men and women for each group). **Functional capacity/endurance** Submax HR: Fit & Firm had significantly greater improvement versus Stretch & Flex **Strength and flexibility** Lift and reach task: Fit & Firm had significantly greater upper body strength than Stretch & Flex. Sit-to-stand: No significant results. Sit-and-reach: Men assigned to Stretch & Flex had significantly greater increases than men in Fit & Firm. No statistical difference in women, but trend for greater improvement for women in Fit & Firm versus. Stretch & Flex. Women in Fit & Firm had significantly greater increases in flexibility at 12 mo than men. **Self-rated physical performance** Significantly greater increases in walking distance and self-efficacy for heavy lifting in Fit & Firm than in Stretch & Flex. **Perceived functioning and well-being** Only pain scale had significantly greater effects for Stretch & Flex (also statistically significant within group) than Fit & Firm.	Community-based physical activity regimens focusing on moderate-intensity endurance and strengthening exercises or flexibility exercises can be delivered through a combination of formats that result in improvements in important functional and quality of life outcomes.	21/24

Table 1: Continued.

Publication country/study type	Objective	Population	Methods	Outcomes	Comments and conclusions	Quality
			energy/fatigue, sleep problems, sense of mastery, and self-esteem. **Analysis** ANOVA, ANCOVA, MANCOVA, Tukey's studentized range test, and least-squares means procedure.			
Lazowski et al. 1999 [13]. Canada. RCT. **Focus** Major muscle groups.	To evaluate group exercise programs in long-term care versus. flexibility control group.	$n = 68$. Age: 80 ± 0.9 yr. 11 male, 57 female. Functional Fitness for long-term care program (FFLTC) group $n = 36$. 7 male, 29 female. Range of motion(ROM) group $n = 32$. 2 male, 30 female. Residents of five long-term care institutions (>3 month) **Inclusion criteria** No recent cardiovascular events, uncontrolled high BP, recent fracture, total blindness, or deafness. Ability to stand with minimal assistance. Walking devices and wheelchairs allowed.	Pre-post 4 mo **Intervention FFLTC group** 45 min, 3 wk^{-1} warm up/stretching (5 min), walking (15 min), progressive upper and lower body strengthening (10 min), balance, and cool down stretching (5 min). **Control group** Seated range of motion group vocal exercises, word/memory games, range of motion exercises (fingers, hands, arms, knees, ankles), and relaxation exercises. **Assessments** Mobility-timed up-and-go (TUG). Functional balance-Berg Scale. Stair climbing power. Functional ability-functional independence measure (FIM). Flexibility-Modified sit and reach test. shoulder flexion. Isometric strength: elbow flexion, shoulder abduction, knee extension, hip abduction/adduction. grip strength. Isotonic Strength: knee extensors.	86% and 79% compliance ROM scored lower on several measures at baseline. Considerable variability within all conditions on all measures. FFLTC led to significant improvements in mobility, balance, flexibility, and various measures of strength. Functional capacity was unchanged in the FFLTC group and decreased in the ROM group. No change in grip strength, gait speed and stair-climbing power for either, group. ROM (control). Increased TUG time. No change in balance or lower body flexibility. Non-significant 3.5% change in shoulder flexion ROM. 21% increase in shoulder abduction strength. Decline in isotonic leg and hip strength.	The FFLTC is suitable for long-term care residents, feasible for staff to deliver, and low-cost. Most importantly, functional outcomes clearly superior to seated ROM program. ROM may improve shoulder-abduction strength, but will not prevent declines in lower body strength, mobility, and balance.	21/24

Table 1: Continued.

Publication country/study type	Objective	Population	Methods	Outcomes	Comments and conclusions	Quality
Stanziano et al. 2009 [14]. USA. RCT. **Focus** Major muscle groups.	To examine impact of an active-assisted (AA) flexibility program on ROM and functional performance variables in older persons living in a residential retirement community (RRC).	$n = 17$. Age: 88 ± 5.4 yr. Experimental group $n = 8$. 90 ± 4.5 yr. 1 male, 7 female. Control group $n = 9$. 88 ± 6.2 yr. 3 male, 6 female. **Inclusion criteria**Living in an RRC, ability to sit upright in a chair for 30 min (no akathisia, neurological, or osteoporotic limitations).	Pre-post 8 wks 2 wk^{-1} **Experimental group** 10 stretches: back scratch (shoulder flexion/abduction), standing thigh (hip hyperextension), side lunge (hip abduction), overhead back (shoulder hyperflexion), overhead side (lateral trunk flexion), cross chest (horizontal shoulder adduction), seated trunk twist (trunk rotation), seated hamstring (trunk/hip flexion), and seated calf (dorsiflexion). 10 repetitions, 4-5 s each. **Control group** Arts and crafts class with limited physical exertion. **Assessment** Conducted 1 wk before and after training period. Flexibility: back scratch test (BS). Modified chair sit and reach test (SR). Supine knee extension test (KE). Modified total body rotation test (BR). Strength/power: 30-sec chair stand (CS). Modified ramp power test (MRPT). 30-sec arm curl (AC). Gallon jug shelf test (GJST). Mobility: 50-foot gait speed test (GS). 8-foot timed up and go (UG). **Analysis** ANCOVA	$n = 13$ **Flexibility** Significant increases in ROM made by experimental group for all measures but left side BS and right side SR. Control group showed no change in any flexibility measure but a significant loss in ROM for right-side knee extension. **Functionality** Experimental group significantly improved CS and MRPT, while control had significant declines. Experimental group significantly improved in AC and the GJST, while control had no change. Experimental group reduced time taken to complete the UG and GS.	Eight weeks of AA stretching may be an effective intervention for improving ROM, mobility, and functional power for older persons living in a RRC. Data provide clear link between flexibility and functional performance in older persons and support the inclusion of flexibility training in interventions designed to increase independence in older persons.	16/24

Table 1: Continued.

Publication country/study type	Objective	Population	Methods	Outcomes	Comments and conclusions	Quality
Raab et al. 1988 [15]. USA. Non-RCT. **Focus** Major muscle groups.	Examine the ability of weighted and nonweighted exercises to increase flexibility in older adults in the hip, shoulder, wrist, ankle, and neck.	$n = 46$. Female. Experimental groups Exercise (no weights, EN). $n = 16$. 70 ± 3.9 yr. Exercise (with weights, EW). $n = 17$. 70 ± 3.2 yr. Control group No exercise. $n = 1371 \pm 8.1$ yr. Healthy, active older adults.	Pre-post 25 wks. **Exercise program** 60 min, 3 days/week; 5–10 min treadmill warm-up; 10 min aerobics at 65% HRmax; 25–30 min whole body strength and flexibility exercises; 10–15 mon cool-down. Exercises involved active and passive stretching held for 20 s, slow circling motions for ROM, and repetitive movements for example, leg curls. EW had gradual introduction of wrist and ankle weights. **Assessments** Shoulder flexion and abduction. Neck rotation. Wrist flexion/extension. Ankle flexion/extension. Hip flexion. **Analysis** Two-way ANOVA, Dunn-planned comparisons with two contrasts, one-and two-tailed t-tests.	Flexibility improved significantly for exercise groups in ankle plantar flexion, shoulder flexion abduction, and cervical rotation to the left. Hip flexion (reflecting hamstring flexibility) increased for all groups, with no between-groups differences. The exercise with no weights groups had nearly 2.5x greater increase in ROM than exercise with weights for shoulder abduction. No other flexibility comparisons in the exercise groups were significant. No functional outcomes.	Exercise can increase flexibility in healthy, older women by improving shoulder flexion and abduction, ankle plantar flexion, and cervical rotation. For shoulder abduction, a nonweighted exercise program can produce greater flexibility gains in older adults than a weighted exercise program, and should be considered if flexibility is the primary goal.	13/23

Table 1: Continued.

Publication country/study type	Objective	Population	Methods	Outcomes	Comments and conclusions	Quality
Bird et al. 2009 [16]. Australia. Randomized Crossover. Tria.l. **Focus** Major muscle groups.	To determine the effect of community-based resistance- versus flexibility-training programs on balance and related measures.	$n = 32$. Age: mean 67 yr. Males = 18, Females = 14. Sedentary. **Inclusion criteria** No history of stroke or other neurological disease or current diabetes, cardiovascular disease, or uncontrolled hypertension. No use of walking aids.	Pre-post 16 wks, 4 wk washout, 16 wks (crossover). **Intervention** Both groups had 3 sessions·wk^{-1} for 16 wks, then 4 wk washout, then switched to other group for 16 wks. **Resistance training (RT)** 2-3 sets of 10–12 reps. **Flexibility training (FT)** 40–45 min with 16–20 stretches; two stretches for each of: hamstrings, quadriceps, back, and chest. **Assessments** Balance, force plate. Timed up-and-go. 10 times sit-to-stand. Step test. Lower limb strength (right and left knee-flexion and extension) with an isokinetic dynamometer. **Analysis** Repeated measures ANOVA	Lower limb strength increased significantly in the RT group, but not in the flexibility group and there was a significant difference between the two groups. Significant improvements were seen in both groups for timed up-and-go, 10 times sit-to-stand, and step test. Significant improvements in medial-lateral sway *range* were seen in the flexibility group only. Significant decreases in sway *velocity* were seen in both conditions.	Significant improvements in balance performance were achieved with both resistance-training and standing flexibility-training programs in healthy untrained older adults. Flexibility program did incorporate some degree of balance training in the nature of the flexibility tasks.	19/24

Table 1: Continued.

Publication country/study type	Objective	Population	Methods	Outcomes	Comments and conclusions	Quality
Swank et al. 2003 [17]. USA. Non-RCT. **Focus** Major muscle groups.	To determine the effects of adding modest hand and ankle weights to whole-body stretching exercise on ROM.	$n = 43$. Age: 55–83 yr. Body Recall (BR). $n = 18$. 68 ± 5.6 yr; 8 male, 10 female. BR + Weights. $n = 14$. 68 ± 3.1 yr. 4 male, 10 female. Control. $n = 11$. 69 ± 6.5 yr. 1 male, 10 female. Participants of body recall older adult low intensity flexibility program. **Inclusion criteria**No overt disease or any severely limiting orthopaedic problems	Pre-post 10 wks. **Intervention** Supervised. BR = pain-free, smooth, rhythmic whole-body movements. **Training group 1 (BR)** 60 minutes, 3 wk^{-1}. **Training group 2 (BR + W)** 60 minutes, 3 $wk^{-1}$with gradual progression of ankle weights and band exercises. **Control group** *No description.* **Assessment** ROM (goniometer) for neck (left and right rotation), hip (flexion and extension), shoulder (flexion and abduction), knee (extension and flexion), and ankle (plantar and dorsiflexion). **Analysis** ANCOVA, Levene's test of equality. Tukey Honestly Significant Difference test, $P = \leq 0.01$.	(pre values not given). Significant differences found for 6 of 10 ROM measures: cervical rotation (left and right), hip extension, ankle flexion/extension and shoulder flexion, for both BR and BR + W in comparison to control BR + W showed significantly greater increases in 4 of 6 measures that showed significant change: cervical rotation (left and right), hip extension, and ankle dorsiflexion versus BR.	Found that the addition of weights enhanced effectiveness of stretching exercise. It is likely that a positive effect was noted for 2 reasons: increased resistance during exercise movement and exercises were performed through full ROM. It seems plausible to hypothesize that greater effects would be shown by addition of weights to stretching routines for nursing home clients or free-living, otherwise sedentary elderly.	14/23

Table 1: Continued.

Publication country/study type	Objective	Population	Methods	Outcomes	Comments and conclusions	Quality
Alexander et al. 2001 [18]. USA. Non-RCT. **Focus** Major muscle groups.	(1) Analyze the biomechanics of rise performance during chair-rise tasks with varying task demand in more disabled older adults. (2) To determine whether a strength-training program might improve chair-rise success and alter chair-rise strategy versus. flexibility control.	$n = 30$ (final). Training Group. $n = 16$. Age: 82 ± 6.0 yr. 4 male, 12 female. Control group. $n = 14$. Age: 84 ± 7.4 yr. 2 male, 12 female. Residents of local housing facility. **Inclusion criteria** >65 yr. No lower extremity hemiplegia or amputations, blindness, acute inflammatory or infectious illness, and no dementia. Must complete the easiest chair-rise task. Cannot be currently involved in formal exercise.	Pre-post 12 wks. **Intervention** **Resistance training** 1 hour/day, 3 days·wk^{-1} using HydraFitness hydraulic equipment for lower body exercise. Also weighted chair rise and weighted ankle flexion/extension. **Control group** Participated in series of seated neck, trunk, arm, leg, and foot flexibility exercises. **Assessment** Seven chair rise tasks, biomechanics of tasks H = using hands NH = without using hands 60/100/140 are seat heights as % of floor to knee heights). **Analysis** Two-way ANOVA, repeated measures ANOVA with pairwise post hoc comparisons (Fisher's PLSD).	Only training group improved ability to complete the most difficult tasks. Controls maintained performances in general, one or two declined. Only significant decrease was in total rise time for both groups at H-100. Centre of Pressure (COP) increased significantly in both groups in all tasks but H-140 (highest seat height). Knee torques increased for both groups significantly for H-100, H-60, NH-100, and NH-100-F. Mean hip torques increased significantly in controls and decreased significantly in training group in H-60.	Subtle, yet significant changes can be demonstrated in chair-rise performance as a result of controlled, short-term resistance training program.	15/23

Table 1: Continued.

Publication country/study type	Objective	Population	Methods	Outcomes	Comments and conclusions	Quality
Takeshima et al. 2007 [19]. Japan. Non-RCT. **Focus** Major muscle groups.	To compare the effects of a walking-based aerobic program, a band-based resistance program, a stretching-flexibility program, a customized balance program, and a Tai Chi program on functional fitness in a group of community older adults.	$n = 117$. 73 ± 6 yr. 64 male, 49 female. Aerobic (AER). $n = 13$. Resistance (RES). $n = 17$. Balance (BAL). $n = 15$.Flexibility (FLEX). $n = 16$. Tai Chi (T-CHI, Yang Style). $n = 31$. Control (CON). $n = 25$. Healthy sedentary. **Inclusion criteria** No meds for hypertension, HRT. No CHD, no regular physical activity.	Pre-post 12 wks. **Intervention** Supervised 2 days wk^{-1} (RES, BAL, FLEX, T-CHI) 3 days per wk (AER). All had 10–15 min warm-up 60–70 min of specific exercise: AER-Outdoor walking RES-Progressive elastic band exercises for all major muscle groups BAL-Eyes open/closed, exercise on floor, on foam mats FLEX-15 static stretches for upper and lower body (15–20 s each). T-CHI- standardized 24 forms. **Assessments** Functional Fitness. 30 s arm curl test. 30 s chair stand time. 8 Ft timed up-and-go. back scratch test. chair sit and reach test. 12 min walk test. **Analysis** ANOVA. Wilk's criterion. Kolomogorov-Smirnov test.	Improvement in cardiorespiratory fitness (12 min walk) was limited to AER (16%) RES, BAL, and T-CHI, resulted in improvements in upper and lower body strength and balance/agility. RES showed greatest upper body strength improvement (31%). BAL showed greatest lower body strength improvement (40%). Balance/agility was similar across RES, BAL, and T-CHI (10%). Functional reach, similar improvements for AER (13%), BAL (16%), RES (15%). No significant changes in either FLEX or CON on any measure.	It is recommended that older adults participate in a well-rounded exercise program vs. single mode. RES, BAL, and TAI CHI cross domains not specifically targeted in their design. AER necessitates aerobic-specific activity to improve cardiorespiratory fitness. With FLEX, lack of improvement suggests that further study is needed to explore the effect of flexibility exercise training in older adults.	18/23

Table 1: Continued.

Publication country/study type	Objective	Population	Methods	Outcomes	Comments and conclusions	Quality
Erickson et al. 2011 [20]. USA. RCT. **Focus** Major muscle groups.	To evaluate whether 1 year of exercise training increases the size of the hippocampus and improves spatial memory using moderate-intensity aerobic exercise versus a stretching and toning exercise program.	$n = 120$. Experimental (exp). $n = 60$. Age: 68 yr. 16 male, 44 female. Control (con). $n = 60$. Age: 66 yr. 24 male, 46 female. Community-dwelling, sedentary. **Inclusion criteria** Aged 55–80 yr, no dementia, healthy less than 30 min. of PA in last 6 mo.	Both EXP and CON groups included same 5 min of stretching, both before and after exercise. Program lasted 1 year. **Aerobic exercise condition (EXP)** Progressed from walking 10 min at 50–60% HRR_{max} to 40 min at 60–75% HRR_{max} by week 7, then maintained until program finished. **Stretching and toning control condition (CON)** 4 muscle toning exercises, 2 balance exercises, one yoga sequence, and one exercise of choice. Told to exercise at RPE of 13–15 on 20 pt Borg scale. **Assessments** VO_2 max MRI for hippocampal volume. Computer-based spatial memory task. **Analysis** Repeated measures ANOVA. *t*-tests.	EXP group VO_2 max increased 7.78% while CON increased 1.11%. EXP group had significant group × time interaction for increased hippocampus size (left + 2.12%, right + 1.97%), while CON group declined (left −1.4%, right −1.43%).	Greater increases in aerobic fitness were associated with greater increased in hippocampal volume, suggesting that larger changes in fitness translate to larger changes in volume. Higher aerobic fitness levels at baseline were associated with better spatial memory. Aerobic exercise-induced increases in BDNF are selectively related to the changes in anterior hippocampal volume. Loss of hippocampal volume in late adulthood is not inevitable and can be reversed with moderate-intensity exercise.	19/24

Table 1: Continued.

Publication country/study type	Objective	Population	Methods	Outcomes	Comments and conclusions	Quality
Ceceli et al. 2009 [21]. Turkey. Non-RCT. **Focus** Major muscle groups.	To determine if performing regular ROM exercises had a beneficial effect on the balance, functional activity, and flexibility of elderly subjects.	$n = 46$. Age: 73 yr. 3 males, 43 females. Group 1. $n = 25$. Age: 74 ± 5.15 yr. 21 female; 3 males. Rest home residents. Group 2 (control). $n = 21$. Age: 72 ± 4.13 yr. Female. Inpatient clinic patients, and sedentary housewives. **Inclusion criteria**>65 yr. Able to ambulate without assistive device. Independent in activities of daily living.	Pre-post; 4 month. **Intervention** Supervised ROM exercises. Supine position with 10 repetitions of each upper and lower extremity joints. 3 wk^{-1}, 20 min. **Flexibility** Lateral trunk flexion (right and left) distance between middle finger at rest and in max lateral flexion. Anterior trunk flexion: distance from middle finger tip to the ground. **Balance** Sharpened Romberg (SR) test. One-legged stance test (OLST). Both tests performed with eyes open then closed. **Functional activity.** 30 m Walking Time. Functional reach test. **Analysis**Mann-Whitney *U* test.	Significant increase in Group 1 versus 2 in left (10.76 to 13.32 cm, $P =$ 0.035) and right (10.47 to 12.88 cm, $P = 0.44$) lateral flexion. No change in anterior flexion (8.66 to 8.24 cm) 30 m walk time decreased significantly from 28.14 to 20 s ($P = 0.001$) in Group 1. Functional reach increased significantly from 15.95 to 19.6 cm ($P = .014$). No significant difference in balance tests.	Authors stated that participating in daily flexibility group exercise increases ROM and causes some improvement in balance. When compared to a randomly selected hospital applied group, the rest home group has better balance, trunk flexibility and functional ability.	11.5/23

Table 1: Continued.

Publication country/study type	Objective	Population	Methods	Outcomes	Comments and conclusions	Quality
Christiansen 2008 [22]. USA. RCT. **Focus** Hips and ankles.	To examine the effects of a hip and ankle static stretching program on freely chosen gait speed of healthy, community-dwelling older people not active in exercise.	$n = 37$. Age: 72 ± 4.7 yr. **Intervention Group.** $n = 18$. Age: 72 ± 4.7 yr. 3 male, 15 female. Control group. $n = 19$. Age: 72 ± 5.0 yr. 5 male, 14 female. Independently living. **Inclusion criteria** In desired age range, healthy, no joint or musculoskeletal pain that limited movement in past month, no diagnosed gait or balance disorder, no falls history, has not participated in formal exercise during the previous 6 month, and has not used an assistive device for walking.	Pre-post 8 weeks. **Intervention group** Hip and ankle stretching. 2 static stretches held for 45 seconds and repeated 3 times alternating sides; total 9 minutes (540 s)/session. Stretches are standing calf stretch and standing hip flexor stretch. **Control group** Ensured no changes in current physical activity. **Assessments** *Passive ROM:* goniometric measurements of hip (hip extension based on Thomas test position) and ankle. *Gait:* shoes on; two walking speeds. **Analysis** Independent t tests or chi-square tests, ICC model 2 and form 1, 2-factor repeated measures ANOVA, separate repeated-measures ANOVA, paired t tests, and Bonferroni adjustment.	85% compliance *Gait*: significant increase in freely-chosen gait speed for intervention group (1.23 to 1.30 m s^{-1}, +0.7m s^{-1}, and $P = 0.016$) versus. control (no change). *joint motion:* peak hip extension and knee flexion increased significantly (59.7 to 66.5°) in intervention group, with no change in control (56.2 to 56.1°). Significant increase in intervention group (7.8 to 11.3°) for passive dorsiflexion, with no change in control. *Other:* No significant changes in stride length or joint angular displacement.	Evidence is provided from the results that joint motion is a modifiable impairment that can be effectively targeted for older people with simple, static stretching home-based intervention.	19/24

Table 1: Continued.

Publication country/study type	Objective	Population	Methods	Outcomes	Comments and conclusions	Quality
Cristopoliski et al. 2009 [23]. Brazil. RCT. **Focus** Hips and ankles.	To determine whether a 4 wk supervised stretching program for lower limbs alters gait kinematics in aged population.	$n = 28$. Female. Experimental Group. $n = 12$. Age: 66 ± 4.2 y.r Control Group. $n = 8$. Age: 65 ± 2.9 yr. **Characteristics** Community dwelling. **Inclusion criteria** Healthy, no gait performance limitations.	Pre-post 4 wks. **Intervention** Experimental group. 3 sessions·wk^{-1}. Supervised. 5 min walking warm-up. Hip extensor/flexor muscles, ankle plantar flexor muscles. Static stretches, 60 s each, 4 times. **Control** no activity. **Assessment** Static ROM of hip extension and flexion and ankle dorsiflexion by photography. Gait performance **Analysis** Repeated measures ANOVA, univariate analysis, post hoc Scheffe.	Static range of motion changed significantly ($P < 0.05$) in both hip and ankle joints for the experimental group, no change in the control group. Hip extension (73 to 91°). Hip uniarticular flexors (6.3 to 2.0°). Hip biarticular flexors (7.0 to 2.7°). Plantar flexor amplitude (39 to 48°). Experimental group showed increased step length, higher velocity, and reduced double support time after-training.	Supervised stretching program is effective to alter a number of gait variables. Aged participants displayed gait parameters which were similar to those of young adults.	17/24

Table 1: Continued.

Publication country/study type	Objective	Population	Methods	Outcomes	Comments and conclusions	Quality
Batista et al. 2009 [24]. Brazil. Experimental (Pre-post within subjects). **Focus** Hamstrings.	To determine if an active stretching program increases knee-flexor torque and flexibility, antagonistic torque, and functional mobility in older adults, and whether the possible adaptations remain after intervention.	$n = 12$. Sex: female. Age: 68 ± 6.4 yr. Participants in geriatric revitalization program for at least 12 month. **Inclusion criteria** >60–80 yrs, no vascular, inflammatory or lower-limb musculoskeletal disorders. No uncontrolled hypertension Flexibility deficit ≥20°.	4 wks without stretching (A1) followed by 4 wks of stretching intervention (B), followed by 4 weeks without stretching (A2). Participants were own controls (A1). **Flexibility intervention (B)** 2 wk^{-1}; 4 wks. Standing in front of table, therapist aligned spine with bar, participant flexed knees and trunk until hands reached table. Then extend knee and tilt pelvis anteriorly to max painless tension Held for 60 s, returned to standing for 30 s. Repeated 7 times ($7 \times 60 = 420$ s). **Assessments** Knee extension ROM deficit (goniometer). Isokinetic torque of knee flexors and extensors. Timed Up-and-Go (TUG), functional capacity. **Analysis** Repeated one-way analysis of variance. Student's Newman-Keuls test.	Significant decrease in knee extension deficit after intervention (24.1° to 14.1°, $P = 0.0001$), but not completely maintained after 4 wks (18.8°). TUG performance improved (8.4 to 7.2 s, $P < 0.05$) and remained at end of program (7.6 s). Significant increase in concentric and eccentric torque of knee flexors and extensors.	The knee flexor stretching program was effective in increasing the flexibility of this muscle group, increasing knee-flexor and extensor torque and improving functional mobility in older adults. Most improvements lasted at least 4 wks after the stretching ceased. The increase in knee ROM is probably a result of adaptation in the connective tissue caused after the knee-flexor program.	13/18

Table 1: Continued.

Publication country/study type	Objective	Population	Methods	Outcomes	Comments and conclusions	Quality
Johnson et al. 2007 [25]. USA. Experimental (Pre-post within subjects). **Focus** Calves.	To investigate the effects of a static calf MTU stretching program on ankle dorsiflexion ROM in healthy adult women 65 years and older.	$n = 13$. Age: 84 ± 4.7 yr. Female. **Inclusion criteria** >65 yr, healthy. No evidence of lower extremity dysfunction (assessed by visual observation of gait). Less than 10° of passive ankle dorsiflexion ROM. Functionally independent.	Pre-post, 6 wks. No control group. **Intervention** Supervised stretching of left and right calf muscle tendon unit (MTU). Standing with shoes on, placed one foot in front of other in comfortable stepping stance with hands on chair. Leaned forward on front leg until stretch felt in rear leg. Held for 60 s and repeated 4x/leg, once daily, 5 days wk^{-1} for 6 wks. **Assessment** Passive ankle dorsiflexion ROM by goniometry. Measured prior to stretching protocol and 3 days after-protocol. Posttesting researcher blind to pretesting data. **Analysis** Paired t-test.	Dorsiflexion ROM increased significantly from −11.1° to 1.2° ($P < 0.001$).	A 6-wk stretching protocol significantly improved ankle dorsiflexion ROM in elderly females. The ROM improvements were maintained 3 days after the last day. Were able to demonstrate a lasting, or plastic change in calf MTU passive ROM.	10/18

TABLE 1: Continued.

Publication country/study type	Objective	Population	Methods	Outcomes	Comments and conclusions	Quality
Gajdosik et al. 2005 [26]. USA. RCT. **Focus** Calves.	(1) To examine the effects of an eight-week stretching exercise program on calf muscle length, and on their length extensibility and passive resistive force properties for older women with limited dorsiflexion ROM. (2) To examine the influence of the stretching program on three functional tests.	$n = 19$. Age: 65–89 yr. Female. Stretching group $n = 10$. Age: 73 ± 6.8 yr. Control Group. $n = 9.75 \pm 8.3$ yr. Community-dwelling. **Inclusion criteria** Active dorsiflexion $\leq 10°$. Had ability to relax calf muscles and tibialis anterior during passive movements of ankle. No history of orthopaedic or neurological disorders. Minimally to moderately active.	Pre-post 8 wks. **Stretching group** Held static stretch for 15 s, 10 repetitions (total 150 s) 3x/wk for 8 wks. **Control group** Did not exercise. **Assessments** (Measured barefoot). **Functional** Timed agility course (modification of timed up-and-go). Timed 10 m walk. Standing forward functional reach. **Passive** Kin-Com ankle-foot apparatus (dorsiflexion) Dorsiflexion range of motion. Passive-electric energy (EMG). Passive resistive forces. **Analysis** Univariate ANOVA, two-way MANOVA, Pillai's Trace, two-way ANOVA for repeated measures, and one-way ANOVAs.	Stretching group significantly increased maximal passive dorsiflexion angle (11.1 to 16.2°, $P < 0.001$) and full stretch ROM (37.1 to 50.0°, $P = 0.005$). No significant changes in control group. Stretching group showed significant improvement in timed agility course (18.26 to 16.88 s, $P = 0.008$) and 10 m walk (6.44 to 5.99 s, $P = 0.030$). No change in control group speed. No change in functional reach test for either group. Stretching group increased both absorbed passive-elastic energy and retained passive-electric energy. MVC: Stretching group increases 14%, while control group increased 3.5% (both nonsignificant).	An 8-week stretching program for short calf muscles of older women increased the maximal DF ROM which indicated increased length of the calf muscles. The stretching program also increased the length extensibility, passive resistive forces and stored and retained passive elastic energy of the calf muscles. These adaptations correspond with decreased agility course and 10m walk times.	19/24

TABLE 1: Continued.

Publication country/study type	Objective	Population	Methods	Outcomes	Comments and conclusions	Quality
Petty et al. 1999 [27]. USA. Time-series, quasi-experimental. **Focus** Calves.	(1) To examine the relationship between maximum ankle dorsiflexion ROM and an individual's ability to move the trunk posteriorly with fixed BOS. (2) To examine intervention designed to increase gastrocnemius length on maximal ankle DF ROM and the ability to move posteriorly with fixed BOS. (3) To examine the contributions of maximum ankle DF ROM, age, and height to performance of volitional posterior trunk movement.	$n = 7$. 82 ± 4.5 yr. 4 male, 3 female. From audience at retirement community lecture. **Exclusion criteria** Any current neurological symptoms, taking any medications that might affect balance, any visual problems interfering with daily function, significant pain during backward lean test. **Inclusion criteria** >65 yr, no greater than 0° ankle DF ROM, at least 90° of shoulder flexion and 0° of elbow extension, ability to stand without external support for 2 min and perform Backward Lean Test properly, and not currently receiving physical therapy.	**Intervention** 4 wk stretching program: gastrocs stretching in "step-standing" position; point of stretch held for 30 s followed by 15 s rest; 4 repetitions per body part, repeated twice per day. **Assessments** Maximal ankle dorsiflexion (knee extended). Backward Lean Test (barefoot). **Analysis** Pearson product moment. correlation coefficient. Paired t test. Multiple regression analysis.	Mean pretest DF ROM: −5.9° ± 2.5° increased to 0.5° ± 2.9° (significant mean change of 6.4° ± 2.2°) Backward Lean pre-test: 5.2 ± 3.5 cm increased to 9.3 ± 3.6 cm (significant mean change of 4.1 ± 2.2 cm).	The Backward Lean test proved useful for assessing changes in dynamic postural control in a posterior direction. The positive correlation between maximal ankle DF ROM and distance of posterior horizontal trunk excursion during Backward Lean may be related to the biomechanical requirements of the BL test. Subjects who performed an exercise program designed to lengthen the gastrocsoleus muscles demonstrated increased range of maximal ankle DF with knee extended and improved ability to lean backward while maintaining a stationary BOS. The significant increase in DF ROM from pretest to posttest supports the efficacy of the stretching protocol. A significant relationship exists between the degree of available maximal ankle DF ROM with the knees extended and the horizontal distance an individual is able to move the trunk posteriorly while maintaining a fixed BOS.	

Table 1: Continued.

Publication country/study type	Objective	Population	Methods	Outcomes	Comments and conclusions	Quality
Kerrigan et al. 2003 [28]. USA. Double-blind RCT. **Focus** Hip flexors.	To test the effect of a hip flexor stretching program on age-related gait changes about the ankle.	$n = 96$. Males = 30. Females = 66. Treatment. $n = 47$. 15 male, 32 women. Control. $n = 49$. 15 men, 34 women. **Inclusion criteria** ≥65 yrs old, healthy.	Pre-post 10 wks. **Protocol** Home exercises. Both groups performed warm-up and cool-down; 30 s stretches alternating limbs for 4 sets/8 stretches in total. 2x per day (approximately 5 min). **Treatment group** Hip stretching exercise. **Control group** Deltoid stretching exercise. **Assessment** Static hip extension range, goniometer. Pelvic and bilateral lower-extremity joint motion and joint kinematics. **Analysis** Unpaired and paired t tests, paired Student t tests, and Bonferroni adjustment.	Only peak ankle dorsiflexion and plantar flexion during swing increased significantly with treatment. Trend for increased in static peak hip extension (6.1 to 7.7°, $P = 0.32$). No major changes with control group. Both groups had similar minor increases in comfortable walking speed.	Tendency toward a reduction in anterior pelvic tilt implies that modest improvement in hip extension range allowed for a slight decrease in anterior pelvic tilt. These findings support the hypothesis that an increase in pelvic tilt in the elderly is a compensation for hip contracture rather than a compensation or a direct result of another impairment. Improvement in peak ankle plantar flexion with hip stretching and a trend toward improved ankle plantar flexor power at comfortable walking speed were found. These results suggest that these outcomes in the elderly may be secondary to proximal impairment rather than to impairment at the ankle or ankle musculature per se.	17/24

Table 1: Continued.

Publication country/study type	Objective	Population	Methods	Outcomes	Comments and conclusions	Quality
Rider & Daly 1991 [29]. USA. RCT. **Focus** Trunk.	To determine if a flexibility training program could positively influence the spinal mobility of older adults and be conducted in such a way as to facilitate the adoption of such a program by the participants as part of their weekly exercise routine.	$n = 20$. Females. Experimental group. $n = 10$. Control group. $n = 10$. Age: mean 72 yr. **Inclusion criteria** No orthopaedic conditions for example, moderate to severe back pain, no osteoporosis or any spinal deconditioning disorders.	Pre-post 10 wks. **Experimental group** Supervised flexibility exercises (sit and reach, knee tuck, pelvic lift, and back extension) 3 times each, held for 10 s each 3 days wk^{-1}. **Control group** Continued current exercise program without flexibility training. **Assessments** Spinal flexion (sit and reach) Spinal extension. **Analysis** Repeated measures ANOVA.	Experimental group showed significant improvement ($P < 0.05$) pre to post for both spinal flexion (28.36 cm to 32.57 cm) and spinal extension (17.87 cm to 25.04 cm).	There is a meaningful positive association between regular flexibility training and spinal mobility in older population studies and may reduce the potential for age-related spinal deconditioning.	14/24

Table 1: Continued.

Publication country/study type	Objective	Population	Methods	Outcomes	Comments and conclusions	Quality
Weng et al. 2009 [30]. Taiwan. RCT (blind assignment). **Focus** Thighs.	To compare the effects of various stretching techniques on the outcomes of isokinetic exercise in patients with knee osteoarthritis (OA).	n = 132. n = 33 in each of 4 groups. Age: 64 ± 7.5 yr. Males = 26, Females = 106. **Inclusion criteria** Bilaterial moderate knee OA (Altman Grade II). No hip joint OA or any other hip problems with ROM limitations.	Pre-post 8 wks. **Intervention** **isokinetic exercise** 3x wk^{-1} for 8 wks at increasing doses. Active-assisted quadriceps and biceps femoris, holding end-point for 30 s, repeat 10x (10 min). *PNF*: HR(hold-relax), CR (contract-relax), CRAC (contract-relax agonist contract), HRAC (hold-relax agonist contract). Group 1: isokinetic muscular strengthening. Group 2: bilateral knee static stretching before isokinetic exercise. Group 3: PNF before isokinetic exercise. Group 4 (control): warm-up only. All groups received 10 min (15 min in control) hot packs and passive ROM on stationary bike. **Assessment** *ROM*: goniometer changes in knee active assisted ROM (flexion and extension). *Pain*: VAS scale. *Disability*: Lequesne's index (LI). *MPT*: flexion and extension with isokinetic dynamometer **Analysis** Weighted kappa statistics, Paired t tests, one-way ANOVA with Tukey's test, and Dunnett's test.	n = 124. Follow-up n = 111. *ROM*: significantly increased in groups II and III. *Pain:* decreased significantly in all groups, but increased in control. Greater decreases in II and greatest in III. *Disability*: average LI scores decreased significantly in all groups, greatest in III. *MPT:* average at 60°/second increased significantly in all measurements for groups II and III. All groups increased significantly more than control.	Stretching therapy is recommended as an adjuvant treatment to isokinetic exercise for patients with knee OA. PNF is more effective than static stretching exercise.	13/24

Yr: year; hr: hour; wk: week; wks: weeks; min: minutes; s: seconds; m: meters; ROM: range of motion; x: times; mo: months; pt: point; HRR: heart rate reserve; cm: centimeters.

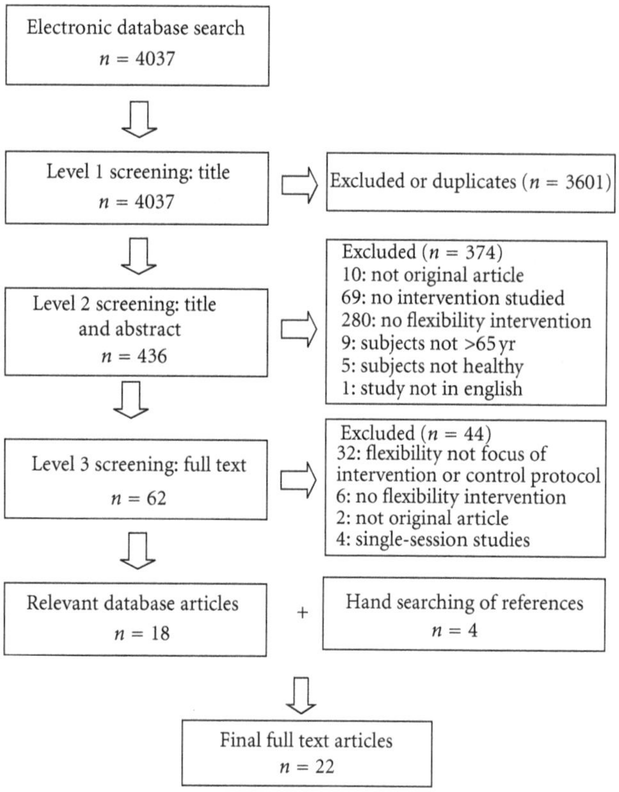

FIGURE 1: Article Screening Flow Chart.

[23, 24], Turkey [21], Australia [9, 16], Taiwan [30], and Canada [13].

3.2. Population. The mean sample age was 74.1 years, ranging from 64 years [30] to 88.8 years [14]. Seven studies included populations that were ≥80 years of age [10, 11, 13, 14, 18, 25, 27]. The number of participants in the articles of this paper ranged from 7 [27] to 132 [30]. There were a total of 1127 participants, 841 of whom were female (75%), while 286 were male. Six studies were female only [15, 23–26, 29]. Twenty studies were based on community-dwelling populations, and two studies involved individuals residing in assisted-living facilities [10, 13].

3.3. Outcome Measures. Outcomes were measured using flexibility measurements, physical ability tests, and questionnaires. One study also used brain imaging for the purposes of identifying changes in hippocampal volume with training [20]. A common outcome measure was simply whether there was a change in range of motion usually assessed by goniometry [15, 17, 20, 24–28, 30]. The inclusion of these studies in the review (although they reported no "functional outcome") was to provide the data for the purpose of determining whether older adults would, in fact, improve range of motion about different joints with various flexibility exercise programs. Functional outcomes were operationally defined as tests or measures designed to reflect abilities for various levels of daily activities and potentially related to maintenance of independence of older adults. In general, these tests assessed ability in a function that involved more than a single fitness component (e.g., not just a strength measure of a weight that could be lifted, but rather a performance that may involve strength and power as well as balance and agility). The most commonly used tests of functional outcome were gait and various walking speeds [11, 13, 14, 19, 21, 22, 26], the sit-and-reach test [10, 12–14, 19, 29], the sit-to-stand test [9, 12, 14, 16, 18, 19], functional reach test [9, 10, 21, 26], step test [9, 16], timed up-and-go (TUG) [10, 13, 14, 16, 19, 24, 26], and Romberg test [11, 21]. Other functional outcome measures were Berg balance scale [13], questionnaires [9, 12], peg board [11], red-light-green-light [11], Lequesne's index of disability [30], the physical performance test (PPT) [11], and the gallon jug shelf test [14]. Gait and walking speed proved to be more positively affected by flexibility training than other outcome measures [14, 19, 21, 22, 26], although this was not entirely consistent [11, 13]. Several studies showed increases in flexibility-related outcomes, but lacked significant changes in other more applicable and generic measures of functionality. Only one study followed up on outcome maintenance after the postintervention measurements. This study found that knee torque and timed up-and-go showed improvements compared to the control group, which persisted for four weeks after intervention [24].

In the sub-group containing eight studies of the very old (≥80 years), frail, and assisted-living populations [10, 11, 13, 14, 18, 21, 25, 27], there were significant improvements seen in functional reach [21], sit-to-stand [10, 14] and 30 m walk times [21], but no changes in the PPT [11] and mixed results for flexibility, strength, balance, and TUG tests. As compared to studies on less aged independently-living populations, the outcomes results of this sub-group were similar, except that the more aged/dependent group had less consistent flexibility outcomes; there were some neutral outcomes and some negative changes following flexibility training.

Six out of the 22 studies included several functional outcome measures and were considered most relevant to this paper [11–14, 16, 19], and are individually reviewed herein. Four of the six conducted randomized control trials (RCT) [11–14], and only two studies reported sample sizes less than 68 participants. Brown et al. [11] conducted a 12-week RCT ($n = 87$), wherein the flexibility trained group demonstrated only flexibility measure improvements and no change in functional outcomes. The measures included were very practical and included the chair stand, picking up a penny, putting on and taking off a coat, and the Romberg balance test. However, it should be noted that this study also showed minor strength and balance losses. In a one year RCT, King et al. [12], similarly, showed no change in most functional outcomes in the flexibility trained group. Functional measures included lift-and-reach, sit-to-stand, sit-and-reach, self-rated physical performance, self-efficacy for physical performance scale, and perceived functioning and well-being. There were only significant increases for the sit-and-reach test in men only (10.4 to 11.9 inches) and decreases in self-rated daily bodily pain scores (by 7.3% for women and 9.4% for men). Lazowski et al. [13] conducted a 16-week RCT ($n = 68$). Timed up-and-go increased (worsened) from 27 to 33 seconds, and no changes were seen in any other functional measures or in the sit-and-reach test. Additional functional measures included strength tests, Berg balance scale, self-paced and fast-paced walk tests, stair-climbing, and the functional independence measure for functional capacity. Stanziano et al. [14] employed an 8-week RCT ($n = 17$), where the experimental flexibility group significantly improved in every measure: chair stand repetitions (11 to 13), modified ramp power (69 W to 86 W), arm curl repetitions (12.9 to 18.8), gallon jug shelf test (13.4 to 11.5 seconds), 8 foot timed up-and-go (8.7 to 7.6 seconds), and 50 foot gait speed (13.9 to 12.3 seconds). The study by Bird et al. [16] was a 32-week randomized cross-over design ($n = 32$) with 16 weeks spent in the flexibility group. Four functional outcomes improved significantly for the flexibility group: TUG (7.6 to 6.6 seconds), sit-to-stand (22.6 to 18.0 seconds), step test (13.5 to 17.6 steps), and mediolateral sway range (eyes open: 4.16 to 2.97 cm; eyes closed: 6.87 to 5.64 cm). Strength was also tested, with no improvement by the flexibility group. In a 12-week non-RCT ($n = 117$), Takeshima et al. [19] reported no improvements for the flexibility trained group in the 12-minute walk, arm curls, chair stand, TUG, functional reach, back scratch, and sit-and-reach. These six studies exemplify the mixed results of the functional outcome measures in this paper. They serve as a strong representation of the lack of consistency of functional outcomes in the literature and therefore, any specific recommendation regarding type or frequency of stretching exercises is premature.

Overall, seven of 22 studies demonstrated mostly positive functional outcomes [9, 10, 14, 16, 21, 23, 29], while six reported mostly negative functional results, that is, no improvement in variables [11–13, 18, 19, 22]. Ten studies showed no functional outcome measures [15, 17, 20, 24–30] and only reported changes in flexibility and ROM (although they purported to relate flexibility to function, and were included for their results related to the ability of older adults to improve flexibility). There were no obvious differences between the characteristics of the studies with positive, negative, or no functional outcomes.

3.4. Intervention Characteristics. Twelve studies used flexibility training as the sole intervention [10, 11, 14, 17, 21–27, 29], four studies used flexibility training as a significant part of an intervention protocol [15, 16, 19, 30], five studies used flexibility as a control group to compare with various other exercise interventions [9, 11–13, 18, 20], and four studies utilized flexibility exercises along with strength or aerobic exercise in the intervention protocol but in the control group, the entire exercise protocol was flexibility exercises [9, 11, 13, 20]. The types of flexibility training methods varied from simple static stretches (19 studies) to different proprioceptive neuromuscular facilitation (PNF) techniques (1 study). Passive static stretching was the most common method used [9, 11–13, 16, 18–29], while passive static stretching with added weights was used once [17], active-assisted (AA) was used twice [14, 30], active and passive were used in conjunction once [15], contract-relax (CR) PNF was used once [30], contract-relax-agonist contract (CRAC) PNF was used once [30], and hold-relax-agonist contract (HRAC) PNF was used once as well [30]. One study compared multiple methods with each other [30]. Active-assisted stretching had positive and sometimes significant improvements in several outcome measures as compared to the inactive control group, but less significant than the improvements seen with the PNF techniques [30]. Weighted flexibility exercises were similar to nonweighted exercises in one study [15], but significantly better than nonweighted exercises in another [17].

Thirteen studies involved whole body flexibility training [9–21], two focused on hips and calves [22, 23], one focused on hamstrings [24], three focused on calves [25–27], one focused on hip flexors [28], one focused on the trunk [29], and one study focused on the quadriceps muscles [30]. Whole body flexibility training showed some minor to significant increases in outcomes; however, most increases were seen in ROM and flexibility measures, per se, and not in other functional outcome measures. These results were consistent with the overall effects of specific isolated stretching interventions on outcome measures for the related specific body parts.

The mean length of the included studies was 14.2 weeks, ranging from 4 weeks to one year [12, 20]. Results did not differ significantly throughout the range of intervention durations. In the three studies of at least 25 weeks in duration [12, 15, 20], no functional outcome measures were improved other than flexibility and ROM. In the four studies with durations of 6 weeks or less [23–25, 27] TUG improved from 8.4 to 7.2 seconds [24], walking velocity increased 1.07 to 1.22 m/s [23], and flexibility and ROM were improved overall.

The mean frequency was 4-exercise sessions per week, ranging from the lowest frequency of twice per week [9, 10, 12, 22, 24] to 14x/week [27, 28]. Two studies did not report exercise frequency [20, 22]. Some results from these studies include a TUG time decrease from 8.4 to 7.2 seconds [24] and a no-change [10], sit-to-stand time decreased from 10.2 to 9.2 seconds [9] and 9.3 to 7.9 seconds [10] and a no-change [12], a step test increased in reps from 16.5 to 20.2 [9], and an increase in freely chosen gait speed from 1.23 to 1.30 m/s [22]. The 5x/week and 14x/week studies did not include functional outcomes similar to the twice weekly studies. The 3x/week studies included results such as an improved TUG time from 7.6 to 6.6 seconds [16] and a worsening time from 26.8 to 33.0 seconds [13], a functional reach improvement of 16.0 to 19.6 cm [21] and two no-changes [19, 26], a sit-to-stand improvement of 22.6 to 18.0 seconds [16], a step test improvement of 13.5 to 17.6 repetitions [16], a 10 m walk time improvement from 6.44 to 5.99 seconds [26], and a 30 m walk time improvement from 28.1 to 20.0 seconds [21]. Although limited in number, these results show that the frequency of the flexibility training interventions had no noticeable differences compare with 2 and 3 times per week.

The mean flexibility exercise session time was 32 minutes, ranging from 30 seconds [29] to 85 minutes [19].

4. Discussion

There are currently scientific discussions regarding the utility of stretching exercises which are regularly recommended and conducted as a part of preexercise protocols to reduce injury and increase performance. Earlier reviews of stretching and flexibility have questioned their value in terms of injury prevention, delayed onset of muscle soreness, and improvement of performance [31, 32]. In fact, what occurs physiologically with stretching remains unknown [32]. Due to equivocal evidence thus far, the current American College of Sports Medicine's guidelines for exercise testing and prescription [33] recommended the removal of static stretching as part of a warm-up routine for strength and power activities. Additionally, based on available evidence, the 2011 ACSM position statement for guidance on prescribing exercise suggests performing flexibility after cardiorespiratory endurance or resistance exercise for general fitness programs. This position stand highlighted the need for further research to ascertain the effects of various flexibility prescriptions for various activities and performance goals. From the present review, there is not enough consistent evidence to make recommendations for any specific prescriptions of type, frequency, duration, or length of program related to flexibility training; particularly no specific recommendations can be made regarding the program or dose response of flexibility training to the focus of the present study, the transfer of flexibility gains to functions of daily life, or ability to live independently. A recent systematic review of 106 articles relating the effects of pre-exercise acute-passive static stretching on maximal muscle performance provided 74 methodologically sound studies providing 104 findings [34]. This paper showed that 50% of the 104 findings reported significant reductions in task performances, and the authors concluded that static muscle stretches totaling less than 45 s can be used in pre-exercise protocols without significant decrement to strength, power or speed type tasks; thus a conclusion was to recommend stretches held for at maximum 45 s to avoid loss of strength. Shrier [35] had also previously reported the potential negative acute effects of stretching on performance, but additionally reviewed the literature regarding regular stretching on performance which indicates that regular stretching improves force, jump height, and speed performance. Both reviews recommend further synthesis of the literature with respect to the effects of other forms of stretching on various performance measures.

The difficulties of the ability of this paper to provide a consensus on flexibility training prescription for healthy older adults include the lack of well-conducted studies focused on flexibility in older adults and the lack of consistency in the flexibility protocols employed, functional outcomes measured, and functional results observed. As such, according to the criteria used to assess level of evidence, to recommend stretching/flexibility exercises as a routine component of an exercise program for older adults to enhance health or functional abilities is Level 4, Grade C. The more influential studies in this paper (based on focused flexibility protocols with clear functional outcomes and relatively large sample sizes) [11–14, 16, 19] showed very comparable effects to the overall outcomes of the 26 studies, namely, an ambivalence in the value of flexibility training on functional outcomes that may be related to maintenance of independence in daily activities of older adults. Of these six studies, 5 were RCTs with an average quality assessment score of 18 out of 24. Only two of the six showed improvement in flexibility and functional outcomes ([14] 16/24; [16] 19/24).

In the sub-group (≥80 years), frail, and assisted-living populations there were significant improvements seen in functional reach, sit-to-stand, and 30 m walk times, but no changes in the PPT, and mixed results were observed for flexibility, strength, balance, and TUG tests. This subgroup was similarly ambivalent in the role of flexibility training with functional outcomes to the rest of the study populations, although this group had less consistency in the flexibility-related outcome measures. Frequency and duration differences between studies showed no noticeable differences in outcomes. When different muscle groups were targeted, the flexibility outcomes were expectedly fairly body-part specific. Regarding the different flexibility training methods, active-assisted (AA) stretching had positive and sometimes significant improvements in several outcome measures as compared to the inactive control group, but less significant than the improvements seen with the PNF techniques. Weighted flexibility exercises were similar to nonweighted exercises in one study, but significantly better than nonweighted exercises in another. One study showed ACR-PNF to be much more effective than CR-PNF and static stretching for both ROM and EMG activity. The overall results point to PNF stretching being more effective than non-PNF techniques for improving flexibility outcomes, but not necessarily functional outcome measures.

While flexibility training interventions synthesized in the present paper have been shown to increase flexibility and joint ROM, no consistent increases in functional outcomes have been observed. Therefore, future studies should consider the relationship that increased flexibility and joint ROM have with functional outcomes to determine if the increased flexibility is beneficial and worthwhile in terms of maintaining or increasing functional capacity for healthy older adults. More research is also needed regarding the relationships between outcome variables (i.e., how one variable such as functional reach would relate to another variable such as the timed up-and-go) and on the relationships between outcome measures and quality of life through self-reported functioning/quality of life questionnaires to best determine the applicability of the outcome measures.

Older adults are less concerned with high performance benefits from increased flexibility and more focused on being safely active and safely performing activities of daily living [36]. Injury and fall prevention are also common motives for recommending flexibility programs to older adults. The 2011 ACSM position statement notes that flexibility training may enhance postural stability and balance when combined with resistance training; however, no consistent link has been shown between regular flexibility exercise and a reduction of musculoskeletal injuries or delayed onset of muscle soreness [4]. However, despite the growing literature describing the relationship of flexibility to injury risk in younger populations [31], there is little research regarding older adults.

5. Conclusions

This paper found that flexibility training interventions in older adults are often effective at increasing joint range of motion in various joints, and various functional outcomes can be improved. However, due to the wide range of intervention protocols, body parts studied, and functional measurements, conclusive recommendations regarding flexibility training and functional outcomes for older adults remain ungrounded. As such, a specific prescription of how long to hold a stretch, how many repetitions of each stretch to conduct, and the type of stretches to do, is not determinable at this point. Because there is conflicting information regarding both the relationship between flexibility training interventions and functional outcomes, and the relationship between improved flexibility and daily functioning and health benefits have not been established, future research studies should attempt to address these issues.

While there is a lack of evidence to recommend stretching routines outside of a rehabilitative context, there is no additional health or functional risk of including flexibility exercises. As such, in light of increases in functional outcomes achieved by other exercise modes (balance, aerobic exercise, and strengthening exercises), stretching exercises can be included as an adjunct to the above, but the current literature would indicate it would add little to the functional benefits of the other exercise modes. Of note, the evidence-based and expert consensus statements of "Physical Activity Guidelines for Older Adults" of the US, the UK, Canada, and the World Health Organization (Global recommendations) have not included flexibility as a component in the recommendations.

Appendix

See Table 2.

Abbreviations

ACSM: American College of Sports Medicine
RCT: Randomized control trial
TUG: Time-Up-and Go
ROM: Range of motion
PNF: Proprioceptive neuromuscular facilitation
CR-PNF: Contract-relax proprioceptive neuromuscular facilitation
EMG: Electromyography
ACR-PNF: Active assisted contract-relax proprioceptive neuromuscular facilitation.

Conflict of Interests

All the authors declare that they have no conflict of interests.

TABLE 2: Sample electronic database search strategy.

	Sample search strategy-PubMed-January 2011	
(1)	Aged	331 611
(2)	Aging	236 732
(3)	Ageing	247 317
(4)	"Older age"	15 622
(5)	"Older adult*"	2 357
(6)	Elderly	3352095
(7)	Senior*	22 086
(8)	"Senior citizens"	734
(9)	(1 OR 2 OR 3 OR 4 OR 5 OR 6 OR 7 OR 8)	3505009
(10)	"Muscle stretching exercises" [Mesh]	420
(11)	"Pliability/physiology" [Mesh]	28
(12)	"Range of motion, Articular/physiology" [Mesh]	8 786
(13)	"Joint motion"	1 420
(14)	"Joint movement"	722
(15)	"Joint mobility"	888
(16)	"Joint range"	491
(17)	"Joint adhesion"	1 825
(18)	"Joint articulation"	42
(19)	"Muscle lengthening"	141
(20)	"Muscle elongation"	35
(21)	"Proprioceptive neuromuscular facilitation"	117
(22)	"Isometric contraction"	12 414
(23)	Yoga	1 483
(24)	"Tai chi"	455
(25)	Pilates	56
(26)	(10 OR 11 OR 12 OR 13 OR 14 OR 15 OR 16 OR 17 OR 18 OR 19 OR 20 OR 21 OR 22 OR 23 OR 24 OR 25)	28 177
(27)	Ability	455 298
(28)	Mobility	94 157
(29)	Frailty	2 112
(30)	Disability	80 338
(31)	Dependen *	1066172
(32)	Independen *	560 960
(33)	Reliance	8 424
(34)	Living	818 389
(35)	Institutionaliz *	12 329
(36)	"Nursing home"	13 615
(37)	"Activities of daily living"	45 277
(38)	"Independent activities of daily living"	3 979
(39)	ADL	4 683
(40)	IADL	1 147
(41)	"Assisted living"	1 197
(42)	"Long-term care"	25 605
(43)	"Long-term care"	25 605
(44)	(27 OR 28 OR 29 OR 30 OR 31 OR 32 OR 33 OR 34 OR 35 OR 36 OR 37 OR 38 OR 39 OR 40 OR 41 OR 42 OR 43)	2738402

TABLE 2: Continued.

Sample search strategy-PubMed-January 2011		
(45)	Control	2295628
(46)	Treatment	6813000
(47)	Modality	165 777
(48)	Adjunct	25 544
(49)	Component	289 484
(50)	Group	1741947
(51)	Subset	76 495
(52)	Subset	446
(53)	Subgroup	55 099
(54)	Subgroup	2 358
(55)	"Exercise" [Mesh]	52 144
(56)	"Exercise prescription"	772
(57)	"Exercise program*"	3 376
(58)	"Exercise treatment"	240
(59)	"Exercise therapy"	20 527
(60)	Activity	1731305
(61)	"Physical activity"	37 516
(62)	"Physical therapy"	38 673
(63)	"Fitness program*"	277
(64)	Dance	2 274
(65)	"Rhythmic exercise"	86
(66)	(45 OR 46 OR 47 OR 48 OR 49 OR 50 OR 51 OR 52 OR 53 OR 54 OR 55 OR 56 OR 57 OR 58 OR 59 OR 60 OR 61 OR 62 OR 63 OR 64 OR 65)	9 702 261
(67)	(9 AND 26 AND 44 AND 66)	2 401
(68)	(67 NOT child NOT children NOT cognit* NOT "alzheimer disease" NOT depression NOT anxiety NOT post-surg* NOT postsurg* NOT surgery NOT surgical NOT cardiac NOT fracture* NOT arthroplasty NOT diabetes NOT diabetic NOT cancer NOT stroke NOT Parkinson* NOT "multiple sclerosis" NOT sclerosis NOT stenosis NOT memory NOT mental NOT coronary NOT cerebral NOT dystrophy NOT polio NOT fibromyalgia)	434

Authors' Contributions

All authors have made substantial contributions to the conception and design of the present systematic review. L. Stathokostas coordinated the conduct of the systematic review. L. Stathokostas and R. M. D. Little were involved in the acquisition and analysis of data. All authors were responsible for the interpretation of data. All authors have been involved in drafting the paper. All authors read and approved the final manuscript for publication.

Disclosure

D. H. P. Paterson is the research director of the Canadian Centre for Activity and Aging and is responsible for evidence-based development of exercise programs for older adults. Recently, DH was a coauthor of a systematic review which resulted in the modification and update of Canada's Physical Activity Guidelines for Older Adults submitted to IJBNPA in 2010. This paper showed that exercise interventions in older adults are effective in maintaining or improving functional abilities. However, it was identified that less is known about the role of flexibility in the maintenance or improvement of functional abilities. As such, the present paper was undertaken.

Acknowledgment

The authors gratefully acknowledge the assistance of Marisa Surmacz, Health Sciences librarian, University of Western Ontario.

References

[1] D. H. Paterson and D. E. R. Warburton, "Physical activity and functional limitations in older adults: a systematic review related to Canada's Physical Activity Guidelines," *International Journal of Behavioral Nutrition and Physical Activity*, vol. 7, article 38, 2010.

[2] W. J. Chodzko-Zajko, D. N. Proctor, M. A. Fiatarone Singh et al., "Exercise and physical activity for older adults," *Medicine and Science in Sports and Exercise*, vol. 41, no. 7, pp. 1510–1530, 2009.

[3] K. P. Speer, *Injury Prevention and Rehabilitation for Active Older Adults*, Human Kinetics, Champaign, Ill, USA, 2005.

[4] C. E. Garber, B. Blissmer, M. R. Deschenes et al., "Quantity and quality of exercise for developing and maintaining cardiorespiratory, musculoskeletal, and neuromotor fitness in apparently healthy adults: guidance for prescribing exercise," *Medicine and Science in Sports and Exercise*, vol. 43, no. 7, pp. 1334–1359, 2011.

[5] U.S. Department of Health and Human Services. 2008 Physical Activity Guidelines for Americans. 29–34. 2008.

[6] D. C. Lau, J. D. Douketis, K. M. Morrison, I. M. Hramiak, A. M. Sharma, and E. Ur, "2006 Canadian clinical practice guidelines on the management and prevention of obesity in adults and children," *Canadian Medical Association Journal*, vol. 176, no. 8, pp. S1–S13, 2007.

[7] S. H. Downs and N. Black, "The feasibility of creating a checklist for the assessment of the methodological quality both of randomised and non-randomised studies of health care interventions," *Journal of Epidemiology and Community Health*, vol. 52, no. 6, pp. 377–384, 1998.

[8] S. C. Gorber, M. Tremblay, D. Moher, and B. Gorber, "A comparison of direct versus self-report measures for assessing height, weight and body mass index: a systematic review," *Obesity Reviews*, vol. 8, no. 4, pp. 307–326, 2007.

[9] C. Barrett and P. Smerdely, "A comparison of community-based resistance exercise and flexibility exercise for seniors," *Australian Journal of Physiotherapy*, vol. 48, no. 3, pp. 215–219, 2002.

[10] D. A. Klein, W. J. Stone, W. T. Phillips, J. Gangi, and S. Hartman, "PNF training and physical function in assisted-living older adults," *Journal of Aging and Physical Activity*, vol. 10, no. 4, pp. 476–488, 2002.

[11] M. Brown, D. R. Sinacore, A. A. Ehsani, E. F. Binder, J. O. Holloszy, and W. M. Kohrt, "Low-intensity exercise as a

modifier of physical frailty in older adults," *Archives of Physical Medicine and Rehabilitation*, vol. 81, no. 7, pp. 960–965, 2000.

[12] A. C. King, L. A. Pruitt, W. Phillips, R. Oka, A. Rodenburg, and W. L. Haskell, "Comparative effects of two physical activity programs on measured and perceived physical functioning and other health-related quality of life outcomes in older adults," *Journals of Gerontology Series A*, vol. 55, no. 2, pp. M74–M83, 2000.

[13] D. A. Lazowski, N. A. Ecclestone, A. M. Myers et al., "A randomized outcome evaluation of group exercise programs in long-term care institutions," *Journals of Gerontology Series A*, vol. 54, no. 12, pp. M621–M628, 1999.

[14] D. C. Stanziano, B. A. Roos, A. C. Perry, S. Lai, and J. F. Signorile, "The effects of an active-assisted stretching program on functional performance in elderly persons: a pilot study," *Clinical Interventions in Aging*, vol. 4, no. 1, pp. 115–120, 2009.

[15] D. M. Raab, J. C. Agre, M. McAdam, and E. L. Smith, "Light resistance and stretching exercise in elderly women: effect upon flexibility," *Archives of Physical Medicine and Rehabilitation*, vol. 69, no. 4, pp. 268–272, 1988.

[16] M. L. Bird, K. Hill, M. Ball, and A. D. Williams, "Effects of resistance- and flexibility-exercise interventions on balance and related measures in older adults," *Journal of Aging and Physical Activity*, vol. 17, no. 4, pp. 444–454, 2009.

[17] A. M. Swank, D. C. Funk, M. P. Durham, and S. Roberts, "Adding weights to stretching exercise increases passive range of motion for healthy elderly," *The Journal of Strength and Conditioning Research*, vol. 17, no. 2, pp. 374–378, 2003.

[18] N. B. Alexander, M. M. Gross, J. L. Medell, and M. R. Hofmeyer, "Effects of functional ability and training on chair-rise biomechanics in older adults," *Journals of Gerontology Series A*, vol. 56, no. 9, pp. M538–M547, 2001.

[19] N. Takeshima, N. L. Rogers, M. E. Rogers, M. M. Islam, D. Koizumi, and S. Lee, "Functional fitness gain varies in older adults depending on exercise mode," *Medicine and Science in Sports and Exercise*, vol. 39, no. 11, pp. 2036–2043, 2007.

[20] K. I. Erickson, M. W. Voss, R. S. Prakash et al., "Exercise training increases size of hippocampus and improves memory," *Proceedings of the National Academy of Sciences of the United States of America*, vol. 108, no. 7, pp. 3017–3022, 2011.

[21] E. Ceceli, F. Gökoğlu, M. Köybaşi, O. Cicek, and Z. R. Yorgancioğlu, "The comparison of balance, functional activity, and flexibility between active and sedentary elderly," *Topics in Geriatric Rehabilitation*, vol. 25, no. 3, pp. 198–202, 2009.

[22] C. L. Christiansen, "The effects of hip and ankle stretching on gait function of older people," *Archives of Physical Medicine and Rehabilitation*, vol. 89, no. 8, pp. 1421–1428, 2008.

[23] F. Cristopoliski, J. A. Barela, N. Leite, N. E. Fowler, and A. L. F. Rodacki, "Stretching exercise program improves gait in the elderly," *Gerontology*, vol. 55, no. 6, pp. 614–620, 2009.

[24] L. H. Batista, A. C. Vilar, J. J. De Almeida Ferreira, J. R. Rebelatto, and T. F. Salvini, "Active stretching improves flexibility, joint torque, and functional mobility in older women," *American Journal of Physical Medicine and Rehabilitation*, vol. 88, no. 10, pp. 815–822, 2009.

[25] E. G. Johnson, B. D. Bradley, K. R. Witkowski et al., "Effect of a static calf muscle-tendon unit stretching program on ankle dorsiflexion range of motion of older women," *Journal of Geriatric Physical Therapy*, vol. 30, no. 2, pp. 49–52, 2007.

[26] R. L. Gajdosik, D. W. Vander Linden, P. J. McNair, A. K. Williams, and T. J. Riggin, "Effects of an eight-week stretching program on the passive-elastic properties and function of the calf muscles of older women," *Clinical Biomechanics*, vol. 20, no. 9, pp. 973–983, 2005.

[27] J. F. Petty, V. S. Mercer, and M. T. Gross, "Relationship between maximum ankle dorsiflexion range of motion and maximal posterior horizontal excursion in standing," *Issues on Aging*, vol. 23, no. 3, pp. 7–14, 1999.

[28] D. C. Kerrigan, A. Xenopoulos-Oddsson, M. J. Sullivan, J. J. Lelas, and P. O. Riley, "Effect of a hip flexor—stretching program on gait in the elderly," *Archives of Physical Medicine and Rehabilitation*, vol. 84, no. 1, pp. 1–6, 2003.

[29] R. A. Rider and J. Daly, "Effects of flexibility training on enhancing spinal mobility in older women," *Journal of Sports Medicine and Physical Fitness*, vol. 31, no. 2, pp. 213–217, 1991.

[30] M. C. Weng, C. L. Lee, C. H. Chen et al., "Effects of different stretching techniques on the outcomes of isokinetic exercise in patients with knee osteoarthritis," *Kaohsiung Journal of Medical Sciences*, vol. 25, no. 6, pp. 306–315, 2009.

[31] S. B. Thacker, J. Gilchrist, D. F. Stroup, and C. D. Kimsey, "The impact of stretching on sports injury risk: a systematic review of the literature," *Medicine and Science in Sports and Exercise*, vol. 36, no. 3, pp. 371–378, 2004.

[32] J. L. Leibesman and E. Cafarelli, "Physiology of range of motion in human joints: a critical review," *Critical Reviews in Physical and Rehabilitation Medicine*, vol. 6, no. 2, pp. 131–160, 1994.

[33] ACSM, *ACSM's Resource Manual for Guidelines for Exercise Testing and Prescription*, Lippincott, Williams & Wilkins, Philidelphia, Pa, USA, 8 edition, 2010.

[34] A. D. Kay and A. J. Blazevich, "Effect of acute static stretch on maximal muscle performance: a systematic review," *Medicine & Science in Sports & Exercise*, vol. 44, pp. 154–164, 2012.

[35] I. Shrier, "Does stretching improve performance? A systematic and critical review of the literature," *Clinical Journal of Sport Medicine*, vol. 14, no. 5, pp. 267–273, 2004.

[36] P. Estabrooks and A. V. Carron, "The conceptualization and effect of control beliefs on exercise attendance in the elderly," *Journal of Aging and Health*, vol. 10, no. 4, pp. 441–457, 1998.

17

Home Features and Assistive Technology for the Home-Bound Elderly in a Thai Suburban Community by Applying the International Classification of Functioning, Disability, and Health

Supawadee Putthinoi,[1] Suchitporn Lersilp,[1] and Nopasit Chakpitak[2]

[1]*Department of Occupational Therapy, Faculty of Associated Medical Sciences, Chiang Mai University, 110 Intawaroroj Rd., Sripoom Subdistrict, Meung, Chiang Mai 50200, Thailand*
[2]*Chiang Mai University International College, Chiang Mai University, 239 Huaykaew Rd., Chiang Mai 50200, Thailand*

Correspondence should be addressed to Supawadee Putthinoi; supawadee.p@cmu.ac.th

Academic Editor: F. R. Ferraro

The ageing population is having an impact worldwide and has created a serious challenge in Thailand's healthcare systems, whereby healthcare practitioners play a major role in promoting independent interaction of their client's abilities, as well as environmental factors. The purpose of this study was to survey features of the home and assistive technology (AT) for the home-bound elderly in the community of Chiang Mai, Thailand. Home evaluation included features inside and outside the home, and AT was based on the International Classification of Functioning, Disability, and Health (ICF) concept. Methods included observation and an interview that were used by the researcher for evaluation. The study found that every home had at least one hazardous home feature such as inappropriate width of the door, high door threshold, tall stair steps, no bedside rail, and inappropriate height of the toilet pan. AT was found in houses as general products and technology for personal use in daily living and for personal indoor and outdoor mobility as well as transportation. Therefore, home features and AT can afford the home-bound elderly independent living within the community. Perspective AT according to the ICF concept could provide a common language for ageing in place benefits.

1. Introduction

Ageing is not merely the passage of time. It is the manifestation of biological events that occur over a time span. It is important to recognize that the ageing body changes differently in different people. Some systems slow down, while others lose their "fine-tuning." As a general rule, slight, gradual changes are common, and most of these are not a problem to people who experience them. However, more dramatic changes might indicate serious health problems, and the United Nations Principles for Older Persons has called for action by luring governments into national programs that cover many areas [1]. The strategy is that active and healthy ageing, older people can remain active and independent that it is a good priority for sustainable management of the effects of global ageing.

Thai society is ageing rapidly due to an increasing elderly population, but active ageing level of Thai older persons is not high [2]. The promotion of healthy, active, and productive ageing services is the challenges and opportunities to implement in Thai context. Chiang Mai in the northern of Thailand has been selected as a pilot project to start implementing a primary healthcare strategy [3]. Additionally, this city is the best practice prototype community and the local administrative unit plays a significant role in promoting the quality of life of older people in the local level [4]. Strengthening the capacity of primary healthcare work is deserved for continuous development to achieve sustainable health for all. Thus, promoting and maintaining good health in the home as well as gaining support from the community are challenging. The problem of elderly people falling is associated with environmental factors and has been of significant importance [5] regarding its potentially high incidence, due to age-related physiological changes [6, 7]. Older people usually spend more time at home [8, 9], where their environment is an important factor in independent living [10]. The home should provide good living conditions that enable the elderly to carry out their daily activities independently. "Ageing in place" is a term that means staying at home or in the community and relates to a sense of identity through independence and autonomy [11]. Successful ageing in place should enable the elderly to carry out basic activities associated with daily living safely and independently participate in social roles and receive personal assistance from caregivers as needed.

The environment is perceived to play a significant role in elderly people experiencing falls [12]. The WHO [7] highlighted that falls can result from environmental hazards and Todd et al. [13] promoted a broad environmental definition encompassing the community in which the elderly live, as well as the environmental challenges they face. The physical environment of a house for the elderly has enormous impact on the safety and functional level of older people. Understanding the risk factors in housing is very important for planning and implementing ageing friendly standards.

The risk of falling relates to personal health and the environment. The elderly have a higher risk of accidents and more severe consequences than younger people, and recovery takes longer for older people after a fall. Therefore, prevention of accidents is the best solution for these people. The environment can facilitate health maintenance and management by supporting health promoting behavior and provision of healthcare services. Environmental modifications, healthcare technologies, and assistive technology (AT) can compensate for limitations in functional abilities by reducing the risk of falling and promoting independent living and well-being [14]. Applying the ageing in place concept leads to the reduction of environmental barriers and paves the way for independent functioning in daily activities. Providing the elderly with a community service is classified as a specific characteristic in each of three groups, that is, healthy elderly, home-bound elderly, and bed-bound elderly [15]. This research focused on the home-bound elderly, who are independent or need partial assistance in performing their daily living activities. This group of elderly also has problems in participating in social activities, while mainly living at home. Environmental modifications can enhance the prevention of home-bound elderly being transformed into bed-bound elderly.

The International Classification of Functioning, Disability, and Health (ICF), which originated from the WHO, intends to specify a useful framework for functioning and disability. The term framework of disability, as specified by the ICF, has focused more on the close connection between the limited experience of disabled people, with their environmental design and structure, and the attitude of the general public in providing a common communicative language [16]. Environmental factors are a component of contextual factors in ICF that act as a facilitator or barrier in the successful functioning of a person [17] and influence individual performance [18–20]. The practical manual of the ICF [21] suggests that a structure can be provided for assessing and managing the home environment of home-bound elderly people.

TABLE 1: Characteristics of the home-bound elderly ($N = 66$).

Areas	Items
Outside the home	Area around the house
	Pathway leading to the house
	Exterior/entrances
Inside the home	Condition of the floor
	Movement around the internal area
	Kitchen
	Bathroom/toilet
	Bedroom
	Living/dining room
	Laundry
	Furniture

Environmental factors in ICF can have the effect of improving or obstructing the body function of an individual and their ability to execute an activity or participate in society. ICF is able to serve as an organizing framework for AT outcomes. However, Smith et al. [22] reported that use of ICF does not quantify AT interventions, and the outcomes lack specificity. When considering environmental factors, assessment tools for the elderly can be applied to evaluate a physically built environment that facilitates a range of activities in the area of mobility, as well as participation in areas of community life. The aim of this study was to evaluate environmental factors of the community-dwelling elderly living in urbanization area by applying AT classification categories of ICF to enable more specific treatment or intervention.

2. Materials and Methods

This study was conducted as pilot study in Chiang Mai, Thailand, between October 2015 and April 2016. This city was selected as the study site because the local administrative units play a significant role to support activities for healthy ageing and arrange home visits for community healthcare undergoing rapid urbanization. Two local communities, Namprae and Sanklang villages, were selected based on the existing structures of primary healthcare program with a significant role of the home visit for the elderly. The study was a cross-sectional survey of people aged 60 years and older. Lists of home-bound elderly people were obtained from the Health Promoting Hospital. Home-bound elderly people were contacted and visited in their homes. All those who agreed to participate in the study were inspected and assessed for home environmental factors and AT. Ethical approval was given by the Ethics Committee of the Faculty of Associated Medical Sciences, Chiang Mai University.

A survey tool was divided into three parts. Part one was the sociodemographic information on age, gender and marital status, condition of health, comorbidities, and physical disability. Part two was a home assessment checklist, using an observation tool with a room assessment technique, in order to evaluate the hazardous features used for elderly and disabled adults living in the community. Finally, part three consisted of an AT checklist completed for the elderly, in

TABLE 2: Categories of the AT checklist under ICF.

El environmental factors	Acceptable consideration related to the home-bound elderly	IOC value
Products or substance for personal consumption (e110)	No	−.40
Products and technology		
For personal use in daily living (e115)	Yes	1
For personal indoor and outdoor mobility and transportation (e120)	Yes	1
For communication (e125)	Yes	1
For education (e130)	No	−.60
For employment (e135)	No	−.60
For culture, recreation, and sport (e140)	Yes	.80
For the practice of religion and spirituality (e145)	Yes	.60
Design, construction, and building products and technology of buildings		
For public use (e150)	No	.00
For private use (e155)	Yes	.60

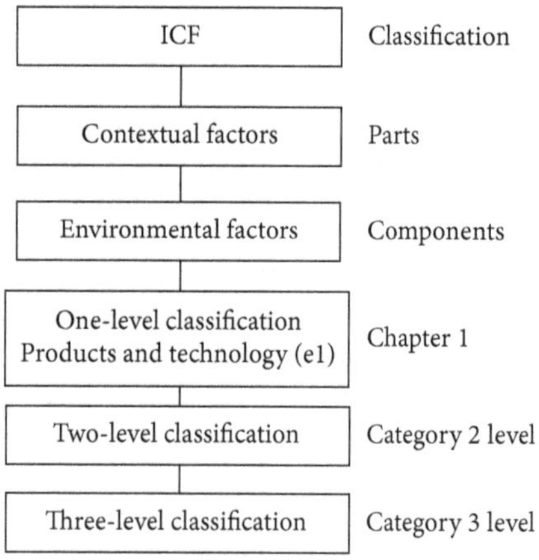

FIGURE 1: AT checklist based on the ICF framework [16].

order to assess the listing of classification categories from the ICF.

Criteria for judging home features were determined by the 2005 ministerial decree, which specifies the facilities in buildings for the disabled/physically handicapped and elderly [23] as well as the minimum standard of housing and environment for the Thai elderly [24]. The categories of home evaluation are shown in Table 1.

The AT checklist was developed as a first version based on the ICF framework under environmental factor components comprising chapter "e1" and a sublevel (category 2 level and category 3 level), as shown in Figure 1. The content validation step was taken by a panel of 3 experts [25], who had at least 5 years qualified experience in teaching and/or practicing in areas of ICF, the community, elderly people, and the environment.

In the first stage to validate the checklist, an expert panel was designed to determine and analyze category variables of the AT of the home-bound elderly. Ten items from all in chapter products and technology were selected. Second stage was carried for rating of agreement by calculating indexes of Item-Objective Congruence (IOC). The value of IOC was higher than 0.5; the item was acceptable. It indicates a good quality for measuring [26]. Finally, six items were validated to be a measurement checklist. The ICF categories are presented in Table 2.

Personal data were collected by face to face interviews with the elderly and/or their family members at home and by direct observation of the home environment. Many techniques were used to complete all of the assessment tools.

3. Results

Home-bound elderly people were investigated in the community at Namprae subdistrict. In all, 66 home-bound elderly people (87% of the target population) agreed to participate. Demographic, home evaluation data, and the AT checklist were analyzed by using descriptive statistics to calculate frequency and percentage. The results were divided into three parts: demographic profile of the home-bound elderly, home evaluation, and AT.

3.1. Sociodemographic Information. All of the home-bound elderly people had chronic health conditions. The majority of 69.70% of them were female and 57.57% had mobility impairment. Characteristics of the participants are presented in Table 3.

3.2. The Home Evaluation. Home evaluation was divided in two parts. The first and second one included assessment outside and inside the home, respectively. The results of home hazard evaluation in the bedroom and bathroom/toilet are shown in Table 4. All of the homes had poor features such as no ramp for a wheelchair and width of the door being smaller than 90 cm. The good features found in the homes were low level floors inside the home and nonslippery floors.

3.3. Assistive Technology (AT) in the Houses. The survey of AT in houses of the home-bound elderly is shown in Table 5. AT

TABLE 3: Characteristics of the home-bound elderly ($N = 66$).

Characteristics	N (%)
Age, years	
60–69	10 (15.16)
70–79	28 (42.42)
>80	28 (42.42)
Gender	
Male	20 (30.30)
Female	46 (69.70)
Marital status	
Single	8 (12.13)
Married	30 (45.45)
Others	28 (42.42)
Chronic health conditions	
No	2 (3.03)
Yes*	64 (96.97)
Rated health	
Excellent	—
Good	2 (3.03)
Fair	34 (51.52)
Poor	30 (45.45)
Physical disabilities	
No disabilities	13 (19.70)
Mobility impairment	38 (57.57)
Visual impairment	13 (19.70)
Hearing impairment	2 (3.03)

*Chronic health conditions include any of the following; heart disease, high blood pressure, arthritis, asthma, or diabetes.

TABLE 4: Home environment of the home-bound elderly ($N = 66$).

Items	N (%)
Outside the home	
Poor features	
No ramp for a wheelchair	66 (100.00)
Uneven/cracked area of ground around the home	10 (15.16)
Good features	
No holes or muddy ground around the home	56 (84.85)
Inside the home	
Poor features	
Width of the door being smaller than 90 cm.	66 (100.00)
High door threshold	64 (96.97)
Tall stair steps	63 (95.45)
No bedside rails	63 (95.45)
Inappropriate height of the toilet pan	61 (92.42)
Door step being higher than 2 cm.	51 (77.27)
Stairs on the staircase being higher than 15 cm.	36 (54.55)
Good features	
Low level floors inside the home	66 (100.00)
Nonslippery floors	62 (93.94)
Adequate lighting	60 (90.91)
No obstacles in the walkway	49 (74.24)
Grab bars in the bathroom	35 (53.03)

Table 5: AT in houses of the home-bound elderly.

Environmental factors: products and technology	Having AT in houses of the elderly
For personal use in daily living (e115)	
General products and technology	
For personal use in daily living (e1150)	Yes
Assistive products and technology	
For personal use in daily living (e1151)	No
Products and technology	
For personal use in daily living, other specifications (e1158)	No
Products and technology	
For personal use in daily living, unspecified (e1159)	No
For personal indoor and outdoor mobility and transportation (e120)	
General products and technology	
For personal indoor and outdoor mobility and transportation (e1200)	No
Assistive products and technology	
For personal indoor and outdoor mobility and transportation (e1201)	Yes
Products and technology	
For personal indoor and outdoor mobility and transportation, other specifications (e1208)	No
Products and technology	
For personal indoor and outdoor mobility and transportation, unspecified (e1209)	No
For communication (e125)	
General products and technology	
For communication (1e 250)	Yes
Assistive products and technology	
For communication (e1251)	No
Products and technology	
For communication, other specifications (e1258)	No
Products and technology	
For communication, unspecified (e1259)	No
For culture, recreation, and sport (e140)	
General products and technology	
For culture, recreation, and sport (e1400)	No
Assistive products and technology	
For culture, recreation, and sport (e1401)	No
Products and technology	
For culture, recreation, and sport, other specifications (e1408)	No
Products and technology	
For culture, recreation, and sport, unspecified (e1409)	No
For the practice of religion and spirituality (e145)	
General products and technology	
For the practice of religion or spirituality (e1450)	No
Assistive products and technology	
For the practice of religion or spirituality (e1451)	No
Products and technology	
For the practice of religion or spirituality, other specifications (e1458)	No
Products and technology	
For the practice of religion or spirituality, unspecified (e1459)	No
For private use (e155)	
For entering and exiting private buildings (e1550)	Yes
For gaining access to facilities in private buildings (e1551)	Yes
For ways of finding path routes and designating locations in private buildings (e1552)	No
For private use, other specifications (e1558)	No
For private use, unspecified (e1559)	No

Table 6: Facilitators and barriers in ICF coding of homes for the home-bound elderly ($N = 66$).

Items Products and technology	Facilitator *N* (%)	Neutral *N* (%)	Barrier *N* (%)	NA *N* (%)
For personal use in daily living				
General products and technology	48 (72.73)	18 (27.27)	—	—
Assistive products and technology	—	—	—	66 (100.00)
Other specifications	—	—	—	66 (100.00)
Unspecified	—	—	—	66 (100.00)
For personal indoor and outdoor mobility and transportation				
General products and technology	—	—	—	66 (100.00)
Assistive products and technology	56 (84.85)	8 (12.12)	—	2 (3.03)
Other specifications	—	—	—	66 (100.00)
Unspecified	—	—	—	66 (100.00)
For communication				
General products and technology	23 (34.85)	—	—	43 (65.15)
Assistive products and technology	—	—	—	66 (100.00)
Other specifications	—	—	—	66 (100.00)
Unspecified	—	—	—	66 (100.00)
For culture, recreation, and sport				
General products and technology	—	—	—	66 (100.00)
Assistive products and technology	—	—	—	66 (100.00)
Other specifications	—	—	—	66 (100.00)
Unspecified	—	—	—	66 (100.00)
For the practice of religion and spirituality				
General products and technology	—	—	—	66 (100.00)
Assistive products and technology	—	—	—	66 (100.00)
Other specifications	—	—	—	66 (100.00)
Unspecified	—	—	—	66 (100.00)
For private use				
For entering and exiting	8 (12.12)	—	58 (87.88)	—
For gaining access to facilities	7 (10.60)	13 (19.70)	—	46 (69.70)
For ways of finding path routes and designating locations	—	—	—	66 (100.00)
For private use, other specifications	—	—	—	66 (100.00)
For private use, unspecified	—	—	—	66 (100.00)

*NA: not applicable.

was found in items e1150, e1201, e125, e1150, and e1151. It did not cover all items of ICF.

AT in homes of the elderly was analyzed in ICF categories as facilitators or barriers as shown in Table 6. Assistive products and technology for personal use in daily living (e1150), and assistive products and technology for personal indoor and outdoor mobility and transportation (e1201), were facilitators for almost all of the participants. The barrier of design, construction, building products, and technology for entering and exiting private buildings (e1550) was found in 87.88% of the homes.

AT device categories listed in ICF categories are presented in Table 7. A majority of 72.73% of the participants had remote controls for a TV, as in the e1150 category. Usability and need were identified as 100% for meeting the need for a walking frame and wheelchair.

4. Discussion

In these findings, most of the home-bound elderly people were over 70 years of age and with chronic health conditions and physical disabilities. Perhaps surprisingly, most of their homes had poor features in areas indoors and outdoors, which were barriers in performing activities of daily living. Furthermore, all homes had multiple risks of hazards in rooms and areas where daily routines are performed, such as the bathroom/toilet, kitchen, bedroom, and areas around the house. A strategy for reducing the problems of physical environmental barriers needs to adapt the home environment to enable people with functional limitations to live in their homes as independently as possible. Home modifications such as handrails, stair glides, or grab bars can reduce the chances of elderly people falling [27, 28]. Intervention could (i) make home modifications to eliminate

Table 7: Assistive technology in the home for the elderly (N = 66).

Assistive devices	N (%)	Usability: None	Scarce	Average	Frequent	Meeting the requirements: Yes	No
For personal use in daily living							
Dentures	23 (34.85)	7 (10.61)	3 (4.55)	3 (4.55)	10 (15.15)	12 (18.18)	11 (16.67)
Remote controls for a TV	48 (72.73)	18 (27.27)	4 (6.06)	13 (19.70)	13 (19.70)	30 (45.45)	18 (27.27)
For personal indoor and outdoor mobility and transportation							
Cane	33 (50.00)	8 (12.12)	8 (12.12)	8 (12.12)	9 (13.64)	25 (37.88)	8 (12.12)
Walking frame	18 (27.27)	—	—	5 (7.57)	13 (19.70)	18 (100.00)	—
Wheelchair	5 (7.57)	—	—	2 (3.02)	3 (4.55)	5 (7.58)	—
For communication							
Spectacles	23 (34.85)	3 (4.55)	10 (15.15)	5 (7.58)	5 (7.58)	18 (27.27)	5 (7.58)
For entering and exiting private buildings							
Portable ramps	8 (12.12)	—	—	—	8 (12.12)	8 (12.12)	—
For gaining access to facilities in private buildings							
Bedside rails	8 (12.12)	—	—	—	8 (12.12)	8 (12.12)	—
Commode chair	7 (10.61)	—	—	—	7 (10.61)	7 (10.61)	—

hazards and (ii) construct purpose-built accommodation, especially with AT, to meet the needs of the elderly. However, to determine whether individuals are at risk of falling, the facilities in each individual household must have a falls risk assessment that relates to the elderly person's abilities. There is evidence that environmental hazards are a particularly important fall risk factor among frail elderly people, whose mobility is unstable [29–32].

In this study, the AT in ICF categories on home visits was evaluated. The results showed that e140 (products and technology for culture, recreation, and sport) and e145 (products and technology for the practice of religion and spirituality) were not found in the homes seen. However, AT devices were not covered in all category 3 levels. Although AT plays a role in facilitating independent living for elderly residents in their own homes [33], the main findings of this study revealed a lack of AT devices in many ICF categories. AT has the potential to improve the quality of life for frail elderly people [31, 34]. Surprisingly low number and types of AT were found. Furthermore, all of the AT products were low-tech devices such as a cane, walking frame, or wheelchair. These devices may have shortcomings and limitations and do not cover the daily life activities of home-bound elderly people. This finding is of great importance to the area of environmental intervention. AT needs to develop intervention for home modification and enable the elderly to live in their home independently and for longer periods of time.

This study generated the solution that it is possible to develop AT devices that cover all ICF categories, thus enhancing ageing in place and quality of life. There is research evidence that applying ICF has the potential to identify underlying facilitators and barriers in its human participants [17, 19, 35, 36]. The environmental factors of ICF categories can be used to address and provide a structure of perspective for assessing AT facilities. If healthcare providers in the community use the ICF framework to communicate in the same direction via tools and approaches, it may be possible to help the home-bound elderly to enhance a healthier lifestyle, while overcoming or reducing the barrier of the environment and their physical limitations.

The study was to developing a better measure of the environmental factors of the home-bound elderly people as new approach that can evaluate as either the facilitators or barrier to functioning in the home. Thus, challenge for future research is to use this assessment as a tool at a strategic-level intervention to facilitate ageing in place.

5. Conclusions

This study presented a strategy to improve understanding by identifying home hazards using the home evaluation process and evaluating AT in the home by applying ICF. AT is a service or tool that helps the home-bound elderly or disabled to perform their daily activities. Nevertheless, assistive devices can be used to meet the demands of a particular task.

Conflicts of Interest

The authors declare that there are no conflicts of interest regarding the publication of this paper.

Authors' Contributions

Supawadee Putthinoi worked in the conception and design, coordinated the data analysis, and contributed to publishing. Suchitporn Lersilp contributed to the data collection and the data analysis. Nopasit Chakpitak designed the research plan.

Acknowledgments

The authors thank all of the subjects for allowing them to do a room-by-room observation evaluation at their houses. They would like to express special thanks to Research Administration Center, Chiang Mai University, for providing valuable impulsion to publish their paper.

References

[1] C. Martin, D. Rodriguez-Pinzon, and B. Brown, *Human Rights of Older People: Universal and Regional Legal Perspectives*, Springer, The Netherlands, 2015.

[2] Md. N. Haque, "Active ageing level of older persons: regional comparison in Thailand," *Journal of Aging Research*, vol. 2016, Article ID 9093018, 9 pages, 2016.

[3] K. S. Kauffman and D. H. Myers, "The Changing role of village health volunteers in Northeast Thailand: an ethnographic field study," *International Journal of Nursing Studies*, vol. 34, no. 4, pp. 249–255, 1997.

[4] W. Suwanrada, W. Pothisiri, V. Prachuabmoh, S. Siriboon, B. Bangkaew, and C. Milintangul, *Community-Based Integrated Approach for Older Persons' Long-Term Care in Thailand*, College of Population Studies, Chulalongkorn University, Bangkok, Thailand, 2014.

[5] National Committee on the Elderly, *Situation of the Thai Elderly 2012*, SS Plus Media Company Limited, Bangkok, Thailand, 2013.

[6] National Council on the Aging, *Falls Free: Promoting a National Falls Prevention Action Plan*, NCOA, Washington, DC, USA, 2005.

[7] World Health Organization, *WHO Global Report on Falls Prevention in Older Age*, WHO Press, France, 2007.

[8] M. Baltes, I. Maas, H.-U. Wilms, M. F. Borchelt, and T. Little, *Everyday Competence in Old and Very Old Age: Theoretical Considerations and Empirical Findings*, ambridge University Press, Cambridge, UK, 1999.

[9] R. Krantz-Kent and J. Stewart, "How do older Americans spend their time?" 2016, https://www.bls.gov/opub/mlr/2007/05/art2full.pdf.

[10] M. Illario, M. Vollenbroek-Hutten, D. W. Molloy et al., "Active and healthy ageing and independent living 2016," *Journal of Aging Research*, vol. 2016, Article ID 8062079, 3 pages, 2016.

[11] J. L. Wiles, A. Leibing, N. Guberman, J. Reeve, and R. E. Allen, "The meaning of "ageing in place" to older people," *Gerontologist*, vol. 52, no. 3, pp. 357–366, 2010.

[12] J. Pynoos, B. A. Steinman, and A. Q. D. Nguyen, "Environmental assessment and modification as fall-prevention strategies for older adults," *Clinics in Geriatric Medicine*, vol. 26, no. 4, pp. 633–644, 2010.

[13] C. J. Todd, C. Ballinger, and S. Whitehead, *A Global Report on Falls Prevention: Reviews of Socio-Demographic Factors Related to Falls and Environmental interventions to Prevent Falls Amongst Older People Living in the Community, World Health Organization*, World Health Organization, Geneva, Switzerland, 2007.

[14] J. Ocepek, Z. Prosic, and G. Vidmar, "Assistive technology and its role among the elderly—a survey," *Informatica Medica Slovenica*, vol. 17, no. 2, pp. 9–15, 2012.

[15] Health Systems Research Institute, *Practice Guidelines for Elderly*, Sahamitr printing & Publishing Co., LTD, Bangkok, Thailand, 2010.

[16] World Health Organizatio, *International Classification of Functioning, Disability and Health: ICF*, World Health Organization, Geneva, Switzerland, 2001.

[17] A. C. Martins, *Facilitators and Barriers to Active and Healthy Aging*, Coimbra University Press, Coimbra, Portugal, 2013.

[18] R. Hamed, "Environmental factors affecting the daily functioning of jordanian individuals with multiple sclerosis," *International Journal of MS Care*, vol. 14, no. 4, pp. 169–178, 2012.

[19] J. H. Rimmer, "Use of the ICF in identifying factors that impact participation in physical activity/rehabilitation among people with disabilities," *Disability and Rehabilitation*, vol. 28, no. 17, pp. 1087–1095, 2006.

[20] K. B. Randström, K. Asplund, and M. Svedlund, "Impact of environmental factors in home rehabilitation—a qualitative study from the perspective of older persons using the International Classification of Functioning, Disability and Health to describe facilitators and barriers," *Disability and Rehabilitation*, vol. 34, no. 9, pp. 779–787, 2012.

[21] World Health Organization, *How to Use the ICF: A Practical Manual for Using the International Classification of Functioning, Disability and Health (ICF): Exposure Draft for Comment*, World Health Organization, Geneva, Switzerland, 2013.

[22] R. O. Smith, C. Jansen, J. Seitz, and K. L. Rust, "The ICF in the context of assistive technology (AT) interventions and outcomes," 2016, http://www.r2d2.uwm.edu/atoms/archive/icf.htm.

[23] Ministry of Interior, *Ministerial Decree Specifying Facilities in Buildings for the Disabled/Physically Handicapped and the Elderly*, Ministry of Interior, Bangkok, Thailand, 2005.

[24] T. Jarutach, J. Kespichayawattana, S. Lormaneenopparat, and K. Chalapati, *A Minimum Standard of Housing and Environment for Thai Elderly*, Thailand Research Fund, Bangkok, Thailand, 2005.

[25] E. K. H. Chan, "Standards and guidelines for validation practices: development and evaluation of measurement instruments," in *Validity and Validation in Social, Behavioral, and Health Sciences*, vol. 54 of *Social Indicators Research Series*, pp. 9–24, Springer International Publishing, Cham, Switzerland, 2014.

[26] R. J. Rovinelli and R. K. Hambleton, "Laboratory of psychometric and evaluative research," Tech. Rep. 24, The University of Massachusetts, Amherst, Mass, USA, 1976.

[27] ECRI Institute, "Falls," 2015, https://www.ecri.org/components/HRC/Pages/SafSec2.aspx?tab=2.

[28] M. D. Keall, N. Pierse, P. Howden-Chapman et al., "Home modifications to reduce injuries from falls in the Home Injury Prevention Intervention (HIPI) study: a cluster-randomised controlled trial," *The Lancet*, vol. 385, no. 9964, pp. 231–238, 2015.

[29] S. Studenski, P. W. Duncan, J. Chandler et al., "Predicting falls: the role of mobility and nonphysical factors," *Journal of the American Geriatrics Society*, vol. 42, no. 3, pp. 297–302, 1994.

[30] S. E. Carter, E. M. Campbell, R. W. Sanson-Fishe et al., "Environmental hazards in the homes of older people," *Age and Ageing*, vol. 26, no. 3, pp. 195–202, 1997.

[31] I. Petersson, M. Lilja, J. Hammel, and A. Kottorp, "Impact of home modification services on ability in everyday life for people ageing with disabilities," *Journal of Rehabilitation Medicine*, vol. 40, no. 4, pp. 253–260, 2008.

[32] B. Sophonratanapokin, Y. Sawangdee, and K. Soonthorndhada, "Effect of the living environment on falls among the elderly in Thailand," *The Southeast Asian Journal of Tropical Medicine and Public Health*, vol. 43, no. 6, pp. 1537–1547, 2012.

[33] Center for Technology and Ageing, "Technologies to Help Older Adults Maintain Independence," SCAN Foundation and Public Health Institute, Oakland, CA, 2009.

[34] W. C. Mann, K. J. Ottenbacher, L. Fraas et al., "Effectiveness of assistive technology and environmental interventions in maintaining independence and reducing home care costs for frail elderly: a randomized controlled trial," *Archives of Family Medicine*, vol. 8, no. 3, pp. 210–217, 1999.

[35] A. Layton, "Barriers and facilitators to community mobility for assistive technology users," *Rehabilitation Research and Practice*, vol. 2012, Article ID 454195, 9 pages, 2012.

[36] U. Schwegler, J. Anner, C. Boldt et al., "Aspects of functioning and environmental factors in medical work capacity evaluations of persons with chronic widespread pain and low back pain can be represented by a combination of applicable ICF Core Sets," *BMC Public Health*, vol. 12, no. 1, p. 1088, 2012.

18

Activation, Inhibition, or Something Else: An Exploratory Study on Response Priming Using Moving Dots as Primes in Middle-Aged and Old Adults

Christina Bermeitinger and Cathleen Kappes

University of Hildesheim, Hildesheim, Germany

Correspondence should be addressed to Christina Bermeitinger; bermeitinger@uni-hildesheim.de

Academic Editor: Jean-Francois Grosset

Response priming refers to the finding that a prime stimulus preceding a target stimulus influences the response to the following target stimulus. With young subjects, using moving dot stimuli as primes indicated faster responses to compatible targets (i.e., prime and target are associated with the same response) with short stimulus onset asynchronies (SOAs). In contrast, with longer SOAs, participants responded faster to incompatible targets. In the present study, we extended the evidence by comparing middle-aged (50–65 years) and old (66–87 years) adults. With two different motion types, the result found in young participants was replicated in the middle-aged adults. In contrast, old adults showed large positive compatibility effects with the short SOA but neither activation nor inhibition effects with the longer SOA. We discuss our findings in light of several theoretical accounts (i.e., inhibitory deficit, deautomatization, evaluation window account, attention, rapid decay).

1. Introduction

There are various kinds of motion surrounding us in our daily life. Perception and discrimination of different kinds of motion represent an important ability, already present in newborns (e.g., [1, 2]). Several research traditions have investigated the special role of motion and moving things in perception and attention (e.g., [3, 4]), and there has been an increased impact of motion research on cognitive theories since common coding approaches to perception and action have been provided (e.g., [5]). In these approaches, it is assumed that perception and action rely on identical cognitive representations. Further, own motion is strongly connected to processes in the motor system as well as to sensory and vestibular feedback. In turn, motor control, sensorimotor functions, motor representations, and general motor performance (for a review, see, e.g., [6]) are subject to age effects, oftentimes studied by functional brain imaging techniques.

Response priming (for a review, see, e.g., [7]) as a behavioral measure investigates the effects of preactivation of motor activations or perceptual/semantic preactivation from a prime event (i.e., a first stimulus) on the processing of a target event (i.e., a second stimulus which has to be categorized). Response priming (please note that, in classical studies on response priming, the same stimuli were used for primes and targets, i.e., in these studies, perceptual priming and response priming cannot be distinguished. However, for the current work, this differentiation is not of central relevance) has mainly been investigated using shape and color stimuli (e.g., [8]). For example, primes and targets are squares and diamonds and the participants' task was to quickly and accurately respond to the shape of the target (e.g., left button press for diamonds and right button press for squares). Reaction times to the target are often reduced when the preceding prime stimulus and the target are associated with the same response (i.e., primes and targets are congruent, consistent, or compatible; e.g., both are squares) compared to targets that are associated with another response (i.e., primes and targets are incongruent, inconsistent, or incompatible; e.g., the prime is a square, the target is a diamond).

Recently, Bermeitinger [9] introduced a variant of response priming in which moving dot rows were used as primes (henceforth "row-of-dots" primes) for static arrow targets to investigate preactivations of directional motions. Bermeitinger [9] found—with young samples—compatibility effects with moving prime stimuli (a row of dots moved leftwards, rightwards, or in a neutral direction (i.e., towards the borders or the center of the screen)) on static arrow targets. The sign of the compatibility effect crucially depended on the stimulus onset asynchrony (SOA) between prime and target. Essentially, with an SOA of 50 ms, no priming was observed. With SOAs of 100 and 150 ms, positive compatibility effects emerged. With SOAs between 250 and 500 ms, negative compatibility effects emerged. This pattern appeared whether the SOA was varied between participants or within participants, independently of prime duration [9, 10], and with forced-choice as well as free-choice tasks [11]. In further experiments utilizing a single moving dot (instead of the row of dots) as a prime, we found the same relative pattern, with positive compatibility effects following shorter SOAs and negative compatibility effects following longer SOAs, but over a different absolute time, we found positive effects up to an SOA of 360 ms and negative effects with SOAs of 800 to 1,200 ms [12].

Although the present research was not concerned with testing theoretical explanations for negative compatibility effects, we shortly summarize the most important explanations of it (for a review, see, e.g., [13]). Schlaghecken, Eimer, and colleagues [14–19] argued that negative priming effects (at least with masked primes) reflect an (self-)inhibition mechanism in low-level motor control. That is, the masked prime initially induces a response tendency corresponding to the action associated with the prime. Thus, positive priming effects are produced. Introducing the mask reduces or eliminates prime visibility. Therefore, early motor activation tendencies are no longer supported by sensory evidence, and positive priming is counteracted by inhibition to prevent premature responding. The results of Bermeitinger [9] can also be explained by this account if one assumes that self-inhibition is released independently of another intervening stimulus (i.e., mask) after some time. The inhibitory motor control always might come into operation when motor activations are classified as unfounded or debilitating. Motion seems to have the capacity to trigger responses rapidly and involuntarily (see also [20], Exp. 4). These response activations resulting from perceived motion have to be inhibited very quickly if they are classified as unfounded. Thus, the general mechanism proposed by Schlaghecken, Eimer, and colleagues could operate in response priming with motion primes, too. There are also alternative accounts which could explain negative compatibility effects (especially with masked primes; e.g., [21–23]; for an attentional account, see [24]).

Interestingly, Schlaghecken and Maylor [25] tested participants in old age (71–83 years) with their subliminal response priming paradigm using static arrows as primes and targets. They found substantial positive compatibility effects with short prime-target SOAs (i.e., 33 ms). However, old participants did not produce significant compatibility effects—neither positive nor negative—with longer SOAs (i.e., between 183 and 483 ms). In contrast, young participants showed clear negative effects with (in their case) the long SOA of 183 ms (there were no significant effects with SOAs of 333 and 483 ms). The authors interpreted their findings of missing negative effects with longer SOAs as evidence that, in old age, self-inhibition at the stage of low-level motor control is impaired (or for some participants at least delayed). According to the inhibitory deficit theory of Hasher and Zacks ([26]; an updated version of the theory is given by Lustig et al. [27]), there are age-related inhibition deficits, mainly associated with decreasing functioning in the frontal lobes. Specific deficits in inhibition are evidenced by several tasks and research methods (for an overview, see, e.g., [27]; for a summary of critics on the inhibitory deficit theory, see also, e.g., [28]). A current point of discussion is whether different inhibition processes (e.g., motor versus sensory, modality-specific, etc.) have to be distinguished and whether these different processes are correlated or not (e.g., [28, 29]). The results of Schlaghecken and Maylor extend the evidence of inhibition deficits to low-level motor control (assumed to be needed for negative compatibility effects with subliminal primes), as low-level motor control is associated with subcortical control structures (e.g., basal ganglia, thalamus, cerebellum).

However, empirical findings, as well as theoretical arguments, are at odds with the initial interpretations of Schlaghecken and Maylor [25]. First, Sumner et al. [30] found clear negative compatibility effects in old age (56–75 years, healthy control group) with SOAs of 150, 200, and 300 ms in manual and saccadic responses (but no, or only slight, positive compatibility effects with an SOA of 500 ms), and Seiss and Praamstra [31, 32] found (reduced) negative compatibility effects in middle-aged adults (51–65 years [31]; approx. 38–64 years [32]). That is, low-level motor control and inhibition still seem to be present in old(er) age. Besides, Schlaghecken, Maylor, and Birak [33, 34] themselves observed negative compatibility effects in old age (63–82 years)—especially when target location and response location (left/right) were incongruent (the authors used a combined Simon and priming procedure; i.e., in incongruent Simon trials, responses are generally slower than in congruent Simon trials) and when individually late responses were analyzed. The authors interpreted their findings and (especially these delayed effects) as evidence for impaired automatic low-level control (i.e., a deautomatization) which is replaced by high-level, automatic control processes.

Verleger [35], however, thought that this is not the most parsimonious interpretation of the data. He relied on the mask-triggered inhibition account of Jaśkowski [36, 37] according to whom the mask induces inhibition (instead of an automatic inhibition according to Schlaghecken and colleagues). Further, Verleger refers to Klauer and Dittrich [38] who presented their "evaluation windows account." Some key assumptions of this account are as follows: (1) participants evaluate all incoming events across a time window, (2) participants learn to partition the stream of incoming evidence into distinct episodes by use of the stimuli occurring during the experiment, (3) the stimulus immediately preceding the target stimulus (this could be the mask or another intervening stimulus, or with unmasked stimuli the prime itself) acts as a go-signal for opening the "evaluation window"—and additionally can be used as temporal marker to close the window due to the prime and cancel activation induced by the prime [35], (4) decisions about stimuli belonging to one of the given (response) categories are influenced by changes in evidence, and (5) negative compatibility effects will result if the prime falls outside the evaluation window, and positive compatibility effects will result if the prime falls inside the evaluation window. Verleger interpreted the findings by Maylor et al. [33] as evidence for "sluggish temporal structuring in the elderly"—that is, older people might have difficulty using the stimuli to segment the incoming stream of events and appropriately open the evaluation window.

In summary, first, there is an ongoing debate on the mechanisms underlying the negative compatibility effect with static stimuli. Second, it is unclear which account is most appropriate for explaining the pattern of results found with motion primes. Third, findings with older adults in response priming are mixed and also the object of theoretical debates. Fourth, until now, there have been no experiments with middle-aged and older adults using motion primes in response priming.

In the present study, we set out to explore some of the open questions. We used motion primes because they afford the opportunity to investigate responses following the same SOA which have led to positive compatibility effects with one prime type (i.e., single-dot motion type) and negative compatibility effects with another prime type (i.e., row-of-dots motion type) in young participants. Therefore, in the present experiments, the same tasks as in Bermeitinger [9] and Bermeitinger and Wentura [12] were used and we tested middle-aged (50–65 years) and old (66–87 years) adults. The division into age groups is based on the normal retirement age in Germany (i.e., between the 65th and 67th birthday for our sample). Participants' task was simply to respond to static target arrows presented at the center of the screen: Participants pressed the left or right key to a left or right arrow with their left or right index finger, respectively. Before each arrow, participants saw one of two motion type primes. Half of the subjects saw a row of 11 dots in the center of the screen (row-of-dots motion type). These dots seemingly moved rightwards, leftwards, to the center, or towards the borders of the screen. The other half of the subjects saw a single dot moving leftwards, rightwards, or alternately left and right (i.e., neutral condition). The shifting of the dots led to the impression of moving dots. The factor Motion Type (row-of-dots versus single-dot) was varied between participants. Further, the stimulus onset asynchrony (SOA) between the first presentation of the dots and the presentation of the arrow was also varied between participants (SOAs of 147 and 360 ms were utilized as these were the most stable SOAs leading to positive compatibility effects (PCEs) with the single-dot as well as the row-of-dots motion, but to negative compatibility effects (NCEs) with the row-of-dots but PCEs with the single-dot motion type, resp.).

Due to the exploratory character of our study, there are several possible outcomes of the experiment. First of all, we expected a main effect of motion type with larger (positive) compatibility effects with single-dot primes than with row-of-dots primes, comparable to the results with young participants in earlier studies [12]. With single-dot primes, we expected no negative compatibility effects at all, as the SOAs used in the current experiments were too short for finding negative effects with this material [12]. Given that negative compatibility effects occurred with an SOA of 360 ms with the row-of-dots motion type [9], we expected at least reduced negative compatibility effects in this SOA condition for the old participants, if they had specific problems regarding inhibition. In contrast, with the single-dot motion type, old adults should show positive compatibility effects in the longer SOA condition comparable to those of young adults [12] if the effects in this SOA condition are independent of inhibition and/or are independent of any kind of automatic decay of activation. Moreover, for the middle-aged age group, we expected either the same pattern as previously found with young participants or a pattern in between young and older participants (e.g., [31]).

2. Method

2.1. Participants. Overall, 85 participants were tested. We had to exclude 6 participants due to technical reasons during recording and 7 participants due to being outliers regarding their mean error rates. From the remaining participants, 33 (19 female) were of the middle-aged age group (range: 50–65; $M = 61.03$ years, $SD = 3.33$) and 39 (21 female) were of the old age group (range: 66–87; $M = 72.31$ years, $SD = 5.03$) (note that the sample sizes of some Age Group × SOA × Motion Type conditions seem rather small. However, power analyses based on our previous experiments (e.g., [12]) showed that some expected effects are very high (e.g., $d = 2.37$ in the 147 ms SOA condition). Thus, the sample size needed to find an effect in this condition is $n = 4$ [39]. Due to the exploratory character of our study, we used the incidental sample that could be recruited via newspaper articles or were guest students. That is, we could not equally assign the age groups to the experimental conditions. Further, we did not measure other cognitive capacities (e.g., general processing capacities or intelligence)). Participants had self-reported normal or corrected-to-normal vision (although all participants reported normal or corrected-to-normal vision, it might be that some older adults did not wear the appropriate glasses for the given task. However, the data speak against an interpretation based on vision problems because reactions times in the SOA 147 ms condition were highly comparable between age groups, which renders the explanation that the older participants needed more time to identify the stimuli improbable) and were right-handed, excepting one who was left-handed and four who were without any dominance. Participants were recruited via newspaper announcements or they were guest students at the University of Hildesheim and could be contacted by email or phone. They received 10 EUR for their participation.

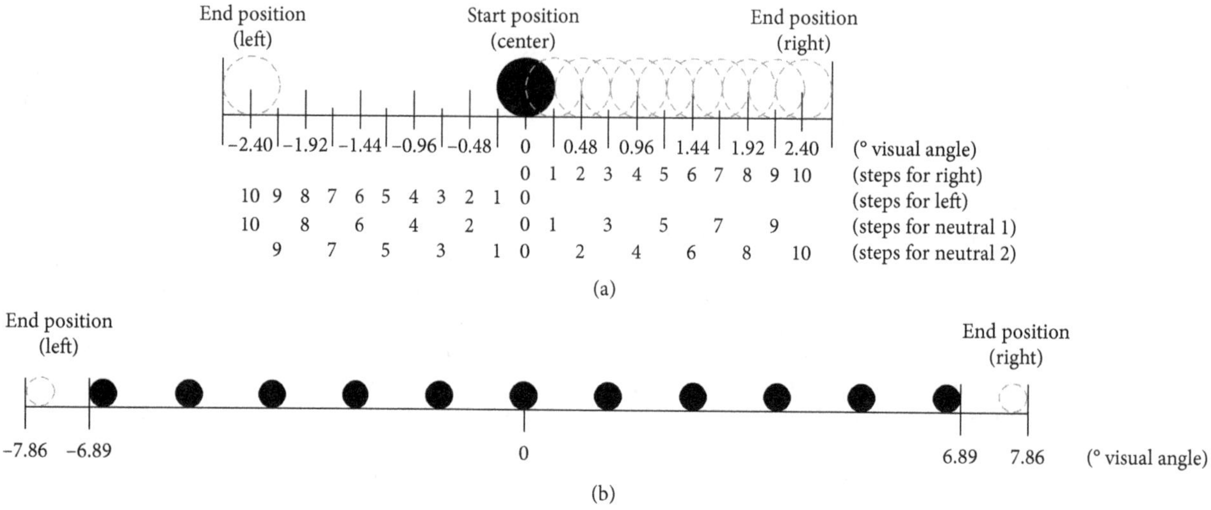

FIGURE 1: Prime stimuli used in the experiment. Black dots represent the original position of each prime at the center of the screen. Gray circles represent motion positions of the dot(s). For the case of a right moving single dot, all possible dot positions are depicted. The last gray circle on the left or right represents the end position of the motion for left or right movements. Each step lasted one refresh cycle (i.e., 13.33 ms). Note that the scale for the single-dot motion type and the scale for the row-of-dots motion type differ. (a) Single-dot motion primes and (b) row-of-dots motion primes.

2.2. Design. A 3 (Motion Direction: rightwards, leftwards, and neutral) × 2 (Arrow Direction: leftwards and rightwards) × 2 (SOA: 147 versus 360 ms) × 2 (Motion Type: single-dot and row-of-dots) × 2 (Age Group: middle-aged and old) design was used. The factors Motion Direction and Arrow Direction were varied within participants, the factors SOA and Motion Type were varied between participants, and the factor Age Group was quasiexperimental. In the tradition of priming experiments, we focused on the compatible (dots moved rightwards and the arrow pointed to the right; dots moved leftwards and the arrow pointed to the left) and incompatible (dots moved rightwards and the arrow pointed to the left; dots moved leftwards and the arrow pointed to the right) conditions. The compatibility effect was computed as the target response time difference between incompatible and compatible trials.

3. Material

All stimuli were presented in black on a white background (see Figure 1 for the primes).

For the row-of-dots motion type, the same material as in Bermeitinger ([9]; see also [12], Exp. 2) was used. Two arrows were used as target stimuli, one pointing to the left and one to the right, and the arrows were approximately 3.34° visual angle (3.5 cm) in length and 0.96° visual angle (1.0 cm) in height. The primes were rows of 10.5, 11, or 11.5 dots; each dot was approximately 0.38° visual angle (0.4 cm) in diameter. The whole row measured approximately 13.78° visual angle (14.5 cm) in length; the distance from one dot to the next dot was approximately 0.96° visual angle (1.0 cm). The prime event started with the presentation of the row at the center of the screen. To instantiate the movement, the dots were shifted from their original position in steps of 0.16° visual angle (0.17 cm) leftwards or rightwards. After six steps, a dot had reached the original position of its neighboring dot and the movement started again from the screen's center (original row position). For each prime event, 11 frames were presented; that is, there were 10 movement steps of the dots. The phenomenal experience is that of a rectangular window that allows a restricted view on an endless chain of moving dots. For the compatible and incompatible conditions, the dots (i.e., the whole row) were moved rightwards or leftwards. For the neutral conditions, the dots were either moved outwards (i.e., the 5.5 left dots of the row moved leftwards and the 5.5 right dots of the row moved rightwards, meaning that the central dot was split into two semicircles that drifted apart) or inwards (i.e., the 5.5 left dots of the row moved rightwards and the 5.5 left dots of the row moved leftwards, meaning that the central dot was split into two semicircles that progressively superimpose; for more details, see [9]).

For the single-dot motion type, the same material as in Bermeitinger and Wentura [12] was used. The target arrows were approximately 2.63° visual angle (2.75 cm) in length and 0.96° visual angle (1.0 cm) in height. A single dot (approximately 0.48° visual angle (0.5 cm) in diameter) was used as the prime. To instantiate the left or right movements, the dot was shifted from its original position in 0.24° visual angle (0.25 cm) steps leftwards or rightwards. In the neutral condition, the dot moved one step to the right (neutral 1) or to the left (neutral 2) and then to the opposite side (i.e., to the left or to the right, resp.); left and right steps alternated successively. For each prime event, 11 frames (each with a single dot) were presented, that is, 10 movement steps of the dot. The end positions of the dots were 2.63° visual angle (2.75 cm) to the left of the original position (i.e., the center) for left movements (and the neutral 1 condition, which started with a right movement) and 2.63° visual angle (2.75 cm) to the right of the original position for right movements (and the neutral 2 condition, which started with a left movement) (please note that these neutral motions are not really neutral; probably, both responses (left and right) are activated, rather than neither. However, a really neutral motion with a single dot seems either impossible or associated with other problems by changing the perceptual properties of the display (e.g., keeping the dot stationary would eliminate not only directional information, but also motion in general; adding a second dot would change the luminance and the number of moving elements). In general, "neutral" conditions are most often not really neutral in each sense. Therefore, the comparison with neutral conditions is usually coupled with some problems).

3.1. Procedure. Participants were individually tested in sound-attenuated chambers. The experiment was run using E-Prime software (version 1.3) with standard PCs and 17″ CRT monitors with a refresh rate of 75 Hz. Stimulus presentation was synchronized with the vertical retrace signal of the monitor. Viewing distance was about 60 cm. Instructions were given on the CRT screen. Participants were requested to quickly and accurately categorize each arrow with regard to its direction (by pressing the right/left key with their right/left index finger for right/left arrows, resp.; response keys were the 3 and 1 key on the numeric pad on which a right or left arrow was pasted, resp.). They were told that the dots are irrelevant to their task. The sequence of each trial in the row-of-dots condition was as follows: first a fixation stimulus (+) appeared at the center of the screen for 1,000 ms. It was followed by the first row of dots, which was presented for one refresh cycle (i.e., approximately 13 ms). Then, the next 10 rows of dots were presented for the next 10 refresh cycles, respectively (i.e., resulting in a prime duration of overall 147 ms) (note, after six refresh cycles, the row sequence started again from the original row). The prime event was followed immediately by the target in the 147 ms SOA condition or by a blank screen of 213 ms in the 360 ms SOA condition, which was then followed by the target. The target remained on the screen until a response was given. The intertrial interval was 400 ms.

In the single-dot condition, the same trial procedure was used as for the row-of-dots condition with the following exceptions. First, the dot moved constantly leftwards or rightwards (instead of repeating from the original position after six cycles) in the compatible and incompatible conditions. Second, in the neutral condition, the dot first moved one step to the right (neutral 1) or to the left (neutral 2) and then to the opposite side (i.e., to the left or to the right, resp.). Left and right steps alternated successively.

Each participant worked through four blocks with 36 trials each. Each block consisted of 12 compatible trials (6 with dots moving rightwards and leftwards, resp.), 12 incompatible trials (6 with dots moving rightwards and leftwards, resp.), and 12 neutral trials (6 with dots moving outwards and inwards, resp.); half of the trials had right arrow targets, and the other half had left arrow targets. There was a short pause after each block. Before the first experimental block, there was a practice phase with 12 trials.

The whole experiment (including instructions, breaks, experimental trials) took about 7 to 10 minutes for each person. Before the response priming experiment, all participants took part in a completely unrelated other response time study with words and a lexical decision task.

4. Results

Mean reaction times (RTs) were derived from correct responses. Outlying RTs that were 1.5 interquartile ranges above the third quartile with respect to the individual distribution [40], were above 1500 ms, or were below 200 ms were discarded. Due to these outlier and error criteria, 3.4% of all trials had to be excluded (0.8% due to errors). As error rates were extremely low, we did not analyze them further.

Mean RTs and mean compatibility effects for each condition are shown in Table 1 and Figure 2.

Mean reaction times were subjected to a mixed analysis of variance (ANOVA) with the within-participants factors Motion Direction (rightwards versus leftwards) and Arrow Direction (leftwards versus rightwards) and the between-participants factors SOA (147 ms versus 360 ms), Motion Type (single-dot versus row-of-dots), and Age Group (middle-aged, old). Results that are not subsequently reported were not significant ($p > 0.10$, two-tailed) (this even holds true for the main effect "Age Group" and the interaction of "Age Group" and SOA, both ps > 0.10).

The main effect Arrow Direction was significant, $F(1, 64) = 4.88$, $p = 0.03$, $\eta_p^2 = 0.07$, indicating slightly faster RTs with the right hand (i.e., arrow pointing to the right) than with the left hand (i.e., arrow pointing to the left). More interestingly, the interaction of Motion Direction and Arrow Direction was significant, $F(1, 64) = 26.31$, $p < 0.001$, $\eta_p^2 = 0.29$, indicating overall a positive compatibility effect. This effect was qualified by significant interactions of Motion Direction, Arrow Direction, and "SOA", $F(1, 64) = 19.86$, $p < 0.001$, $\eta_p^2 = 0.24$; of Motion Direction, Arrow Direction, and Motion Type, $F(1, 64) = 22.93$, $p < 0.001$, $\eta_p^2 = 0.26$; and, most interestingly, of Motion Direction, Arrow Direction, "SOA," Motion Type, and "Age Group," $F(1, 64) = 5.23$, $p = 0.025$, $\eta_p^2 = 0.08$ (these effects were also (at least marginally) significant if we included the neutral condition into analysis). Therefore, we further conducted mixed ANOVAs with the factors Arrow Direction, Motion Direction (both within-subjects), Motion Type, and Age Group (both between-subjects) separately for each SOA condition.

4.1. 147 ms SOA Condition. For the 147 ms SOA condition, we found a significant Arrow Direction × Motion Direction interaction, $F(1, 31) = 52.32$, $p < 0.001$, $\eta_p^2 = 0.63$, and a significant interaction of Arrow Direction, Motion Direction, and Motion Type, $F(1, 31) = 20.25$, $p < 0.001$, $\eta_p^2 = 0.40$: there were stronger positive compatibility effects with single-dot primes ($M = 49$ ms, SE = 5.2, $t(15) = 9.45$, $p < 0.001$) than with row-of-dots primes ($M = 11$ ms, SE = 5.8, $t(18) = 1.91$, $p = 0.07$), independent of age group (compatibility effects in both age groups were of comparable size).

TABLE 1: Mean response times (in ms; SD in parentheses) of the compatible, the incompatible, and the neutral conditions as well as the compatibility effects (incompatible–compatible; in ms; SE in parentheses; discrepancies due to rounding differences) for each SOA (147 versus 360 ms) × Motion Type (single-dot versus row-of-dots) × Age Group (middle-aged, old) condition. Additionally, the effects of young participants (MED_{age} = 22 years, ranging from 18 to 47) in the single-dot ([12], Exp. 1, 147 and 360 ms SOA conditions) and row-of-dots ([9], Exp. 3) conditions from experiments published in previous papers with the same conditions as in the current experiment are presented for a direct comparison.

	Young (results from previous papers)		Middle aged								Old age							
	Single-dot motion type	Row-of-dots motion type	Single-dot motion type				Row-of-dots motion type				Single-dot motion type				Row-of-dots motion type			
	Effect	Effect	Compatible	Incompatible	Neutral	Effect	Compatible	Incompatible	Neutral	Effect	Compatible	Incompatible	Neutral	Effect	Compatible	Incompatible	Neutral	Effect
147 ms SOA	37 (3.9)	11 (3.6)	429 (66.3)	467 (73.3)	452 (63.3)	38 (4.7)	466 (53.2)	476 (37.4)	466 (38.7)	10 (7.9)	429 (64.8)	485 (47.6)	457 (53.3)	56 (7.2)	464 (63.0)	475 (59.4)	464 (66.5)	12 (8.7)
360 ms SOA	16 (6.6)	−11 (3.2)	406 (31.7)	431 (30.9)	421 (32.6)	26 (6.4)	440 (34.6)	424 (27.9)	434 (27.5)	−15 (5.8)	456 (30.9)	456 (39.0)	447 (33.2)	0 (10.7)	465 (47.2)	463 (61.5)	473 (61.4)	−2 (8.7)

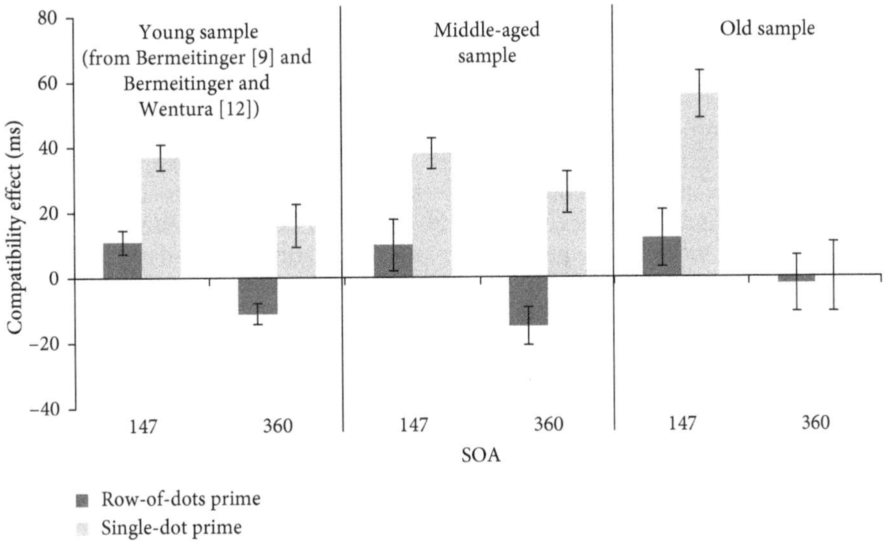

FIGURE 2: Mean compatibility effects (mean RT incompatible–mean RT compatible) from the 147 and 360 ms SOA condition, separately depicted for the middle-aged and old samples. For reasons of comparison, we added the corresponding priming effects from young samples from experiments published in previous papers with the same conditions as in the current experiment (for the single-dot condition from [12], Exp. 1; for the row-of-dots condition from [9], Exp. 3); error bars represent the standard error of the mean.

(Positive) benefits are defined as the facilitation in compatible trials compared to neutral trials, and (positive) costs are defined as the slowing in incompatible trials compared to neutral trials (i.e., negative benefits = faster neutral than compatible trials; negative costs = faster incompatible than neutral). Compatibility effects (incompatible versus compatible trials) might be made up of benefits and costs. In fact, the positive compatibility effect in short SOAs splits into significant benefits, $F(1, 31) = 18.52$, $p < 0.001$, $\eta_p^2 = 0.374$–$F < 1$ for the moderation by age and $F(1, 31) = 17.23$, $p < 0.001$, $\eta_p^2 = 0.357$ for the moderation by motion type, with benefits with single-dot primes and no benefits with row-of-dots primes, and significant costs, $F(1, 31) = 39.07$, $p < 0.001$, $\eta_p^2 = 0.448$–$F < 1$ for the moderation by age and $F(1, 31) = 4.24$, $p = 0.04$, $\eta_p^2 = 0.125$ for the moderation by motion type, with larger costs with single-dot primes than with row-of-dots primes. Compatibility effects at the short SOA thus were composed of facilitation after compatible row-of-dots primes and deceleration after both incompatible motion type primes.

A further analysis evaluated the correlation between mean reaction time and the size of the compatibility effect in the 147 ms SOA condition, yielding a trend towards a negative correlation ($r(n = 35) = -0.31$, $p = 0.07$). That is, faster participants showed a slightly larger positive compatibility effect (note that age and mean RT are not correlated, $r(n = 35) = 0.09$, $p = 0.61$).

4.2. 360 ms SOA Condition. In the 360 ms SOA condition, we found a significant main effect of Arrow Direction, $F(1, 33) = 4.79$, $p = 0.04$, $\eta_p^2 = 0.13$, and a significant main effect of "Age Group," $F(1, 33) = 6.55$, $p = 0.02$, $\eta_p^2 = 0.17$: participants of the old age group responded more slowly than participants of the middle-aged age group. Further, we found significant interactions of Arrow Direction, Motion Direction, and Motion Type, $F(1, 33) = 5.84$, $p = 0.02$, $\eta_p^2 = 0.15$, as well as of Arrow Direction, Motion Direction, Motion Type, and "Age Group," $F(1, 33) = 4.60$, $p = 0.04$, $\eta_p^2 = 0.12$: we found no compatibility effect in the old age group (neither with single dot, $M = 0$ ms, SE = 10.7, $t(7) = 0$, $p = 1.0$, nor with row of dots, $M = -2$ ms, SE = 8.7, $t(10) = 0.28$, $p = 0.79$). In contrast, in the middle-aged age group, we found the same pattern as found in previous experiments with young participants in the 360 ms SOA condition (see [9, 12]): there was a positive compatibility effect with single-dot primes ($M = 26$ ms, SE = 6.4, $t(12) = 4.06$, $p = 0.002$) and a negative compatibility effect with row-of-dots primes ($M = -15$ ms, SE = 5.8, $t(4) = 2.64$, $p = 0.058$) (to further substantiate these findings, we additionally conducted regression analyses in which age was treated as continuous variable. Compatibility effects of each condition (SOA × Motion Type) were linearly regressed on age. In the 147 ms SOA condition with single-dot primes, there was a trend towards a positive association between age and the compatibility effect, $\beta = 0.46$, $t(14) = 1.92$, $p = 0.076$: with each year, the compatibility effect increases by 1.56. In the 360 ms SOA condition with single-dot primes, there was a negative association between age and the compatibility effect, $\beta = -0.44$, $t(19) = -2.13$, $p = 0.046$: with each year, the compatibility effect decreases by 1.44. In the 147 ms SOA condition with row-of-dots primes, there was no association between age and the compatibility effect, $\beta = 0.11$, $t(17) = -0.30$, $p = 0.77$. In the 360 ms SOA condition with row-of-dots primes, there was a trend towards a positive association between age and the compatibility effect, $\beta = 0.45$, $t(14) = 1.89$, $p = 0.08$: with each year, the negative compatibility effect decreases by 1.65).

With regard to benefits and costs at the longer SOA, we analyzed the effects separately for age groups. The benefits and costs in middle-aged subjects were moderated by motion type, $F(1, 16) = 9.09$, $p = 0.008$, $\eta_p^2 = 0.362$ for benefits and $F(1, 16) = 8.59$, $p = 0.01$, $\eta_p^2 = 0.349$ for costs: there were positive benefits and positive costs with single-dot primes and negative benefits as well as negative costs with row-of-dots primes. Thus, the positive compatibility effect with single-dot primes at the longer SOA for middle-aged subjects is composed of facilitation after compatible primes and deceleration after incompatible primes, and the negative compatibility effect with row-of-dots primes is composed of deceleration after compatible primes and facilitation after incompatible primes. The benefits and costs in old subjects were moderated (at least by trend) by motion type, $F(1, 17) = 3.15$, $p = 0.09$, $\eta_p^2 = 0.156$ for benefits and $F(1, 17) = 3.14$, $p = 0.09$, $\eta_p^2 = 0.156$ for costs: there were negative benefits and positive costs with single-dot primes and positive benefits as well as negative costs with row-of-dots primes.

4.3. Correlation between Mean Reaction Time and Compatibility Effect. A further analysis evaluated the correlation between mean reaction time and the size of the compatibility effect, yielding no correlation ($r(n = 21) = -0.16$, $p = 0.48$) in the single-dot condition and a trend towards a positive correlation ($r(n = 16) = 0.44$, $p = 0.09$) in the row-of-dots condition. That is, in this condition, faster participants showed a larger negative compatibility effect (note that age and mean RT are correlated in the 360 ms conditions, $r(n = 21) = 0.51$, $p = 0.02$, and $r(n = 16) = 0.63$, $p = 0.01$, for the single-dot and row-of-dots condition, resp.).

5. Discussion

In the present study, we conducted a response priming task using moving dots as primes for static arrow targets. We tested two different motion types (single-dot primes and row-of-dots primes) at SOAs of 147 ms and 360 ms with middle-aged (50–65 years) and old (66–87 years) participants. In summary, for middle-aged adults, we found the same pattern of results as with younger participants of previous studies: there were positive compatibility effects with single-dot primes independent of SOA, positive compatibility effects with row-of-dots primes in the short SOA condition, and negative compatibility effects with row-of-dots primes in the longer SOA condition. Further, as expected, in the short SOA condition, middle-aged and old participants showed the same pattern of results with positive effects in both motion type conditions and the age groups showed impressively similar reaction times in the motion type conditions (Table 1). Importantly, there was a difference between middle-aged and old participants in the longer SOA condition: old participants showed no compatibility effects, neither a positive effect with single-dot primes nor a negative effect with row-of-dots primes. That is, separate things seem to happen after 147 ms in middle-aged and old adults. In the following, we discuss these main findings of our experiment.

First, as expected [12], we found overall larger compatibility effects with the single-dot motion type than with the row-of-dots motion type. This could be further evidenced that different motion types trigger initial activation processes differently. The single-dot primes seem to release larger and/or more directed and focused activation than row-of-dots primes. When looking at benefits and costs, compatibility effects with single-dot primes are composed of facilitation and deceleration. In contrast, (positive) compatibility effects with row-of-dots primes solely are based on deceleration. There is an ongoing debate on the relationship between activation and inhibition processes. Generally, it is assumed that inhibition is released only when a high level of internal activation is reached (e.g., [41]). However, in our case, activation after row-of-dots primes might be more blurred—as might be the case with masked primes, too. Thus, the requirement of inhibition might be stronger after row-of-dots primes. A further explanation might be that single dot and row of dots are differently suitable as triggers for opening the evaluation window [38]. According to this account, negative compatibility effects will result if the prime falls outside the evaluation window and positive compatibility effects will result if the prime falls inside the evaluation window. In turn, row-of-dots primes might lead to a later opening of the evaluation window which does not include the prime, resulting in negative compatibility effects. In contrast, single-dot primes might act as a signal to open the evaluation window with their start (or vice versa, they might be less distinguishable from the entire stream of incoming events and not act as a signal to open the evaluation window with their *end*), resulting in positive compatibility effects. In either case (impaired inhibition and evaluation windows account), our results again showed that the role of a mask (e.g., Jaśkowski, 2007, 2008) [35] is not decisive—as we had no mask at all.

Second, we found exactly the same pattern in the middle-aged age group as with young participants in previous studies [9, 12]: there were positive compatibility effects with both motion types in the short SOA condition (as expected, larger effects with the single-dot motion type than the row-of-dots motion type) and positive compatibility effects in the longer SOA condition with the single-dot motion type, but negative effects with the row-of-dots motion type. This pattern can be seen as evidence that middle-aged participants have no obvious relevant impairments of activation, inhibition, attention, and/or decay processes, as compared to young participants. Our finding is somewhat different to that of Seiss and Praamstra [31] who found only reduced negative compatibility effects with middle-aged participants. Probably, motion has a generally higher salience than static symbols. Additionally, directional motion is closely related to spatial attention (e.g., [42]), again also due to the fact that motion is a nonsymbolic prime which might trigger an own motion directly, whereas static stimuli (e.g., shapes, colors, words) represent symbolic and abstract information which has to be transformed from the symbol to task-specific requirements in a first step (we thank Friederike Schlaghecken for suggesting this point). Thus, activation and following inhibition can be released faster than with static stimuli.

Third, in the short SOA condition, we found comparable positive compatibility effects in middle-aged and old participants (for both motion types) with even slightly larger compatibility effects in the old than the middle-aged age group with single-dot primes. That is, participants of both age groups preactivated the response tendency associated with the prime (at least after single-dot primes), resulting in faster responses to compatible than incompatible targets. This finding perfectly matches previous findings showing sustained or even enhanced activation [25, 27]. In neuroimaging studies, larger and/or more distributed activation in older compared to younger persons has oftentimes been found (for a review, see, e.g., [43]). There is ongoing debate as to whether the activation patterns in old age reflect compensation or inappropriate processing (for reviews, see, e.g., [44, 45]). Overall, we see the pronounced positive compatibility effects in the short SOA condition as evidence that there are no general activation deficits, especially not in the old age group. This is comparable to other findings in which there was no age-related decrement in initial activation (e.g., [25]).

Fourth and most interesting, there are differences between the age groups in the longer SOA conditions—here, middle-aged participants showed positive compatibility effects with single-dot primes and negative compatibility effects with row-of-dots primes. This mirrors the effects for young adults. In contrast, we found no compatibility effects in old participants in the longer SOA conditions. First, the lack of negative compatibility effects with row-of-dots primes matches expectations based on other findings and can be explained with reduced inhibition and impaired low-level motor control (e.g., [25]), as well as with the evaluation windows account [38] and the assumption of a more sluggish temporal processing in old age [35]. According to the deautomatization account by Maylor et al. [33], we would have expected larger negative compatibility effects with longer response times in the longer SOA condition (especially for row-of-dots primes). However, our correlation analysis showed—by trend—the opposite pattern: shorter response times are associated with larger negative compatibility effects (but note that age and response times are also correlated here). Second, according to previous findings and theoretical ideas, we should have found positive compatibility effects with single-dot primes (comparable to young and middle-aged participants), as activation processes are not assumed to be reduced in older age (e.g., [27]). The lack of (positive) compatibility effects with single-dot primes in the longer SOA is thus surprising.

How can this be explained? We again may refer to the theories already mentioned above. Perhaps, with larger initial activations in old people, the requirement of faster/earlier inhibition is given. Thus, the finding of no compatibility effect might reflect an intermediate state and lead subsequently to a negative compatibility effect with longer SOAs which might be an interesting question for future research. Note that, for young participants and single-dot primes, negative compatibility effects may only occur with rather long SOAs (above 800 ms). Alternatively, the deautomatization of low-level control could lead to controlled inhibition with the same time course independently of material and initial activation resulting in the same null effect with row-of-dots and single-dot primes. Last, but not least, we propose a further explanation whereby our results are evidence that activation processes change with age (in contrast to the inhibitory deficit theory; e.g., [27]).

Accordingly, a plausible alternative assumption is that, in older adulthood, activation processes are also altered, or more specifically, there might be a lack of (preceding) sustained activation in longer SOAs. Thus, inhibition is not initiated due to this lack of sustained activation. As found in other studies (e.g., [27, 46]), there is larger initial activation in older age, often interpreted as reflecting compensatory processes. Rapid decay of activation, in turn, could be caused by such compensatory processes. Such processes might limit the capacity to sustain the initial activation. Thus, no positive compatibility effects occur with the longer SOA of 360 ms after an initially large positive compatibility effect with the short SOA of 147 ms in the old age group. However, the results of Schlaghecken and Maylor [25] seem to stand at odds with this interpretation as they found positive priming effects (i.e., activation) in older adults, but not negative priming effects (i.e., inhibition). However, they tested positive and negative compatibility with different SOAs, of course (i.e., 33 ms for PCEs and 183 ms for NCEs, see above). Due to differences in timing caused by different SOAs and resulting in different time distances between prime presentation/initial activation release and target presentation/response execution, it is unclear whether the lack of compatibility effects in old age is caused by impaired automatic inhibition or whether there is a more rapid activation decay than in younger persons (please note that this explanation will not conflict with the deautomatization account, e.g., [33]). That is, it could be that, in old age, (1) activation decays rapidly without the necessity to initiate inhibition processes, or (2) no initiation of automatic inhibition processes is actually possible. Both explanations would result in a lack of negative compatibility effects with longer SOAs, even after a high level of initial activation (expressed in positive priming effects with shorter SOAs). With our paradigm, it was possible to compare conditions in which positive and negative priming effects occur at the same SOA of 360 ms (single-dot primes: positive priming effects; row-of-dots primes: negative priming effects) in young age. Thus, the results with old participants can also be explained by a rapid decay of initial activation, which removed the need for the release of inhibitory processes. Thus, we propose the interpretation that the lack of compatibility effects can be seen as evidence for a rapid decay of initial activation.

Additionally, we would like to propose a further argument for our point that the lack of negative compatibility effects in old age is not (fully) caused by impaired automatic inhibition. In contrast to some response priming experiments, we included a neutral condition in which the prime is associated with neither the left nor the right response; thus, no specific directional preactivation is possible. With the row-of-dots motion type in the short SOA condition, we found no differences between compatible and the neutral conditions, neither in the middle-aged age group, nor in the old age group, nor in comparable experiments with young age groups ([9], Exp. 1, Exp. 3). In contrast, the positive compatibility effects result from response time differences between the incompatible and the neutral condition (i.e., costs)—we found slower responses in incompatible than neutral trials. That is, some kind of inhibition process was released for incompatible targets, slowed the responses to them, and caused the overall positive compatibility effect. As there is no difference between age groups, this kind of inhibition also occurs in the old age group. We take this as evidence that inhibition is not generally impaired (in response priming tasks) in old age. Further, with single-dot primes, the missing compatibility effect in old participants is the result of decelerations after both compatible and incompatible primes (compared to neutral). That is, each kind of directional activation seems to be downregulated or decayed. With row-of-dots primes, the compatibility effect is also cancelled out by equally high facilitation after compatible and incompatible primes (compared to neutral).

Finally, as already pointed out by Bermeitinger [9], our pattern of results also matches results from another background, that is, from attention research (see also [24]). This is especially relevant as we used somewhat unusual targets that were slightly larger than the region of foveal vision. Research on spatial attention shows that when responding to a target stimulus, people are typically slower when it appears at least approximately 200 ms later at the same location as a previous event (up to 200 ms, benefits often are found). The phenomenon is often called inhibition of return (IOR; for a review, see, e.g., [47]). Castel et al. [46] investigated the time course of IOR in young and old participants. The results showed larger initial facilitation at shorter SOAs in older than in younger participants—comparable to our findings here—and 300 ms delayed IOR effects in older than in younger participants—comparable to the findings of, for example, Maylor et al. [33]. Castel et al. did not try to explain their results, except for the comment that there might be changes in the temporal dynamics of inhibition with age. Overall, it is open to future research how far IOR and priming research could and should be considered together.

To conclude, the patterns (at least parts of them) found in our study can be explained with recourse to several theories (i.e., impaired low-level motor control, evaluation windows account, attention theories) and even as evidence for a rapid decay of initial activation and not (or not exclusively) impaired inhibition in older age. Our study had the advantage that we could measure positive and negative compatibility effects at the same SOA by means of two different motion types as primes. Different elapsed time between prime and target as well as explanations relying on some kind of mask can be excluded as explanations for differences in compatibility effects and our results in general. Thus, the specific material and task are suitable for future research to study further differences between age groups and activation, inhibition, timing, and/or decay processes. Future research should also test some of the explanations in direct comparison with each other which was not the in the scope of the current (exploratory) study.

Conflicts of Interest

The authors declare that they have no conflicts of interest.

Acknowledgments

The authors thank Heidi Femppel, Mareike Walther, Svenia Prinzhorn, Luise Maier, Laura Flatau, and Nicolas Salzer for their help in data collection. Many thanks go to Ryan Hacklaender who improved the readability of the article. The authors also thank Christian Frings, Friederike Schlaghecken, Bernhard Hommel, Stuart Klapp, Dirk Wentura, Markus Janczyk, and Wilfried Kunde for their helpful comments on the project and on some data the paper is related to.

References

[1] T. Farroni, S. Massaccesi, D. Pividori, F. Simion, and M. H. Johnson, "Gaze following in newborns," *Infancy*, vol. 5, no. 1, pp. 39–60, 2004.

[2] F. Simion, L. Regolin, and H. Bulf, "A predisposition for biological motion in the newborn baby," *Proceedings of the National Academy of Sciences*, vol. 15, no. 2, pp. 809–813, 2008.

[3] S. Bosbach, W. Prinz, and D. Kerzel, "Movement-based compatibility in simple response tasks," *European Journal of Cognitive Psychology*, vol. 17, no. 5, pp. 695–707, 2005.

[4] H. E. Egeth and S. Yantis, "Visual attention: control, representation, and time course," *Annual Review of Psychology*, vol. 48, no. 1, pp. 269–297, 1997.

[5] B. Hommel, J. Müsseler, G. Aschersleben, and W. Prinz, "The theory of event coding (TEC): a framework for perception and action planning," *Behavioral and Brain Sciences*, vol. 24, no. 5, pp. 849–937, 2001.

[6] R. D. Seidler, J. A. Bernard, T. B. Burutulo et al., "Motor control and aging: links to age-related brain structural, functional, and biochemical effects," *Neuroscience and Biobehavioral Reviews*, vol. 34, no. 5, pp. 721–733, 2010.

[7] F. Schmidt, A. Haberkamp, and T. Schmidt, "Dos and don'ts in response priming research," *Advances in Cognitive Psychology*, vol. 7, no. 1, pp. 120–131, 2011.

[8] M. Eimer and F. Schlaghecken, "Links between conscious awareness and response inhibition: evidence from masked priming," *Psychonomic Bulletin and Review*, vol. 9, no. 3, pp. 514–520, 2002.

[9] C. Bermeitinger, "Response priming with apparent motion primes," *Psychological Research*, vol. 77, no. 4, pp. 371–387, 2013.

[10] R. Hacklaender, D. Eckert, and C. Bermeitinger, "Visual processing: the role of importance," in *Advances in Visual Perception Research*, T. Heinen, Ed., pp. 1–28, Nova Publishing, New York, NY, USA, 2015.

[11] C. Bermeitinger and R. P. Hackländer, "Response priming with motion primes: negative compatibility or congruency effects, even in free-choice trials," *Cognitive Processing*, 2018, In press.

[12] C. Bermeitinger and D. Wentura, "Moving single dots as primes for static arrow targets: negative effects at very long SOAs," *Experimental Psychology*, vol. 63, no. 2, pp. 127–139, 2016.

[13] A. Kiesel, W. Kunde, and J. Hoffmann, "Mechanisms of subliminal response priming," *Advances in Cognitive Psychology*, vol. 3, no. 1, pp. 307–315, 2007.

[14] F. Schlaghecken, H. Bowman, and M. Eimer, "Dissociating local and global levels of perceptuo-motor control in masked

priming," *Journal of Experimental Psychology: Human Perception and Performance*, vol. 32, no. 3, pp. 618–494, 2006.

[15] F. Schlaghecken and M. Eimer, "Motor activation with and without inhibition: evidence for a threshold mechanism in motor control," *Perception & Psychophysics*, vol. 64, no. 1, pp. 148-162, 2002.

[16] F. Schlaghecken and M. Eimer, "Active masks and active inhibition: a comment on Lleras and Enns (2004) and on Verleger, Jaśkowski, Aydemir, van der Lubbe, and Groen (2004)," *Journal of Experimental Psychology: General*, vol. 135, no. 3, pp. 484–494, 2006.

[17] F. Schlaghecken, L. Rowley, S. Sembi, R. Simmons, and D. Whitcomb, "The negative compatibility effect: a case for self-inhibition," *Advances in Cognitive Psychology*, vol. 3, no. 1, pp. 227–240, 2007.

[18] S. T. Klapp, "Two versions of the negative compatibility effect: comment on Lleras and Enns (2004)," *Journal of Experimental Psychology: General*, vol. 134, no. 3, pp. 431–440, 2005.

[19] P. Sumner, "Negative and positive masked-priming–implications for motor inhibition," *Advances in Cognitive Psychology*, vol. 3, no. 1, pp. 317–326, 2007.

[20] L. Machado, N. Wyatt, A. Devine, and B. Knight, "Action planning in the presence of distracting stimuli: an investigation into the time course of distractor effects," *Journal of Experimental Psychology: Human Perception and Performance*, vol. 33, no. 5, pp. 1045–1061, 2007.

[21] P. Jaśkowski, A. Białuńska, M. Tomanek, and R. Verleger, "Mask- and distractor-triggered inhibitory processes in the priming of motor response: an EEG study," *Psychophysiology*, vol. 45, no. 1, pp. 70–85, 2008.

[22] A. Lleras and J. T. Enns, "Negative compatibility or object updating? A cautionary tale of mask-dependent priming," *Journal of Experimental Psychology: General*, vol. 133, no. 4, pp. 475–493, 2004.

[23] R. Verleger, P. Jaśkowski, A. Aydemir, R. H. J. van der Lubbe, and M. Groen, "Qualitative differences between conscious and nonconscious processing? On inverse priming induced by masked arrows," *Journal of Experimental Psychology: General*, vol. 133, no. 4, pp. 494–515, 2004.

[24] G. G. Cole and G. Kuhn, "What the experimenter's prime tells the observer's brain," *Attention, Perception, and Psychophysics*, vol. 72, no. 5, pp. 1367–1376, 2010.

[25] F. Schlaghecken and E. A. Maylor, "Motor control in old age: evidence of impaired low-level inhibition," *Journal of Gerontology Series B: Psychological Sciences and Social Sciences*, vol. 60, no. 3, pp. P158–P161, 2005.

[26] L. Hasher and R. T. Zacks, "Working memory, comprehension, and aging: a review and a new view," in *The Psychology of Learning and Motivation*, G. H. Bower, Ed., vol. 22, pp. 193–225, Academic Press, New York, NY, USA, 1988.

[27] C. Lustig, L. Hasher, and R. T. Zacks, "Inhibitory deficit theory: recent developments in a "new view," in *Inhibition in Cognition*, D. S. Gorfein and C. M. McLeod, Eds., pp. 145–162, American Psychological Association, Washington, DC, USA, 2007.

[28] J. R. Jennings, D. N. Mendelson, M. S. Redfern, and R. D. Nebes, "Detecting age differences in inhibition processes with a test of perceptual and motor inhibition," *Experimental Aging Research*, vol. 37, no. 2, pp. 179–197, 2011.

[29] J. A. Anguera and A. Gazzaley, "Dissociation of motor and sensory inhibition processes in normal aging," *Clinical Neurophysiology*, vol. 123, no. 4, pp. 730–740, 2012.

[30] P. Sumner, P. Nachev, P. Morris et al., "Human medial frontal cortex mediates unconscious inhibition of voluntary action," *Neuron*, vol. 54, no. 5, pp. 697–711, 2007.

[31] E. Seiss and P. Praamstra, "The basal ganglia and inhibitory mechanisms in response selection: evidence from subliminal priming of motor responses in Parkinson's disease," *Brain*, vol. 127, no. 2, pp. 330–339, 2004.

[32] E. Seiss and P. Praamstra, "Time-course of masked response priming and inhibition in Parkinson's disease," *Neuropsychologia*, vol. 44, no. 6, pp. 869–875, 2006.

[33] E. A. Maylor, K. S. Birak, and F. Schlaghecken, "Inhibitory motor control in old age: evidence for de-automatization?," *Frontiers in Psychology*, vol. 2, p. 132, 2011.

[34] F. Schlaghecken, K. S. Birak, and E. A. Maylor, "Age-related deficits in efficiency of low-level lateral inhibition," *Frontiers in Human Neuroscience*, vol. 6, 2012.

[35] R. Verleger, "Slowing of mask-triggered inhibition in the elderly," *Frontiers in Psychology*, vol. 2, p. 138, 2011.

[36] P. Jaśkowski, "The effect of nonmasking distractors on the priming of motor responses," *Journal of Experimental Psychology: Human Perception and Performance*, vol. 33, no. 2, pp. 456–468, 2007.

[37] P. Jaśkowski, "The negative compatibility effect with nonmasking flankers: a case for mask-triggered inhibition hypothesis," *Consciousness and Cognition*, vol. 17, no. 3, pp. 765–777, 2008.

[38] K. C. Klauer and K. Dittrich, "From sunshine to double arrows: an evaluation window account of negative compatibility effects," *Journal of Experimental Psychology: General*, vol. 139, no. 3, pp. 490–519, 2010.

[39] F. Faul, E. Erdfelder, A. G. Lang, and A. Buchner, "G*Power 3: a flexible statistical power analysis program for the social, behavioral, and biomedical sciences," *Behavior Research Methods*, vol. 39, no. 2, pp. 175–191, 2007.

[40] J. W. Tukey, *Exploratory Data Analysis*, Addison-Wesley, Reading, MA, USA, 1977.

[41] G. Houghton and S. P. Tipper, "Inhibitory mechanisms of neural and cognitive control: applications to selective attention and sequential action," *Brain and Cognition*, vol. 30, no. 1, pp. 20–43, 1996.

[42] Y. Xu, S. Suzuki, and S. L. Franconeri, "Shifting selection may control apparent motion," *Psychological Science*, vol. 24, no. 7, pp. 1368–1370, 2013.

[43] N. S. Ward, "Compensatory mechanisms in the aging motor system," *Ageing Research Reviews*, vol. 5, no. 3, pp. 239–254, 2006.

[44] M. N. Rajah and M. D'Esposito, "Region-specific changes in prefrontal function with age: a review of PET and fMRI studies on working and episodic memory," *Brain*, vol. 128, no. 9, pp. 1964–1983, 2005.

[45] P. A. Reuter-Lorenz and C. Lustig, "Brain aging: reorganizing discoveries about the aging mind," *Current Opinion in Neurobiology*, vol. 15, no. 2, pp. 245–251, 2005.

[46] A. D. Castel, A. L. Chasteen, C. T. Scialfa, and J. Pratt, "Adult age differences in the time course of inhibition of return," *Journal of Gerontology Series B: Psychological Sciences*, vol. 58, no. 5, pp. P256–P259, 2003.

[47] J. Lupiáñez, R. M. Klein, and P. Bartolomeo, "Inhibition of return: twenty years after," *Cognitive Neuropsychology*, vol. 23, no. 7, pp. 1003–1014, 2006.

19

The Effect of Age on Fracture Risk: A Population-Based Cohort Study

Wenbin Liang and Tanya Chikritzhs

National Drug Research Institute, Curtin University, GPO Box U1987, Perth, WA 6845, Australia

Correspondence should be addressed to Wenbin Liang; w.liang@curtin.edu.au

Academic Editor: F. R. Ferraro

Aim. To precisely estimate the effect of age on the risk of fracture hospitalisation among the Western Australia population over the life course. *Methods.* This population-based cohort study used hospital data on fractures for the period January 1991 to January 2013 among Western Australians born between 1915 and 1990. *Results.* The average incidence rates (per 10,000 person-years) of fracture hospitalisation (95% confidence interval) were 50.12 (49.90, 50.35), 55.14 (54.82, 55.48), and 45.02 (44.71, 45.32) for both males and females, males only, and females only, respectively. The age-specific rate of fracture hospitalisation (in natural logarithm form) in adults (>18 years) was well predicted by age at its 1st, 2nd, and 3rd power in males with an adjusted R-squared of 0.98 and $p < 0.001$. For females, the trend was also well predicted by its 1st and 2nd powers (the 3rd power term of age was removed due to its p value > 0.8) with an adjusted R-squared of 0.99 and $p < 0.001$. *Conclusions.* Overall trends in age and gender specific risk of fracture among the Western Australian population were similar to estimates reported from previous studies. The trend in fracture hospitalisation risk over the life course can be almost fully explained by age.

1. Introduction

Injuries are a major cause of morbidity and mortality in both developing and developed countries, while fractures account for a substantial proportion of injuries [1–3]. Fractures not only cause temporary or permanent physical disability but may also impair the overall life quality and mental health of affected individuals [4, 5] and lead to significant burden on healthcare systems as well as family carers [1, 5–7]. Age and gender are important factors that influence the risk of fractures [8]. A number of European epidemiological studies have focused on the effects of age and gender among adult [9–14] and child [15–18] populations. There are limited data available on the overall lifetime incidence rate of fracture among the general Australian population [19, 20], and the majority of Australian studies have focused on site specific fractures [20–22]. In this study, we aim to investigate the effect of age and gender on the risk of fracture among the Western Australian population and apply age to model fracture risk over the life course with good precision.

2. Method

This population-based cohort study used hospital separation data on injuries and fractures due to injuries for the period January 1991 to January 2013 among Western Australians (WA) born between 1915 and 1990 (participants are 75–0 years old at baseline). Data were extracted from the WA Hospital Morbidity Data System by the WA Department of Health. The WA Hospital Morbidity Data System included separations from all WA public and private acute hospitals [23]. Hospitalisation records were coded using ICD-9 between 1990/91 and 1998/99 (fiscal year) and ICD-10 classification system from 1999/00. In this study primary diagnosis, codes including ICD-9 codes (800–829) and ICD-10 codes (S12, S22, S32, S42, S52, S62, S72, S82, S92, T02, T08, T10, and T12) were used to identify fracture cases, whereas External Causes of Injury and Poisoning (ICD-9) and External Causes of Morbidity and Mortality (ICD-10) were used to define hospitalisations due to injuries (rather than pathologic causes). Annual estimates of WA gender and age-specific residential populations over the

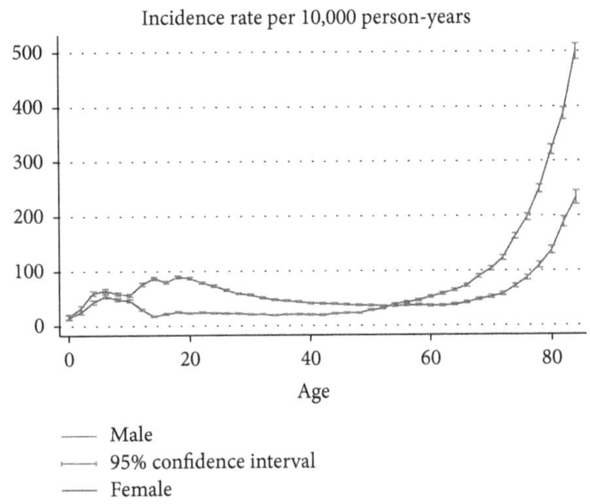

FIGURE 1: Gender-age-specific incidence rates of fracture hospitalisation.

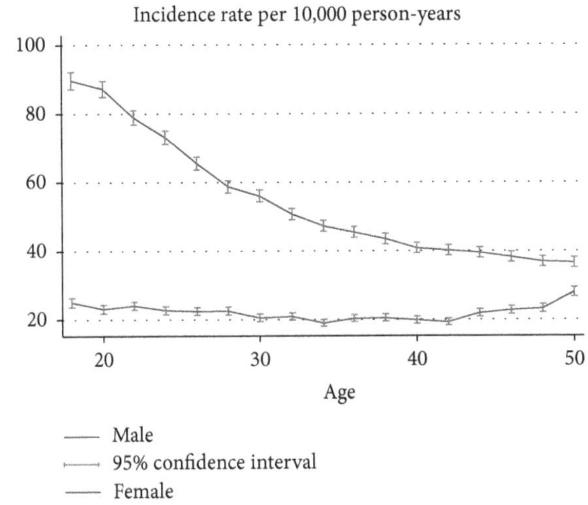

FIGURE 2: Gender-age-specific incidence rates of fracture hospitalisation for the age between 18 and 50 years.

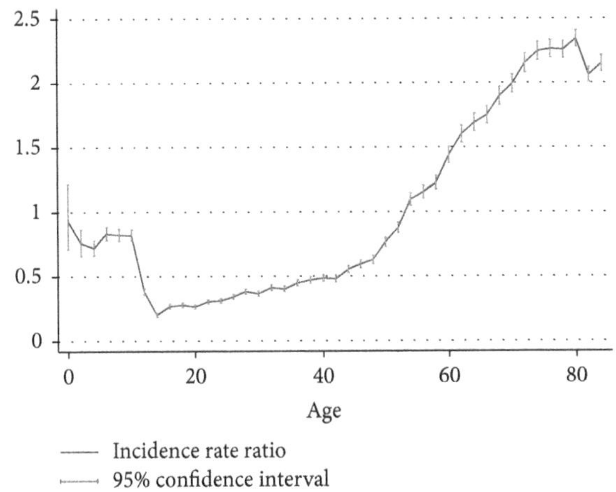

FIGURE 3: Age-specific female-to-male incidence rate ratios of fracture hospitalisations.

observation period were provided by the Australian Bureau of Statistics (ABS).

3. Data Analysis

In the descriptive analysis, overall and age-specific incidence rates of fracture were estimated by age between 0 and 85 years in 2-year intervals, separately for males and females. The age-specific incidence rates were then used to compute the cumulative risk of having at least one fracture hospitalisation for males and females. The risk of hospitalisation due to any injury (including nonfracture cases) was also described using gender and age-specific incidence rates. To investigate how the effects of gender may change over the lifetime, age-specific female-to-male incidence rate ratios were estimated. Log-linear models with age, age to the power of 2, and age to the power of 3 as predictors were fitted based on the age-specific risk of fracture for ages 18 to 85, separately for males and females.

4. Results

Overall 193,434 cases of fracture hospitalisation arose from 38,591,627 person-years of observation. The average incidence rates (per 10,000 person-years) of fracture hospitalisation (95% confidence interval) were 50.12 (49.90, 50.35), 55.14 (54.82, 55.48), and 45.02 (44.71, 45.32) for both males and females, males only, and females only, respectively. The incidence rates (per 10,000 person-years) for overall injury hospitalisations (95% confidence interval) were 151.24 (150.85, 151.63), 168.82 (168.2, 169.40), and 133.37 (132.85, 133.89) for both males and females, males only, and females only, respectively. The overall fracture-to-injury risk ratio was about 1 to 3.

The gender-age-specific incidence rates of fracture hospitalisation are shown in Figure 1. Figure 2 provides a close-up illustration of the risk pattern for ages 18–50 years. Overall, the risk of fracture increased continuously up to 8 years of age and remained unchanged between 6 and 11 years for both genders. From the age of 12, the risk of fracture increased gradually until the age of 19 in males, whereas the risk of fracture decreased over adolescent period for females. The risk of fracture declined in males from age 20 years through to the late 40s; among females, however, the risk of fracture began increasing from about the age of 42 years. Up to the age of 54 years, the incidence rate of fracture was consistently higher for males compared to females; thereafter, female rates exceeded male rates and remained higher to the end of the observation period. Accordingly, the age-specific female-to-male incidence rate ratios of fracture increased from the age of 20 (Figure 3). The pattern of age-specific injury hospitalisation rates appeared to be similar between the two genders, except for ages 55 to 65, when the risk of injury continuously increased in females but remained largely unchanged in males (Figure 6).

The age-specific rate of fracture (in natural logarithm form) in adults (>18 years) was well predicted by age at its

TABLE 1: log-linear model of age-specific fracture hospitalisation rates.

Gender	Model and estimated coefficients
Male	$\ln(\text{risk of fracture}) = 4.648261 + 0.0158851 \times \text{age} - 0.0017527 \times \text{age}^2 + 0.0000198 \times \text{age}^3$
Female	$\ln(\text{risk of fracture}) = 4.405889 - 0.0843678 \times \text{age} + 0.0012531 \times \text{age}^2$

ln: natural logarithm.

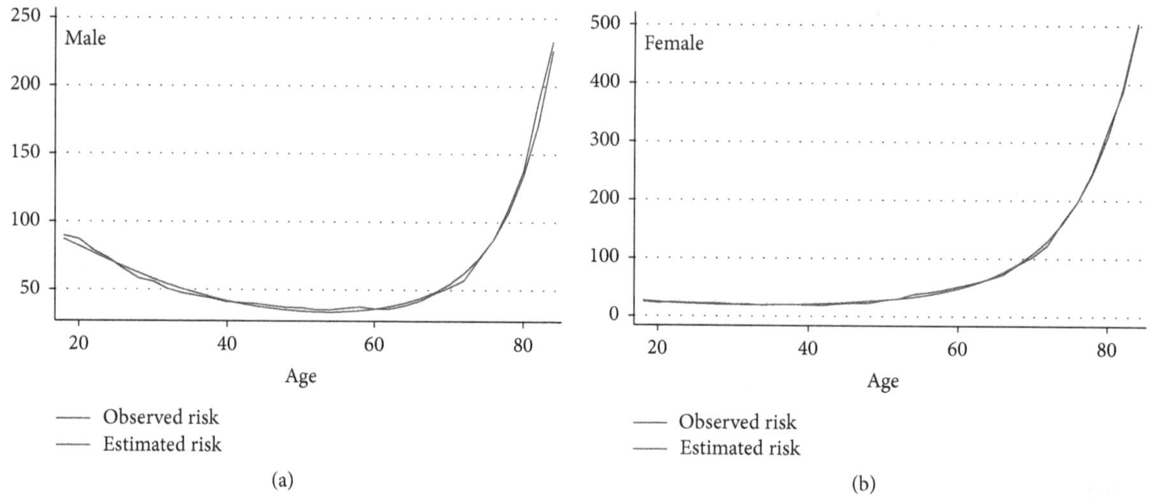

FIGURE 4: Comparison between observed gender-age-specific incidence rates of fracture hospitalisation and estimates from log-linear model (per 10,000 person-years).

1st, 2nd, and 3rd power in males with an adjusted R-squared of 0.98 ($p < 0.001$). For females, the trend was also well predicted by its 1st and 2nd powers (the 3rd power term of age was removed due to its p value > 0.8) with an adjusted R-squared of 0.99 ($p < 0.001$) (see Table 1). Comparison between the observed incidence rates of facture and estimates from the model are shown in Figure 4.

For males and females, respectively, the cumulative risk of having at least one fracture hospitalisation due to injury was 11.8% and 6.3% by the age of 18 years, increased to 23.8% and 11.4% by the age of 45 years and increased again to 37.4% and 37.6% by 80 years (Figure 5).

5. Discussion

This study provided a detailed picture of the risk of fracture hospitalisations among the Western Australia population. Overall trends in age and gender specific risk of fracture were similar to observations from previous studies conducted on other populations [9–14, 20, 24]. The relative increase in fracture risk among females compared to males throughout the 20s and 30s (Figure 3) was also evident although this has not been explored in detail in some of the earlier studies [12, 13, 19]. This increasing trend of female-to-male fracture incidence rate ratios appears to be driven by a decrease in risk for males and stable risk for females in that age period (Figure 2). However, the age-specific risk of all injuries appeared to decrease at a similar rate for the two genders (Figure 6), and therefore the increase in female-to-male incidence rate ratio in the 20s and 30s is unlikely to be entirely due to reductions in involvement of injury-related activities among males as they mature. The observed gender difference in the age-specific trend of fracture over this age period may be due to sex-specific changes in musculoskeletal fitness. This study also showed that the changes in the probability of fracture in adults over the life course can be expressed as a function of age. This suggests that the variation in fracture risk at different life stages is driven by risk factors (causes) that are determined or strongly associated with age. There is good evidence suggesting that the progression of osteoporosis [6, 25], changes in musculoskeletal fitness [2, 26], probability of involvement in injury-related behaviours [26, 27], and having certain health conditions [8, 28] are dependent on age; however, it is unclear what other factors may underpin the strong association between fracture risk and age, and further research is required.

This study has some limitations. The analyses relied entirely on hospitalisation cases, which do not include fractures that are treated by outpatient services (such as at Emergency Departments and GP clinics) and which may be relatively less severe. In addition, the study is unable to distinguish first ever and secondary fractures. However, strengths of the study include its very large population-based sample, long follow-up period, application of a number of statistical methods, and the provision of detailed estimates of the absolute risks and cumulative risk of facture from birth to 85 years. In addition, this study showed that the trend in

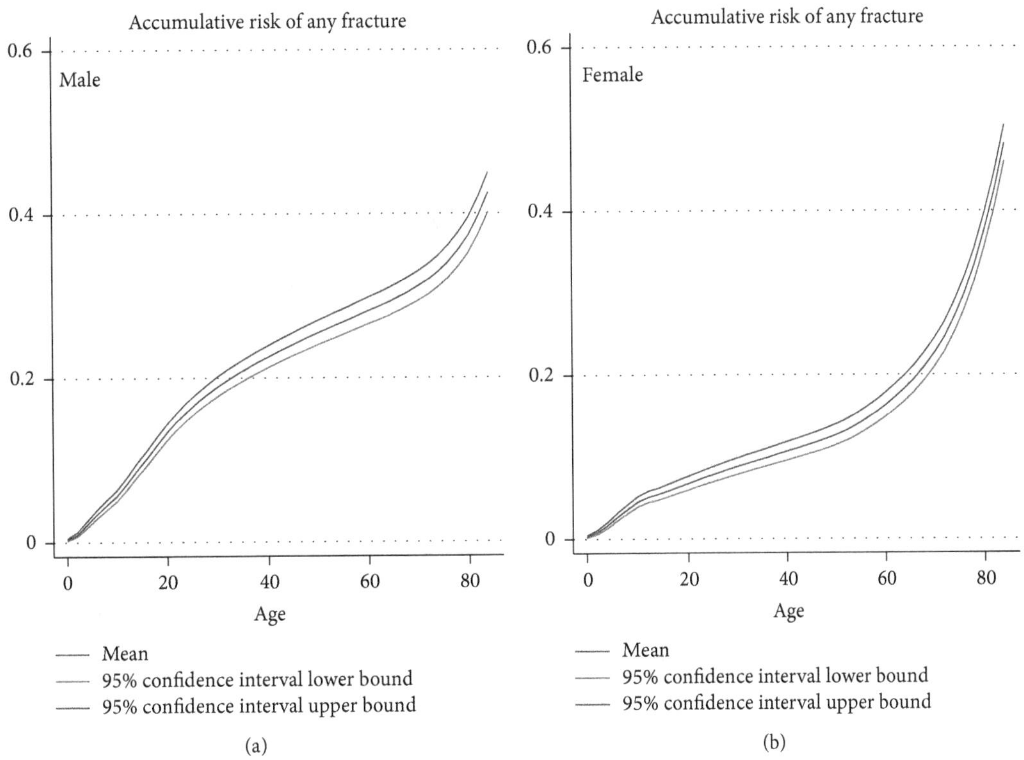

FIGURE 5: Cumulative risk of having any fracture hospitalisation since birth.

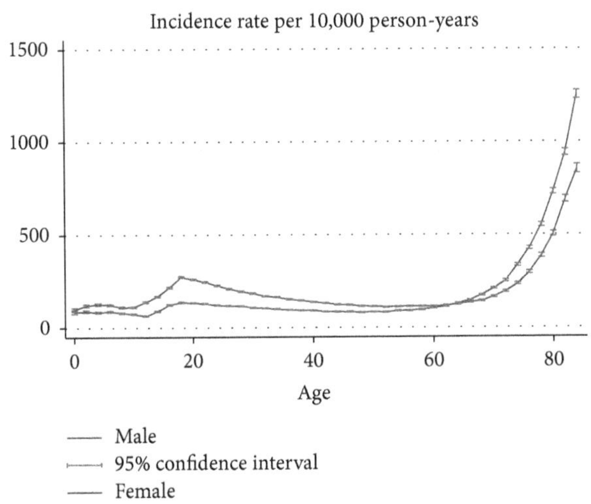

FIGURE 6: Gender-age-specific overall injury hospitalisations rates.

fracture risk over the life course can be almost fully explained (i.e., predicted) by age.

6. Conclusion

Overall trends in age and gender specific risk of fracture among the WA population were similar to estimates reported from previous studies. There is a relative increase in fracture risk among females compared to males throughout their 20s and 30s which could not be explained by reductions in injury-related activities among males. The trend in fracture risk over the life course can be almost fully explained by age.

Ethical Approval

This study has been approved by Department of Health Western Australia Human Research Ethics Committee and by Human Research Ethics Committee, Curtin University (approval number NDRI-04-2013).

Competing Interests

The authors declare that there is no conflict of interests regarding the publication of this paper.

Acknowledgments

This work was supported by the Australian Government Department of Health and Ageing under the National Drug Strategy's funding of the National Drug Research Institute. This work was also supported by Healthway and the Drug and Alcohol Office, Western Australia. The authors thank the Western Australia Department of Health and Australian Bureau of Statistics for providing the data used in this study.

References

[1] S. Polinder, W. J. Meerding, S. Mulder et al., "Assessing the burden of injury in six European countries," *Bulletin of the World Health Organization*, vol. 85, no. 1, pp. 27–34, 2007.

[2] C. Mock and M. N. Cherian, "The global burden of musculoskeletal injuries: challenges and solutions," *Clinical Orthopaedics and Related Research*, vol. 466, no. 10, pp. 2306–2316, 2008.

[3] T. Vos, A. D. Flaxman, M. Naghavi et al., "Years lived with disability (YLDs) for 1160 sequelae of 289 diseases and injuries 1990–2010: a systematic analysis for the Global Burden of Disease Study 2010," *The Lancet*, vol. 380, no. 9859, pp. 2163–2196, 2012.

[4] I. A. Harris, J. M. Young, B. B. Jalaludin, and M. J. Solomon, "The effect of compensation on general health in patients sustaining fractures in motor vehicle trauma," *Journal of Orthopaedic Trauma*, vol. 22, no. 4, pp. 216–220, 2008.

[5] S. Boufous and A. Williamson, "Work-related injury in NSW hospitalisation and workers' compensation datasets: a comparative analysis," *Australian and New Zealand Journal of Public Health*, vol. 27, no. 3, pp. 352–357, 2003.

[6] A. D. Woolf and B. Pfleger, "Burden of major musculoskeletal conditions," *Bulletin of the World Health Organization*, vol. 81, no. 9, pp. 646–656, 2003.

[7] P. Mujuru, L. Singla, J. Helmkamp, J. Bell, and W. Hu, "Evaluation of the burden of logging injuries using West Virginia workers' compensation claims data from 1996 to 2001," *American Journal of Industrial Medicine*, vol. 49, no. 12, pp. 1039–1045, 2006.

[8] J. A. Kanis, H. Johansson, A. Oden, and E. V. McCloskey, "Assessment of fracture risk," *European Journal of Radiology*, vol. 71, no. 3, pp. 392–397, 2009.

[9] M. R. Brinker and D. P. O'Connor, "The incidence of fractures and dislocations referred for orthopaedic services in a capitated population," *The Journal of Bone & Joint Surgery—American Volume*, vol. 86, no. 2, pp. 290–297, 2004.

[10] B. R. Singer, G. J. McLauchlan, C. M. Robinson, and J. Christie, "Epidemiology of fractures in 15,000 adults: the influence of age and gender," *The Journal of Bone & Joint Surgery—British Volume*, vol. 80, no. 2, pp. 243–248, 1998.

[11] L. J. Donaldson, A. Cook, and R. G. Thomson, "Incidence of fractures in a geographically defined population," *Journal of Epidemiology and Community Health*, vol. 44, no. 3, pp. 241–245, 1990.

[12] C. M. Court-Brown and B. Caesar, "Epidemiology of adult fractures: a review," *Injury*, vol. 37, no. 8, pp. 691–697, 2006.

[13] T. P. van Staa, E. M. Dennison, H. G. M. Leufkens, and C. Cooper, "Epidemiology of fractures in England and Wales," *Bone*, vol. 29, no. 6, pp. 517–522, 2001.

[14] D. Fife and J. I. Barancik, "Northeastern Ohio trauma study III: incidence of fractures," *Annals of Emergency Medicine*, vol. 14, no. 3, pp. 244–248, 1985.

[15] E. M. Hedström, O. Svensson, U. Bergström, and P. Michno, "Epidemiology of fractures in children and adolescents: increased incidence over the past decade: a population-based study from northern Sweden," *Acta Orthopaedica*, vol. 81, no. 1, pp. 148–153, 2010.

[16] P.-H. Randsborg, "Fractures in children: aspects on health service, epidemiology and risk factors," *Acta Orthopaedica*, vol. 84, no. 350, pp. 1–24, 2013.

[17] P.-H. Randsborg, P. Gulbrandsen, J. Saltyte Benth et al., "Fractures in children: epidemiology and activity-specific fracture rates," *The Journal of Bone & Joint Surgery—American Volume*, vol. 95, no. 7, article e42, 2013.

[18] L. Rennie, C. M. Court-Brown, J. Y. Mok, and T. F. Beattie, "The epidemiology of fractures in children," *Injury*, vol. 38, no. 8, pp. 913–922, 2007.

[19] G. Jones and H. M. Cooley, "Symptomatic fracture incidence in those under 50 years of age in southern Tasmania," *Journal of Paediatrics and Child Health*, vol. 38, no. 3, pp. 278–283, 2002.

[20] K. M. Sanders, E. Seeman, A. M. Ugoni et al., "Age- and gender-specific rate of fractures in Australia: a population-based study," *Osteoporosis International*, vol. 10, no. 3, pp. 240–247, 1999.

[21] S. Boufous, C. Finch, S. Lord, J. Close, T. Gothelf, and W. Walsh, "The epidemiology of hospitalised wrist fractures in older people, New South Wales, Australia," *Bone*, vol. 39, no. 5, pp. 1144–1148, 2006.

[22] A. A. Fisher, E. D. O'Brien, and M. W. Davis, "Trends in hip fracture epidemiology in Australia: possible impact of bisphosphonates and hormone replacement therapy," *Bone*, vol. 45, no. 2, pp. 246–253, 2009.

[23] C. D. J. Holman, A. J. Bass, I. L. Rouse, and M. S. T. Hobbs, "Population-based linkage of health records in Western Australia: development of a health services research linked database," *Australian and New Zealand Journal of Public Health*, vol. 23, no. 5, pp. 453–459, 1999.

[24] R. E. Gibson, M. Harden, J. Byles, and J. Ward, "Incidence of falls and fall-related outcomes among people in aged-care facilities in the Lower Hunter region, NSW.," *New South Wales Public Health Bulletin*, vol. 19, no. 10, pp. 166–169, 2008.

[25] J. A. Pasco, E. Seeman, M. J. Henry, E. N. Merriman, G. C. Nicholson, and M. A. Kotowicz, "The population burden of fractures originates in women with osteopenia, not osteoporosis," *Osteoporosis International*, vol. 17, no. 9, pp. 1404–1409, 2006.

[26] R. Bahr and T. Krosshaug, "Understanding injury mechanisms: a key component of preventing injuries in sport," *British Journal of Sports Medicine*, vol. 39, no. 6, pp. 324–329, 2005.

[27] J. M. Conn, J. L. Annest, and J. Gilchrist, "Sports and recreation related injury episodes in the US population, 1997–99," *Injury Prevention*, vol. 9, no. 2, pp. 117–123, 2003.

[28] L. Z. Rubenstein, "Falls in older people: epidemiology, risk factors and strategies for prevention," *Age and Ageing*, vol. 35, supplement 2, pp. ii37–ii41, 2006.

20

Optimism and Mortality in Older Men and Women: The Rancho Bernardo Study

Ericha G. Anthony,[1,2] Donna Kritz-Silverstein,[1] and Elizabeth Barrett-Connor[1]

[1]*Department of Family Medicine and Public Health, University of California San Diego, La Jolla, CA 92093-0628, USA*
[2]*Graduate School of Public Health, San Diego State University, San Diego, CA 92182, USA*

Correspondence should be addressed to Ericha G. Anthony; ericha_anthony@yahoo.com

Academic Editor: Barbara Shukitt-Hale

Purpose. To examine the associations of optimism and pessimism with all-cause, cardiovascular disease (CVD), coronary heart disease (CHD), and cancer mortality in a population-based sample of older men and women followed ≤12 years. *Methods.* 367 men and 509 women aged ≥50 from the Rancho Bernardo Study attended a 1999–2002 research clinic visit when demographic, behavioral, and medical history were obtained and completed a 1999 mailed survey including the Life Orientation Test-Revised (LOT-R). Mortality outcomes were followed through 2012. *Results.* Average age at baseline was 74.1 years; during follow-up (mean = 8.1 years), 198 participants died, 62 from CVD, 22 from CHD, and 49 from cancer. Total LOT-R, optimism and pessimism scores were calculated. Participants with the highest optimism were younger and reported less alcohol use and smoking and more exercise. Cox proportional hazard models showed that higher total LOT-R and optimism, but not pessimism scores, were associated with reduced odds of CHD mortality after adjusting for age, sex, alcohol, smoking, obesity, physical exercise, and medication (HR = 0.86, 95% CI = 0.75, 0.99; HR = 0.77, 95% CI = 0.61, 0.99, resp.). No associations were found for all-cause, CVD, or cancer mortality. *Conclusions.* Optimism was associated with reduced CHD mortality in older men and women. The association of positive attitudes with mortality merits further study.

1. Introduction

Numerous studies report significant associations between optimism or pessimism and various health outcomes including cardiovascular disease (CVD), coronary heart disease (CHD), myocardial infarction, and cancer; most report that optimism is protective whereas pessimism is associated with increased risk of disease [1–6]. The few clinical studies that examined the association between optimism or pessimism and mortality report less consistent results. For example, a study of 238 US male and female cancer patients aged 30 years and older suggested that pessimism was a mortality risk factor only for younger patients [7], while a predominantly male French cohort of 101 cancer patients, aged 35 to 81 years, reported greater risk of death for pessimistic as compared to optimistic patients one year after diagnosis [6]. A recent study by Chang et al. showed statistically significant sex differences in the reporting of psychological outcomes: men were more inclined to report positive psychological outcomes for *self rather than for others* and also more likely to report negative psychological outcomes for *others rather than for self* [8].

Only two population-based studies have reported the association of optimism or pessimism with mortality. Among 97,253 women aged 50 to 79 years from Women's Health Initiative who were followed up by mail for eight years, optimism was associated with a reduction of 14% for total, 24% for CVD, and 30% for CHD-related mortality after adjusting for traditional and lifestyle risk factors such as age, hypertension, BMI, smoking, alcohol use, and physical activity [4]. The Arnhem Elderly Study of 999 Dutch men and women aged 65 to 85 years followed up for nine years reported protective effects of optimism on all-cause and CVD mortality in men after adjusting for risk factors, including lifestyle and medical history, whereas, after adjusting for the same risk factors in women, the protective effect of optimism was found only for CVD mortality [9]. Analysis of a 15-year follow-up of men only from the Zutphen Study showed that optimism was associated with lower risk of cardiovascular death [10] as well as healthier lifestyle and dietary habits, suggesting that lower levels of optimism may influence behavioral choices leading to cardiovascular death [11]. However, there has been no US population-based study of both older men and women who were followed up for 10–12 years.

The purpose of this report was to examine the association of optimism and pessimism with all-cause and cause-specific mortality in the Rancho Bernardo Study, a large population-based sample of community-dwelling older men and women. Given the associations of optimism and pessimism with multiple diseases and the inconsistency in the literature relating to mortality, it is important to determine how optimism and pessimism are associated with mortality and whether there are sex differences in these associations.

2. Materials and Methods

2.1. Participants. Between 1972 and 1974, the Rancho Bernardo Heart and Chronic Disease Study enrolled 82% (n = 6629) of residents aged 30 to 79 years from the Southern California community of Rancho Bernardo. These participants have been followed up with periodic clinic visits and yearly mailed surveys; death certificates were obtained for all decedents. Between 1999 and 2002, 463 men and 678 women (n = 1141) participated in a follow-up research clinic visit. In 1999, a mailed survey including the Life Orientation Test-Revised (LOT-R) questionnaire used to assess optimism and pessimism was mailed to all participants. Participants for this study were members of the Rancho Bernardo cohort who attended the 1999–2002 clinic visits, responded to the 1999 mailed LOT-R questionnaire, and were followed up through 2012. After excluding the 78 men and 145 women (n = 223) who did not complete the LOT-R questionnaire, 8 men and 21 women (n = 29) missing two or more LOT-R responses, 10 men and 2 women (n = 12) younger than age 50 at the time of this clinic visit, and 1 woman missing a death certificate, there remained a total of 367 men and 509 women (n = 876) who formed the cohort for this report. Participants were followed up through 2012, the last year for which complete mortality data was available; at that time, 102 men and 96 women (n = 198) were deceased; 265 men and 413 women (n = 678) were alive (Figure 1).

This study was approved by the Human Research Protections Program at the University of California, San Diego. All participants gave written informed consent prior to participation.

2.2. Procedures. At the 1999–2002 clinic visit, height and weight were measured in participants wearing light clothing without shoes and used for calculation of body mass index (BMI, kg/m^2) as an estimate of obesity. Waist circumference was measured at the bending point and hip girth was measured at the widest point for calculation of waist-hip ratio (WHR) as an estimate of central adiposity. Two blood pressure measures were obtained 5 minutes apart by a nurse trained in the Hypertension Detection and Follow-up Program (HDFP) protocol after participants had been seated quietly for five minutes, using the average of the two systolic and diastolic measures [12].

A trained interviewer used a standardized interview to obtain information on current marital status (no/yes), cigarette smoking history (never/past/current), and exercise 3 or more times per week (no/yes). Alcohol use during an average week (grams/week) was calculated based on the number of beers and glasses of wine and drinks of hard liquors and liqueurs per week. Participants were asked about their medical history including physician's diagnosis of hypertension, diabetes, heart attack, transient ischemic attack (TIA), stroke, angina, and cancer. Participants were also queried about current medication use including antihypertensives and angina treatment and cholesterol-lowering and diabetes medications. Women were also asked about hormone replacement therapy (HRT) use and duration. Current medications were validated by a nurse who examined pills and containers brought to the clinic for that purpose. The Medical Outcomes Short-Form Health Survey (SF-12) is a 12-item, self-report measure of functional health and well-being from the participant's point of view [13]. This scale has been reported to have test-retest (2-week) correlations of 0.89 and 0.76, respectively, for the 12-item Physical Component Summary and the 12-item Mental Component Summary [13].

In 1999, a mailed survey included the Life Orientation Test-Revised (LOT-R), a widely used, 10-item, validated questionnaire assessing dispositional optimism that consists of 3 items assessing optimism, 3 items assessing pessimism, and 4 filler items [14]. The total LOT-R score takes into account the relative contributions of optimism and pessimism whereas all of the subscales only assess a single dimension. Responses are given on a 0–4 scale ranging from Strongly Agree to Strongly Disagree [14]. An example of an optimism question is, "In uncertain times, I usually expect the best" and an example of a pessimism question is, "If something can go wrong for me, it will" [14]. This scale has been reported to have internal reliability of 0.78 and test-retest reliability of 0.79 at 28 months [14]. Internal consistency for total LOT-R in this sample was 0.73 based on Cronbach's α coefficient. In addition to the total LOT-R score, the authors also separately examined the 3 optimism items (optimism subscale) and the 3 pessimism items (pessimism subscale) to determine whether there were differences across these subscales and the total score.

Death certificates were obtained for all decedents and cause of death was coded by a certified nosologist using the International Classification of Disease, Ninth Revision (ICD-9). Cancer deaths included codes 140–239, CVD deaths included codes 401–414, 426–438, and 440–448, and CHD deaths included codes 410–414.

2.3. Statistical Analysis. Total LOT-R score was calculated by reverse scoring the three optimism items and adding this value to the sum of the three pessimism items to obtain a score ranging from 0 to 24; higher total LOT-R scores indicate greater optimism [15]. Filler items were not used when calculating the total score. A separate subscale score

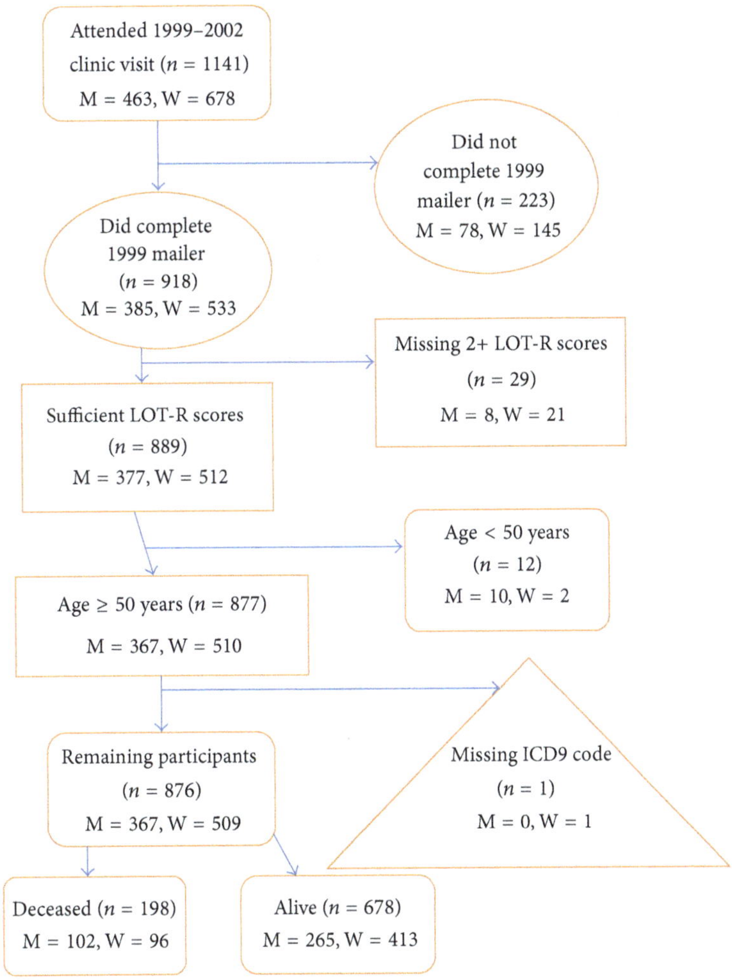

FIGURE 1: Study participant flow chart.

for optimism was calculated by summing the three reverse scored optimism items and a separate subscale score for pessimism was calculated by summing the scores for the three pessimism items. For both optimism and pessimism subscales, if one item was unanswered, it was given the mean value of the two answered optimism or pessimism items; higher scores indicated greater optimism or pessimism. The total LOT-R score measures the balance of optimism versus pessimism whereas the optimism subscale measures optimism only and the pessimism subscale measures pessimism only. Based on data distributions, total LOT-R scores were divided into quartiles and the subscales were each divided into tertiles. Data were analyzed for both sexes combined and also stratified by sex. Descriptive statistics were calculated and reported as rates for categorical data and means (± standard deviations) for continuous data. Comparisons were performed for categorical variables using chi-square tests and for continuous variables using independent t-tests. LOT-R scores were divided into quartiles of increasing optimism based on the total sample (0–15, 16-17, 18-19, and 20–24); comparisons between quartiles were made for age, behaviors such as exercise, alcohol use, smoking, and other potential confounders using age-adjusted univariate logistic regression for categorical variables and age-adjusted univariate linear regression for continuous variables. Because all analyses yielded similar results for men and women, only the results using data from both sexes combined are shown. Variables for which differences between quartiles were obtained where $p < 0.20$ were included as covariates in later multivariable analyses. Forward stepwise Cox proportional hazard models were used to assess the association between continuous total LOT-R score and each of four main mortality outcomes: all-cause, cancer, CVD, and CHD mortality. For variables that did not meet the proportional hazards assumption (p value ≤ 0.05), the time/variable interaction term was also included in the final model. Time was measured from date of 1999–2002 clinic visit to date of last contact or date of death. Model 1 examined the unadjusted associations of total LOT-R score with each mortality outcome. Model 2 included total LOT-R and age. Model 3 included Model 2 variables with sex added as a covariate. Model 4 included Model 3 variables with average alcohol use per week, smoking status, WHR, and exercise added. Model 5 included Model 4 variables plus angina, cholesterol-lowering, and diabetic

TABLE 1: Unadjusted comparison of LOT-R scores and behaviors and other covariates for men and women, Rancho Bernardo, CA, 1999–2002 ($N = 876$).

	All ($n = 876$) Mean (SD)	Men ($n = 367$) Mean (SD)	Women ($n = 509$) Mean (SD)	p value*
Age (yr)	74.1 (9.7)	74.3 (9.3)	74.1 (10.1)	0.78
Follow-up (yr)	8.1 (2.7)	7.8 (2.9)	8.3 (2.5)	0.01
Alcohol use (avg g/wk)	62.7 (78.9)	79.6 (92.0)	50.6 (65.4)	**<0.001**
Duration of smoking (yr)	23.7 (15.9)	23.7 (15.5)	23.8 (16.2)	0.96
WHR	0.87 (0.09)	0.95 (0.05)	0.81 (0.06)	**<0.001**
BMI (kg/m^2)	26.3 (4.2)	27.0 (3.7)	25.7 (4.5)	**<0.001**
SBP (mmHg)	139.7 (20.3)	138.9 (20.3)	140.3 (20.3)	0.33
DBP (mmHg)	78.2 (9.5)	78.8 (10.1)	77.7 (9.0)	0.09
Duration HRT (yr)	—	—	14.8 (12.3)	—
LOT-R total	17.1 (3.2)	17.1 (3.3)	17.1 (3.2)	0.99
Optimism subscale	8.5 (1.7)	8.5 (1.7)	8.6 (1.7)	0.69
Pessimism subscale	3.5 (1.9)	3.4 (1.9)	3.5 (1.9)	0.71
	N (%)	N (%)	N (%)	
Mortality, all-cause	198 (22.6)	102 (27.8)	96 (18.9)	**<0.001**
Cancer	49 (5.6)	24 (6.5)	25 (4.9)	0.85
CVD	62 (7.1)	31 (8.4)	31 (6.1)	0.76
CHD	22 (2.5)	16 (4.4)	6 (1.2)	**0.04**
HRT (ever)	—	—	264 (51.9)	—
Smoking status				**0.003**
Never	394 (45.0)	141 (38.4)	253 (49.7)	
Past	446 (50.9)	211 (57.5)	235 (46.2)	
Current	36 (4.1)	15 (4.1)	21 (4.1)	
Exercise ≥ 3x/wk (% yes)	632 (72.1)	274 (74.7)	358 (70.3)	0.16
Marital status (% yes)	615 (70.2)	310 (84.5)	305 (59.9)	**<0.001**
BP low meds (% yes)	302 (34.5)	134 (36.5)	168 (33.0)	0.27
Angina meds (% yes)	25 (2.9)	19 (5.2)	6 (1.2)	**0.001**
Chol low meds (% yes)	230 (26.3)	119 (32.4)	111 (21.8)	**<0.001**
Diabetes meds (% yes)	40 (4.6)	24 (6.5)	16 (3.1)	**0.02**
Hypertension (% yes)	561 (64.0)	244 (66.5)	317 (62.3)	0.18
Diabetes (% yes)	55 (6.3)	27 (7.4)	28 (5.5)	0.22
Heart attack (% yes)	33 (3.7)	17 (4.6)	16 (3.1)	0.17
TIA (% yes)	58 (6.6)	35 (9.5)	23 (4.5)	**0.002**
Stroke (% yes)	10 (1.1)	9 (2.5)	1 (0.02)	**0.001**
Angina (% yes)	50 (5.7)	38 (10.4)	12 (2.4)	**<0.001**
Cancer (% yes)	189 (21.6)	84 (22.9)	105 (20.6)	0.26

*Reference: sex differences: t-test is used for continuous variables; χ^2 is used for categorical variables; bold indicates p value ≤ 0.05.

medications. Hazard ratios, 95% confidence intervals, and p values are reported. All analyses were conducted using SAS version 9.2 (SAS Institute, NC); p value ≤ 0.05 was considered statistically significant. The sample size of 876 participants had greater than 80% statistical power for detecting an association with 95% confidence [16].

3. Results

Table 1 shows descriptive statistics for men and women combined and separately for each sex. Average age was 74.1 ± 9.7 years (men 74.3 ± 9.3 years and women 74.1 ± 10.1 years). Compared to women, men had significantly higher average alcohol consumption per week (50.6 g versus 79.6 g, $p < 0.001$, resp.) and higher rates of medication use for angina ($p = 0.001$), cholesterol ($p < 0.001$), and diabetes ($p = 0.02$). Participants were followed up for up to 12 years for an average of 8.1 years. There were no significant differences in total LOT-R score or optimism and pessimism subscale scores between men and women ($p = 0.99$). During follow-up there were 198 deaths due to all causes, 49 due to cancer, 62 due to CVD, and 22 due to CHD. All-cause mortality and CHD mortality were significantly higher in men than in women (27.8% versus 18.9%, $p < 0.001$, and 4.4% versus 1.2%,

Table 2: Age and age-adjusted covariates comparison by LOT-R score quartiles in both sexes, Rancho Bernardo, CA, 1999–2002 ($N = 876$).

	Q1 (0–15) ($n = 242$) Mean	Q2 (16-17) ($n = 234$) Mean	Q3 (18-19) ($n = 230$) Mean	Q4 (20–24) ($n = 170$) Mean	p value
Age (yr)	76.6	74.4	73.8	70.9	**<0.001**$^{+}$
Follow-up (yr)	7.7	7.8	8.3	8.7	0.06
Alcohol use (avg g/wk)	64.4	56.9***	75.6***	50.8	**0.02**
Duration of smoking (yr)	24.8	24.3	24.6	19.4	0.15
WHR	0.86	0.87	0.87	0.87	0.75
BMI (kg/m^2)	26.0	26.7	26.0	26.3	0.26
SBP (mmHg)	140.5	141.7	139.3	136.6	0.41
DBP (mmHg)	77.3	78.8	77.9	78.8	0.59
SF-12					
PCS	43.2$^{\wedge\wedge *}$	44.7*	47.5	50.8	**<0.001**
MCS	51.7$^{\wedge *}$	53.0$^{*\wedge\wedge}$	55.7	57.7	**<0.001**
	%	%	%	%	
Sex (male)	44.2	35.5***	43.9	44.7	0.14
Smoking status (ever)	55.4	61.1***	55.2	45.9	**0.05**
Exercise ≥ 3x/wk (% yes)	68.6	68.8	75.2	77.6	0.14
Marital status (% yes)	69.8	68.4	70.9	72.4	0.62
BP low meds (% yes)	38.8	33.9	33.3	28.2	0.82
Angina meds (% yes)	6.6	2.6	0.01	0	0.06
Chol low meds (% yes)	23.1	30.3	30.4***	19.4	**0.02**
Diabetes meds (% yes)	2.5	7.7**	4.3	3.5	0.06
Hypertension (% yes)	68.6	65.4	61.7	58.8	0.93
Diabetes (% yes)	5.0	9.0	6.1	4.7	0.29
Heart attack (% yes)	5.4	3.0	3.5	2.9	0.75
TIA (% yes)	5.8	6.8	6.5	7.6	0.77
Stroke (% yes)	0.01	0.02	0.01	1.2	0.83
Angina (% yes)	6.2	4.3	7.4	4.7	0.43
Cancer (% yes)	19.4	22.6	23.0	21.2	0.88

Reference: compared to Q3 only $^{\wedge}p < 0.001$, $^{\wedge\wedge}p < 0.01$, and compared to Q4 only $^{*}p < 0.001$, $^{**}p < 0.01$, and $^{***}p < 0.05$; $^{+}$unadjusted age; total LOT-R scored 0–24 by increasing optimism by quartile; bold indicates p value < 0.05.

$p = 0.04$). There were no significant sex differences in cancer (6.5% versus 4.9%, $p = 0.85$) or CVD mortality (8.4% versus 6.1%, $p = 0.76$). Other comparisons for men and women are shown in Table 1.

Age and age-adjusted comparisons of covariates by quartile of LOT-R scores for men and women combined are presented in Table 2. There were significant differences in age by quartile of total LOT-R; those with the highest quartile had the lowest mean age while those with the lowest quartile had the highest mean age ($p \leq 0.001$). There were significant differences by quartile of total LOT-R in rates of smoking ($p = 0.05$), use of cholesterol-lowering medications ($p = 0.02$), and average alcohol use per week ($p = 0.02$).

Figures 2(a)–2(c) show unadjusted comparisons of all-cause, cancer, CVD, and CHD mortality percentages by quartile of total LOT-R and by tertiles of optimism and pessimism subscales scores. All-cause, CVD, and CHD mortality decreased with increasing quartile of total LOT-R (Figure 2(a)) and increasing tertile of optimism subscale score (Figure 2(b)). There were significant differences for all-cause, cancer, and CHD mortality between the lowest and highest quartiles of total LOT-R and significant differences between the lowest and highest tertiles of the optimism subscale scores for cancer and CHD deaths. Conversely, CHD mortality increased with increasing tertile of pessimism subscale (Figure 2(c)), with significant differences between the lowest and highest tertile of pessimism subscale for all-cause mortality.

Table 3 shows the associations of total LOT-R and optimism and pessimism subscale scores with mortality, after adjusting for covariates. Prior to adjusting for covariates, there were significant associations between total LOT-R score and lower rates of all-cause ($p = 0.002$), CVD ($p = 0.004$), and CHD mortality ($p = 0.003$). After adjusting for age, odds of CHD mortality were 15% lower for those with higher optimism (HR = 0.85, 95% CI = 0.74, 0.97), a difference that remained significant after further adjustment for sex, alcohol use, smoking status, waist-hip ratio (WHR), exercise status, and use of angina treatment and cholesterol-lowering and/or

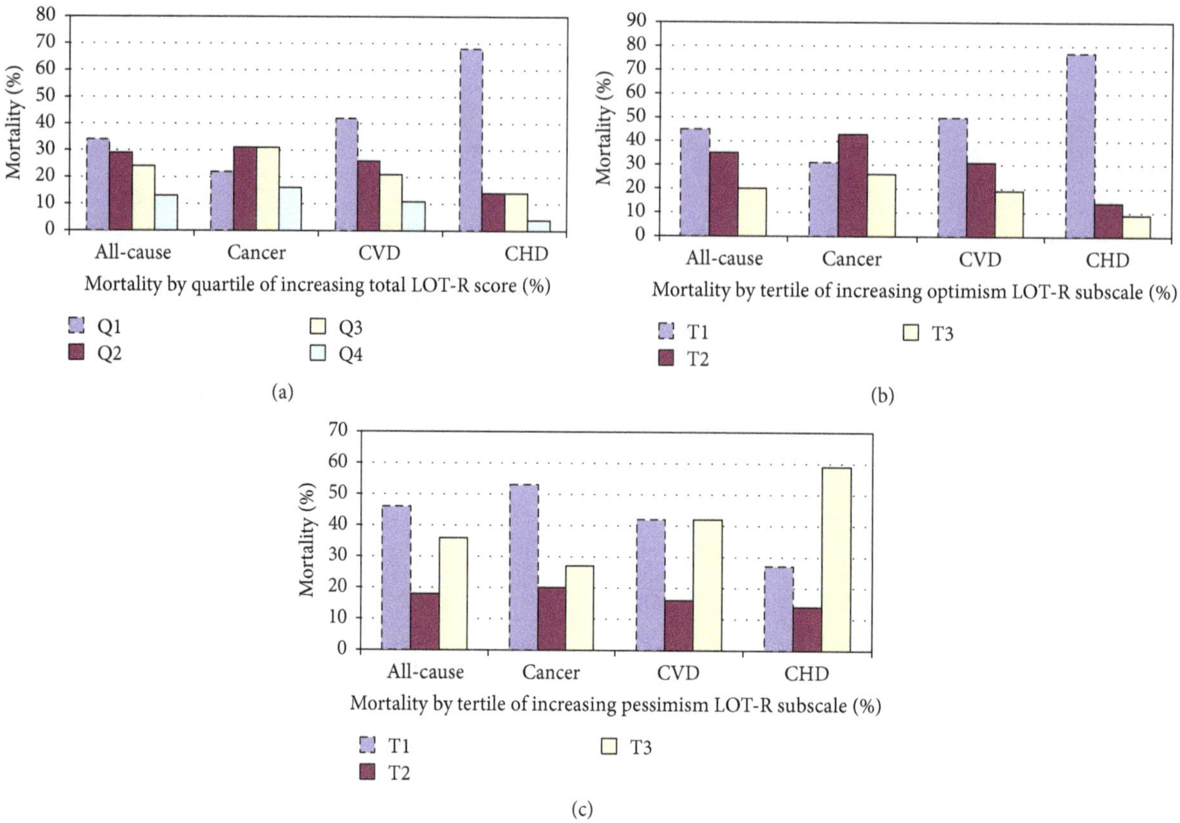

FIGURE 2: (a) Unadjusted comparisons of overall and cause-specific mortality+ by quartile of total LOT-R; Rancho Bernardo, CA, 1999–2012 ($n = 876$). *Reference*: all-cause mortality, $p = 0.01$ when Q1 compared to Q4; cancer mortality, $p = 0.05$ when Q1 compared to Q4; CHD mortality, $p = 0.001$ when Q1 compared to Q4; +all-cause, cancer, CVD, and CHD mortality are present among those who died. (b) Unadjusted comparisons of overall and cause-specific mortality+ by tertile of optimism subscale score; Rancho Bernardo, CA, 1999–2012 ($n = 876$). *Reference*: cancer mortality, $p = 0.03$ when T1 compared to T3; CHD mortality, $p = 0.003$ when T1 compared to T3. (c) Unadjusted comparisons of overall and cause-specific mortality+ by tertile of pessimism subscale score; Rancho Bernardo, CA, 1999–2012 ($n = 876$). *Reference*: all-cause mortality, $p = 0.002$ when T1 compared to T3.

diabetic medications (HR = 0.86, 95% CI = 0.75, 0.99). Associations of total LOT-R with all-cause and CVD mortality became nonsignificant after adjustment for age. There were no significant associations between total LOT-R and cancer mortality either before or after adjustment for covariates. Similar patterns were found for the optimism subscale score, which was significantly associated with decreased risk of CHD before and after adjustment for age, sex, alcohol use, smoking status, WHR, exercise status, and use of angina, cholesterol-lowering, and/or diabetic medications (HR = 0.77, 95% CI = 0.61, 0.99). The optimism subscale score was not significantly associated with all-cause, cancer, or CVD mortality. The pessimism subscale score also was not associated with odds of all-cause or cause-specific mortality after adjusting for age and/or other covariates.

4. Discussion

In both sexes, higher optimism, whether based on total LOT-R score or based on optimism subscale score, was associated with 14% and 23% lower risk, respectively, of CHD mortality. Although participants with higher optimism had healthier lifestyle behaviors, these associations were independent of age, sex, lifestyle variables (alcohol use, smoking status, obesity, and exercise), and medication use; adjustment for these variables did not alter the results. After adjustment for covariates there was no association of optimism with CVD, all-cause, or cancer mortality and no association of pessimism with all-cause or cause-specific mortality. Results of this study are important, as, to our knowledge, this is the largest population-based US study of optimism and mortality that includes both older men and women.

These results are in accord with those from Women's Health Initiative, which reported a significant association between higher levels of optimism based on total LOT-R and a 30% reduction in CHD mortality for white women after adjusting for age and other potential confounders [4]. However, our study included both sexes and found similar reductions of ~14% for CHD mortality for analyses including both men and women and in other analyses stratified by sex.

In contrast to results from Women's Health Initiative, our study did not find an association between higher levels of optimism and reduced odds of all-cause and CVD mortality [4], nor was pessimism associated with increased odds of

TABLE 3: Associations of continuous LOT-R score with mortality in both sexes, Cox proportional hazard modeling, Rancho Bernardo, CA, 1999–2002 ($N = 876$).

	All-cause mortality		Cancer mortality		CVD mortality		CHD mortality	
	HR (95% CI)	p value	HR (95% CI)	p value	HR (95% CI)	p value	HR (95% CI)	p value
Total LOT-R score								
Model 1	**0.94 (0.90, 0.98)**	**0.002**	1.00 (0.92, 1.09)	0.99	**0.90 (0.84, 0.97)**	**0.004**	**0.85 (0.77, 0.95)**	**0.003**
Model 2	0.98 (0.93, 1.02)	0.32	1.03 (0.94, 1.13)	0.53	0.94 (0.87, 1.02)	0.14	**0.85 (0.74, 0.97)**	**0.02**
Model 3*	0.98 (0.94, 1.02)	0.36	1.03 (0.94, 1.13)	0.53	0.94 (0.87, 1.02)	0.16	**0.86 (0.76, 2.98)**	**0.02**
Model 4	0.99 (0.94, 1.03)	0.50	1.03 (0.94, 1.13)	0.48	0.95 (0.88, 1.03)	0.22	**0.87 (0.76, 0.99)**	**0.04**
Model 5	0.99 (0.94, 1.03)	0.53	1.04 (0.94, 1.14)	0.46	0.94 (0.87, 1.03)	0.16	**0.86 (0.75, 0.99)**	**0.04**
LOT-R optimism subscale								
Model 1	0.96 (0.89, 1.04)	0.30	1.13 (0.95, 1.33)	0.17	0.91 (0.79, 1.04)	0.16	**0.77 (0.62, 0.95)**	**0.01**
Model 2	0.98 (0.90, 1.07)	0.64	1.15 (0.97, 1.36)	0.12	0.92 (0.80, 1.07)	0.29	**0.75 (0.59, 0.95)**	**0.02**
Model 3*	0.99 (0.91, 1.08)	0.83	1.15 (0.97, 1.36)	0.11	0.94 (0.81, 1.08)	0.38	**0.78 (0.62, 0.98)**	**0.03**
Model 4	1.00 (0.92, 1.09)	1.00	1.15 (0.97, 1.37)	0.11	0.94 (0.81, 1.08)	0.38	**0.77 (0.61, 0.97)**	**0.03**
Model 5	1.00 (0.92, 1.09)	1.00	1.16 (0.97, 1.38)	0.10	0.92 (0.80, 1.07)	0.30	**0.77 (0.61, 0.99)**	**0.04**
LOT-R pessimism subscale								
Model 1	**1.16 (1.09, 1.25)**	**<0.001**	1.09 (0.95, 1.26)	0.23	**1.24 (1.10, 1.39)**	**<0.001**	**1.31 (1.08, 1.58)**	**0.007**
Model 2	1.05 (0.97, 1.13)	0.23	1.03 (0.88, 1.19)	0.74	1.10 (0.96, 1.25)	0.16		
Model 3*	1.05 (0.98, 1.13)	0.18	1.03 (0.89, 1.20)	0.71	1.11 (0.97, 1.26)	0.13	1.22 (0.98, 1.52)	0.07
Model 4	1.04 (0.97, 1.12)	0.27	1.02 (0.88, 1.18)	0.80	1.08 (0.95, 1.23)	0.23	1.18 (0.95, 1.47)	0.13
Model 5	1.04 (0.96, 1.12)	0.33	1.02 (0.88, 1.19)	0.79	1.10 (0.96, 1.25)	0.19	1.20 (0.95, 1.50)	0.13

Reference: (1) Model 1: it includes LOT-R, Model 2: it includes Model 1 + age, Model 3: it includes Model 2 + sex, Model 4: it includes Model 3 + lifestyle variables (average week alcohol use, smoking status, waist-to-hip ratio, and exercise status), Model 5: it includes Model 4 + medication variables (angina meds, cholesterol-lowering meds, and diabetic meds), and Model 6: it includes Model 5 + SF-12 variables (PCS, MCS). (2) All-cause mortality ($n = 198$), cancer mortality ($n = 49$), CVD mortality ($n = 62$), and CHD mortality ($n = 22$). (3) *LOT-R and sex interaction is not statistically significant. Bold indicates p value ≤ 0.05.

cancer mortality as shown in some prior clinical studies [6, 7]. However, participants in our study were older, had higher socioeconomic status, and had health insurance compared to previous studies. Associations of pessimism with poor outcomes disappeared after adjusting for age and other covariates, suggesting a relatively large role of age and lifestyle factors on all-cause or CVD deaths. Our results also differed from both the Arnhem Elderly Study where optimism was protective for all-cause and CVD mortality and the Zutphen Study where optimism was protective for CVD mortality, but this is most likely due in part to the fact that scales other than the LOT-R were used to assess dispositional optimism [9–11].

Results of this study have clinical utility as they suggest that a personality characteristic, namely, optimism, is protective against CHD mortality. The biological and psychological mechanism of action between optimism, pessimism, and mortality are complex and not fully understood. Our participants with higher optimism scores had healthier behaviors; those in the highest optimism quartile were younger, drank less per week, smoked less, and exercised more, and a greater proportion were married compared to participants in the three lower optimism quartiles. Thus, optimism may exert indirect effects on health via a healthier lifestyle or marital status. However, optimism also had an effect on health independent of lifestyle and other covariates. Participants in the highest optimism quartile also had lower systolic blood pressure and lower rates of hypertension, diabetes, and heart disease, and fewer reported taking medications for hypertension, angina, and cholesterol. Others have shown that optimism is associated with lower levels of inflammation [17] and stress and negative emotions [18, 19]. Thus, it is plausible that optimism exerts a beneficial effect by improved physiologic parameters such as reduced inflammation [17] or biological side effects of stress (such as hypertension, diabetes, and heart disease), and negative emotions, thereby contributing to reduced mortality in more optimistic persons [18, 19]. While recent studies have shown associations between increased levels of inflammatory biomarkers and increased risk of CHD [20, 21], it is not clear if this is unique to CHD or applies to CVD in general [21].

Several limitations and strengths of this study must be considered. Given the older age of our study participants, it is conceivable that an association of optimism or pessimism with mortality was missed because participants had died before the follow-up assessment. Our study included participants who completed both the clinic visit and the mailed survey. Comparisons showed that those who did not complete the mailed survey had a higher proportion of men (65%), fewer married individuals (63.7% versus 70.2%), and lower rates of exercise (64.1% versus 72.1%) and drank on average less alcohol per week (53.9 g versus 67.2 g). Thus, survival bias cannot be excluded. Self-reported responses on the LOT-R introduce the possibility of misreporting. Due to the small number of cases in each analyzed mortality subgroup, we cannot exclude the possibility that low power may have reduced the ability to detect differences in mortality, although the association of optimism with reduced CHD mortality argues against this. Participants from the Rancho Bernardo Study are white and middle-class with relatively good access to healthcare. Thus, these results may not be generalizable to different ethnicities, lower socioeconomic status, or limited healthcare. On the other hand, this homogeneity means that the associations of optimism and pessimism with mortality may be less confounded by these differences. A major strength of this study includes its prospective design with follow-up for mortality over 10–12 years.

5. Conclusion

In conclusion, participants with higher optimism had healthier behaviors, but optimism was associated with reduced risk of CHD mortality independent of age, sex, and behaviors including alcohol use, smoking status, obesity, exercise, and medication use. These associations suggest similar direct and indirect effects of optimism on CHD mortality in men and women. Additional studies including both men and women with longer follow-up are necessary to further explore both sex and cause-specific nature of these associations.

Conflict of Interests

The authors declare that there is no conflict of interests regarding the publication of this paper.

Acknowledgment

This study was supported by Grants nos. AG07181 and AG028507 from the National Institute on Aging, National Institutes of Health.

References

[1] Y. Chida and A. Steptoe, "Positive psychological well-being and mortality: a quantitative review of prospective observational studies," *Psychosomatic Medicine*, vol. 70, no. 7, pp. 741–756, 2008.

[2] H. N. Rasmussen, M. F. Scheier, and J. B. Greenhouse, "Optimism and physical health: a meta-analytic review," *Annals of Behavioral Medicine*, vol. 37, no. 3, pp. 239–256, 2009.

[3] M. F. Scheier, G. J. Magovern, R. A. Abbott et al., "Dispositional optimism and recovery from coronary artery bypass surgery: the beneficial effects on physical and psychological well-being," *Journal of Personality and Social Psychology*, vol. 57, no. 6, pp. 1024–1040, 1989.

[4] H. A. Tindle, Y.-F. Chang, L. H. Kuller et al., "Optimism, cynical hostility, and incident coronary heart disease and mortality in the women's health initiative," *Circulation*, vol. 120, no. 8, pp. 656–662, 2009.

[5] L. R. Yanek, B. G. Kral, T. F. Moy et al., "Effect of positive well-being on incidence of symptomatic coronary artery disease," *The American Journal of Cardiology*, vol. 112, no. 8, pp. 1120–1125, 2013.

[6] P. J. Allison, C. Guichard, K. Fung, and L. Gilain, "Dispositional optimism predicts survival status 1 year after diagnosis in head and neck cancer patients," *Journal of Clinical Oncology*, vol. 21, no. 3, pp. 543–548, 2003.

[7] R. Schulz, J. Bookwala, M. Scheier, J. E. Knapp, and G. M. Williamson, "Pessimism, age, and cancer mortality," *Psychology and Aging*, vol. 11, no. 2, pp. 304–309, 1996.

[8] E. C. Chang, L. J. Sanna, J. M. Kim, and K. Srivastava, "Optimistic and pessimistic bias in European Americans and Asian Americans: a preliminary look at distinguishing between predictions for physical and psychological health outcomes," *Journal of Cross-Cultural Psychology*, vol. 41, no. 3, pp. 465–470, 2010.

[9] E. J. Giltay, J. M. Geleijnse, F. G. Zitman, T. Hoekstra, and E. G. Schouten, "Dispositional optimism and all-cause and cardiovascular mortality in a prospective cohort of elderly Dutch men and women," *Archives of General Psychiatry*, vol. 61, no. 11, pp. 1126–1135, 2004.

[10] E. J. Giltay, M. H. Kamphuis, S. Kalmijn, F. G. Zitman, and D. Kromhout, "Dispositional optimism and the risk of cardiovascular death: the Zutphen Elderly study," *Archives of Internal Medicine*, vol. 166, no. 4, pp. 431–436, 2006.

[11] E. J. Giltay, J. M. Geleijnse, F. G. Zitman, B. Buijsse, and D. Kromhout, "Lifestyle and dietary correlates of dispositional optimism in men: The Zutphen Elderly Study," *Journal of Psychosomatic Research*, vol. 63, no. 5, pp. 483–490, 2007.

[12] Hypertension Detection and Follow-up Program Cooperative Group, "The hypertension detection and follow-up program," *Preventive Medicine*, vol. 5, no. 2, pp. 207–215, 1976.

[13] J. E. Ware Jr., M. Kosinski, and S. D. Keller, "A 12-item short-form health survey: construction of scales and preliminary tests of reliability and validity," *Medical Care*, vol. 34, no. 3, pp. 220–233, 1996.

[14] M. F. Scheier, C. S. Carver, and M. W. Bridges, "Distinguishing optimism from neuroticism (and trait anxiety, self-mastery, and self-esteem): a reevaluation of the life orientation test," *Journal of Personality and Social Psychology*, vol. 67, no. 6, pp. 1063–1078, 1994.

[15] M. F. Scheier and C. S. Carver, "Optimism, coping, and health: assessment and implications of generalized outcome expectancies," *Health Psychology*, vol. 4, no. 3, pp. 219–247, 1985.

[16] HyLown Consulting LLC, "Power and Sample Size," 2016, http://powerandsamplesize.com/Calculators/Test-Time-To-Event-Data/Cox-PH-Equivalence.

[17] B. Roy, A. V. Diez-Roux, T. Seeman, N. Ranjit, S. Shea, and M. Cushman, "The association of optimism and pessimism with inflammation and hemostasis in the Multi-Ethnic Study of Atherosclerosis (MESA)," *Psychosomatic Medicine*, vol. 72, no. 2, pp. 134–140, 2010.

[18] M. E. P. Seligman, "Optimism, pessimism, and mortality," *Mayo Clinic Proceedings*, vol. 75, no. 2, pp. 133–134, 2000.

[19] P. Salovey, A. J. Rothman, J. B. Detweiler, and W. T. Steward, "Emotional states and physical health," *American Psychologist*, vol. 55, no. 1, pp. 110–121, 2000.

21

The Factors Influencing the Sense of Home in Nursing Homes

M. D. Rijnaard,[1,2] J. van Hoof,[1,2] B. M. Janssen,[3] H. Verbeek,[4] W. Pocornie,[5] A. Eijkelenboom,[5] H. C. Beerens,[4] S. L. Molony,[6] and E. J. M. Wouters[1,2]

[1] *Fontys University of Applied Sciences, Institute of Allied Health Professions, Dominee Theodor Fliednerstraat 2, 5631 BN Eindhoven, Netherlands*
[2] *Fontys University of Applied Sciences, Fontys EGT-Centre for Health Care and Technology, Dominee Theodor Fliednerstraat 2, 5631 BN Eindhoven, Netherlands*
[3] *Fontys University of Applied Sciences, Fontys School of People and Health Studies, Dominee Theodor Fliednerstraat 2, 5631 BN Eindhoven, Netherlands*
[4] *CAPHRI School for Public Health and Primary Care, Department of Health Services Research, Maastricht University, Duboisdomein 30, 6229 GT Maastricht, Netherlands*
[5] *EGM Architecten, Wilgenbos 20, 3311 JX Dordrecht, Netherlands*
[6] *Quinnipiac University School of Nursing, North Haven Campus, Office MNH 470P, 275 Mount Carmel Avenue, Hamden, CT 06518-1908, USA*

Correspondence should be addressed to J. van Hoof; joost.vanhoof@fontys.nl

Academic Editor: F. R. Ferraro

Purpose. To provide an overview of factors influencing the sense of home of older adults residing in the nursing home. *Methods*. A systematic review was conducted. Inclusion criteria were (1) original and peer-reviewed research, (2) qualitative, quantitative, or mixed methods research, (3) research about nursing home residents (or similar type of housing), and (4) research on the sense of home, meaning of home, at-homeness, or homelikeness. *Results*. Seventeen mainly qualitative articles were included. The sense of home of nursing home residents is influenced by 15 factors, divided into three themes: (1) psychological factors (sense of acknowledgement, preservation of one's habits and values, autonomy and control, and coping); (2) social factors (interaction and relationship with staff, residents, family and friends, and pets) and activities; and (3) the built environment (private space and (quasi-)public space, personal belongings, technology, look and feel, and the outdoors and location). *Conclusions*. The sense of home is influenced by numerous factors related to the psychology of the residents and the social and built environmental contexts. Further research is needed to determine if and how the identified factors are interrelated, if perspectives of various stakeholders involved differ, and how the factors can be improved in practice.

1. Introduction

For older people who can no longer age in place, nursing homes provide an alternative place of residence where care and assistance are offered by professionals [1]. Nursing home residents no longer live in their "own home." Because a nursing home has a dual nature as an institution and as a home, many health care organizations try to provide living arrangements that focus on "the good life" and the creation of an environment that is like a home to its residents, instead of a health care facility in which they reside [2, 3]. At the same time, the prevalence of dementia and care dependency in nursing homes increases (e.g., Schüssler et al. [4]). However, delivering both good (clinical) care and a homelike environment is challenging. In the near future, the demand for care of nursing home residents will increase as residents deal with the effects of dementia or severe physical limitations. At the same time, there is a trend towards small-scaled and homelike accommodations. To date, the exact elements that shape the physical, social, and organization contexts are largely unknown.

Health care organizations across The Netherlands are responsible for providing the basic furnishing of a room within a nursing home. With all basic clinical requirements a room should fulfill [5–7], the question about how to provide residents of nursing homes with a sense and feeling of home remains. Admission to a nursing home is a major life event, as most individuals do not wish to leave the home they have been living in for a long time in order to move to a nursing home [8]. Nevertheless, "*there seem to be good reasons to assert that living in an institution and being 'at home' is not a contradiction in terms*" [9, p. 221].

In the second half of the 20th century, the quality of the nursing home building was often expressed in terms of technological, functional, and economic requirements [10]. Hence, requirements related to the personal preferences of the residents were given less attention. A more holistic vision of health care is currently emerging and considers the consequences of the built environment on the well-being of the residents [10]. For instance, Van Steenwinkel et al. [10] conducted a study focusing on how the built environment contributes to a sense of home of older people living in different contexts in Belgium. Van Steenwinkel et al. [11] investigated the sense of home among permanent and temporary residents of nursing homes in The Netherlands. Both studies concluded that a sense of home is a multifactorial phenomenon which is highly influenced not only by the (built) environment, but also by social and personal characteristics. A sense of home is related to personal experiences and emotions and does not come into existence overnight but is gradually developed by the person in whom independence, security, and the source of own identity, choice, and controls, as well as memories, are essential [12–16]. Fully understanding the experienced sense of home of nursing home residents from both the insider and a holistic perspective might have important implications for the development of policy of health care organizations and the innovations in nursing homes of the future [17]. Conceptual frameworks and constructs concerning a sense of home that have been developed and researched from these perspectives are assumed to be relevant to this effort. According to Duyvendak [18], there are two situations that support the process of feeling at home: "haven" (a place that is secure, comfortable, and predictable; a place where one can feel at ease) and "heaven" (a place where you can be who you are and feel connected with like-minded people) [18].

The objective of this study is to systematically review which factors contribute to a sense of home for older people living in residential care facilities. To date, a list of specific factors contributing to the sense of home experienced by nursing home residents is not yet available to nursing home organizations, family members, architects, and other stakeholders. An understanding of these factors is necessary to build and test hypotheses that may predict and eventually improve experiences of home in residential care facilities.

2. Methodology

2.1. Search Strategy. A systematic literature search was performed in May and June 2015. In order to scan the literature for factors which contribute to the sense of home for older people living in nursing homes, five databases (CINAHL, PsycINFO, PubMed, Scopus, and Web of Science) were searched using a combination of two groups of keywords: (1) "meaning of home", "sense of home", and synonyms for these terms; (2) "care home" OR "nursing home" and similar search terms. Truncation was used when variations of the used nouns were commonly used in the literature. The full list was ("at-homeness" OR "meaning of home" OR "sense of home" OR "feeling of home" OR homelike OR homeliness or "experience of home") AND ("care home*" OR "nursing home*" OR "institutional care" OR "long-term care" OR "long term care" OR "care institution*" OR "residential care" OR "residential home*" OR "assisted living" OR "small scale setting*" OR "small scale living" OR "small scale facilit*" OR "shared housing arrangement*" OR "special care facilit*" OR "institutionali*" OR "sheltered housing" OR "small scale group accommodation*" OR "elderly hous*" OR "elderly home*" OR "special care unit"). Furthermore, references of the included articles were checked for additional articles eligible for this review (snowball method).

2.2. Article Selection. Titles, abstracts, and full articles were subsequently screened by the principal investigator [M. D. Rijnaard] for the inclusion criteria mentioned in the following list. In case of doubt, three authors [M. D. Rijnaard, E. J. M. Wouters, and J. van Hoof] discussed the selection first and consulted the project group if consensus was not reached.

Inclusion and Exclusion Criteria

Inclusion criteria include the following:

(i) Original and peer-reviewed articles written in English.

(ii) Data collected from residents living in nursing homes and other stakeholders.

(iii) Aiming at investigating factors that influence the sense of home, meaning of home, at-homeness, or homelikeness.

(iv) Data collected from studies which aimed to find out what contributes to a sense of home for the residents through the eyes of residents, family, or care staff.

(v) Being qualitative, quantitative, and mixed-method studies.

Exclusion criteria include the following:

(i) Short stay in nursing home.

(ii) Assisted living or congregate living.

(iii) Studies not written in English.

Note

(i) No exclusion criterion is based on country, continent, age of the study, residents' age, and year of publication.

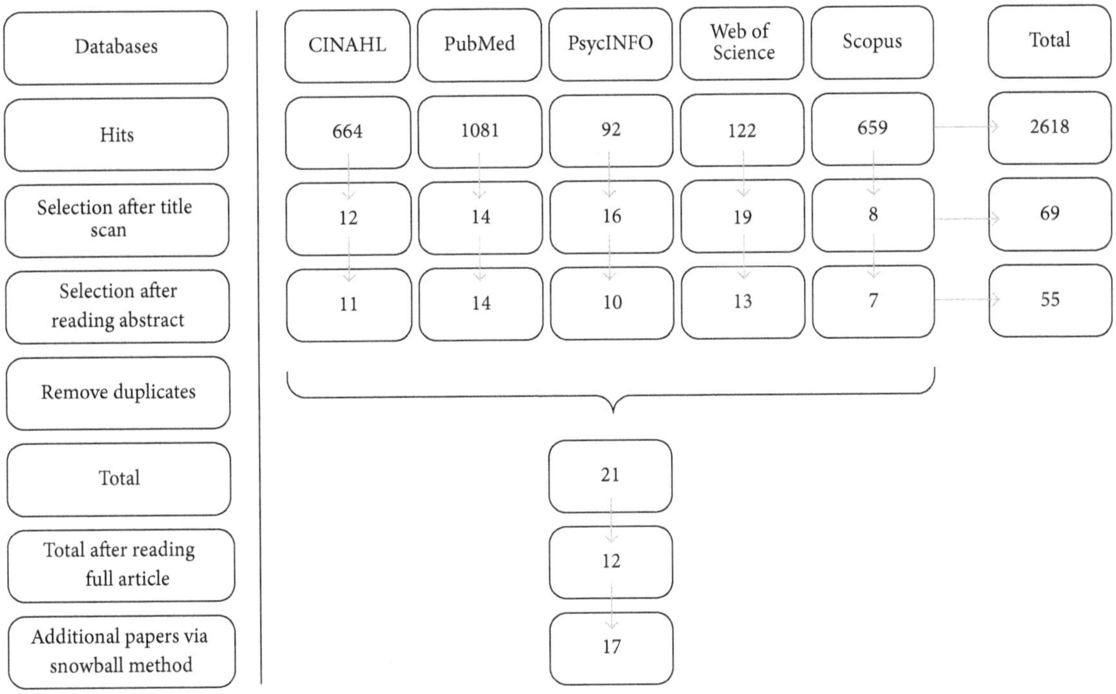

FIGURE 1: Flow diagram of the article selection process.

2.3. Data Extraction and Analysis. Thematic synthesis was used to synthesize data into factors. Prior to the literature search, a meeting was held during which the strategy of the literature search was set out. Choices were made about which databases to screen, which key terms to use, and what inclusion and exclusion criteria would be.

One author [M. D. Rijnaard] read all articles and extracted data which described a relationship with sense of home. Four other authors [J. van Hoof, B. M. Janssen, E. J. M. Wouters, and H. Verbeek] each read part of the papers and also extracted data, which described a relationship with sense of home. Next, M. D. Rijnaard paired up with each of the four authors mentioned before, and they together reached consensus on the extracted data, that is, open codes. The data extraction identified a large number of quotes which are used in the Results section as a presentation of the data to exemplify the meaning of a specific factor. After this open coding, multiple sessions were held to group factors derived from the reviewed articles (axial coding). The first meeting of axial coding involved four authors [M. D. Rijnaard, B. M. Janssen, W. Pocornie, and H. Verbeek], and three subsequent meetings each involved two authors [M. D. Rijnaard and J. van Hoof; M. D. Rijnaard and W. Pocornie]. Additionally, several sessions were held [M. D. Rijnaard and J. van Hoof] and an additional session was held [M. D. Rijnaard, J. van Hoof, and W. Pocornie] to create a conceptual model as an expression of the thematic synthesis, which shows the relationships between themes.

3. Results

The search in five databases generated a total of 2,618 results (Figure 1). The selection process initially led to the inclusion of 21 articles. After reading the full text, 12 articles remained. The snowball method added five articles, bringing the total number of articles included in this review to 17. The characteristics of these studies are described in Table 1. Of these studies, six were conducted in The Netherlands, four in USA, two each in Sweden and Norway, and one each in New Zealand, Ireland, and Australia. From these studies, 15 factors were identified that impact the sense of home of nursing home residents (Figure 2). Some of these factors have a certain degree of overlap, as boundaries are not sharp but gradually blend into each other. As a consequence of the process of clustering of factors, three main themes emerged as follows:

(a) Psychological aspects, which include behavioral, cognitive, and emotional components.

(b) Social aspects, which include home as a place of connection and socialization.

(c) The built environment, which includes the layout of a space, its interior design, and the surroundings.

3.1. Theme: Psychological Factors. Among the factors constituting the psychological aspects of the sense of home are the sense of acknowledgement, the preservation of one's habits and values, autonomy, and control, and coping.

3.1.1. Sense of Acknowledgement. There are numerous factors within the theme of sense of acknowledgement that contribute to a sense of home among nursing home residents. Molony et al. [27] identified a relationship with staff who "really cared" and having fun with staff and other residents among the relevant factors associated with at-homeness. Fun and friendship and laughing with one another are important

TABLE 1: Characteristics of the 17 reviewed articles.

Author (year) [reference]	Design and number of participants	Setting	Goal of study	Notes
Bland (2005) [12]	Interview (n = 1).	Nursing home, psychogeriatric ward in New Zealand.	To provide insight into how people in New Zealand feel at home in a nursing home.	
Carboni (1990) [19]	Hybrid model of field observations and theoretical analysis. Unstructured interviews (n = 2).	Nursing home with 120 beds in the USA.	To study if residents feel "at home" (and how this is defined for the participants) and if this has a specific meaning.	It is hard to differentiate between the field observations and theoretical analysis. It is not clear if any of the residents have a psychogeriatric background.
Cooney (2012) [15]	Unstructured interviews with residents (n = 61).	Public and private long-term care settings in Ireland.	To understand older people's perceptions of "being at home" in long-term care settings and the factors that influence these perceptions.	
de Veer and Kerkstra (2001) [20]	Quantitative study with 686 residents (with both mental and physical health problems) or significant others of residents.	36 nursing homes in the Netherlands.	To examine the determinants of "feeling at home" in nursing homes	
Falk et al. (2013) [21]	Qualitative study comprised of interviews (n = 25).	Several care institutions in Sweden.	To understand the strategies creating a sense of home.	
Fleming et al. (2015) [22]	Focus groups (FG) with family caregivers of people with dementia (FG1) and people with dementia and family caregivers of people with dementia (FG2) and practitioners caring for people with dementia nearing or at the end of their lives (FG3) (n = 4 + 9 + 5).	Focus groups were conducted among people suffering from dementia in three big cities in NSW, Australia.	To explore the views of people with dementia, family caregivers, and professionals on what aspects of the physical environment would be important to support a good quality of life to the very end.	There is no clear distinction if participants of focus groups 1 and 2 lived at home or in a nursing home. Focus group 3 included a care home manager, a dementia care educator, and a palliative care nurse researcher. Their work experience could be obtained at home or in the nursing home.
Hauge and Heggen (2008) [23]	Participant observation and interviewing (n = 24).	Two Norway based long-stay units with 12 residents in each unit.	To study how and to what extent the ideas of a nursing home as a home have been realized.	
Jonsson et al. (2014) [24]	Interviews (n = 12).	Three nursing homes in Stockholm, Sweden.	To explore the relationship between furniture and people.	
Klaassens and Meijering (2015) [25]	Observations, in-depth interviews, and diaries. Study includes both caregivers and residents. All 20 residents were observed. Interviews were held with 5 residents and 3 caregivers.	Korsakov ward of within larger nursing home in the Netherlands.	To gain insight into (1) the features of home and institution as experienced by residents and caregivers of a secured ward in a nursing home and (2) how interventions implemented on the ward can contribute to a more homelike environment.	
Lewinson et al. (2012) [26]	Qualitative, photovoice method (n = 10).	A large assisted living facility in Atlanta, GA, USA.	To explore home through residents' eyes.	

TABLE 1: Continued.

Author (year) [reference]	Design and number of participants	Setting	Goal of study	Notes
Molony et al. (2011) [27]	Mixed-methods study, $N = 25$ nursing home residents.	100-bed nursing home in USA. A descriptive, longitudinal mixed-methods design with four waves of repeated measures was used to achieve study aims. Interviews were conducted after residents made the decision to stay or move (baseline) and at 1, 3, and 6 months after the person relocated to the small-scale nursing home.	To examine trajectories of *at-homeness* over time in two groups of older adults who were given a choice to move to a small house nursing home or stay in their existing residence, a usual care nursing home to provide insight into the complex relationships between individual needs and desires, the LTC environment, at-homeness, and health.	The qualitative examples illustrate the individualized nature of at-homeness and the necessity of smooth integration of both the "social model" and the "medical model" of care.
Nakrem et al. (2013) [28]	Interview with 15 residents.	4 small-, medium-, and large-sized nursing homes in both urban and rural areas in Norway. The nursing homes had mixed populations according to medical diagnosis, physical and cognitive functioning, and age.	To study life in nursing homes in relationship to quality of care.	
Robinson et al. (2010) [29]	Interviews and focus groups with 29 family caregivers.	2 nursing homes in USA.	To study the meaning of home according to family of people with dementia.	
van Dijck-Heinen et al. (2014) [2]	Interviews and focus group session ($n = 10$, of which $n = 4$ permanent residents and $n = 6$ temporary residents).	One nursing home organization in the Netherlands.	To investigate the sense of home and its constituent factors among both permanent and temporary residents.	Study included 6 temporary residents (rehabilitation).
van Hoof et al. (2016) [16]	Interviews with 27 residents.	5 nursing homes in the Netherlands	To find out which personal possessions were most important and if they contribute to a sense of home.	
van Hoof et al. (2015) [30]	A photo production study. Interviews with 12 residents.	2 wards of 1 nursing home in the Netherlands for residents with physical limitations and gerontopsychiatric health problems.	To investigate which factors in the physical and social environment correlate with the sense of home of the residents and which environmental factors are most meaningful.	
van Zadelhoff et al. (2011) [31]	Observations and interviews with residents, their family, and nursing staff ($n = 5 + 4 + 5$).	Two group living units, located on the grounds of a traditional large-scale nursing in the Netherlands.	To investigate experiences of residents, their family caregivers, and nursing staff in group living homes for older people with dementia and their perception of the care process.	

too. Robinson et al. [29, pp. 498-499] stated that "*knowing the person 'underneath' the dementia*" and "*enhanced family access to staff as regular conversations occurred in the midst of everyday activities*" are important for the creation of a sense of home in small-scaled group accommodations for people with dementia. de Veer and Kerkstra [20] also underlined the need for resident-centered attitudes of staff. These positive interactions with staff members and other residents were also mentioned by Lewinson et al. [26, pp. 750-751]. Having things in common with other residents contributes to establishing new relationships [12]. Feeling respected and feeling known by the people in a facility make it a home [26, p. 751].

In addition, the style of working of care professionals has an influence [25, p. 96].

> *What the caregivers did change was their style of working. They provided the residents with more control and choice within the daily routines by listening more carefully and by consulting the residents.*

Cooney [15, p. 192] also stressed the aspects of feeling known and valued as an individual. The identity of residents was strongest when their sense of their own value and uniqueness and other people's (particularly staff) actions that communicated their worth matched.

3.1.2. Preservation of One's Habits and Values. Engaging in domestic chores and trying to live in the same manner as one always had were experienced as moments of privacy imperative for feelings of being at home [21, p. 1002]. Within the private sphere, residents should be able to engage in domestic chores. Nakrem et al. [28] added that women in particular felt that their role had been uncomfortably altered when admitted in a nursing home, as the engagement in old habits was impaired. There seemed to be a tension between the necessary institutional routines and the residents' personal habits, which resident should be able to continue. Nakrem et al. [28] mentioned the positive effects of support in self-activation which could make a great difference to the resident, by exploiting one's own strengths.

In addition, Robinson et al. [29, p. 500] found that there were competing demands for staff who were charged with creating a "homely atmosphere" in nursing home cottages, in which they had to choose between carrying out household activities and addressing serious health care needs. Through respecting the residents' wishes, the caregivers provide room for residents' self-determination [25, p. 97]. Continuity in activities from one's previous home-life is important too [25]. Items related to practicing a hobby are important even though many of the hobby activities were too complicated to carry out in the nursing home, because of impairments and limitations [16]. Cooney [15, p. 191] found that the continuity in normal activities and day-to-day activities and rituals are important for experiencing a sense of home. This is illustrated by a quote about the route of a facility by Cooney [15, p. 192].

> *What was noticeable was that more residents with an 'inward gaze' resided in settings where the [clinical] routine was dominant.*

Cooney [15, p. 191] stated that the degree to which participants could maintain personal routines mirrored the degree to which they were able to exert control over their day-to-day life. Carboni [19], Nakrem et al. [28], and Bland [12] stressed the negative impact of routines, rules, lack of control, and intrusions to privacy. Cooney [15, p. 193] continued by stating that residents' life experiences, values, and expectations of long-term care shaped both their initial response to long-term care and their long-term experience. Fleming et al. [22, p. 6] further added the engagement with one's senses (sounds, sunshine, and scents) and spiritual engagement as a way of nurturing one's core self to the aforementioned factors. Fleming et al. [22] also concluded that it is important to respect a person's dignity while carrying out care and that it is important for care professionals to see residents as unique individuals.

3.1.3. Autonomy and Control. Autonomy and control are frequently mentioned factors in relation to having a sense of home in a nursing home environment [2, 16, 29, 30]. van Dijck-Heinen et al. [2, p. 65] described autonomy as being able to do what you want to do, even though not everyone will develop a sense of home when given full autonomy.

> *You feel like home when you can do whatever you want to do. Grab your own belongings, or a book whenever you want to read. Or play music when you want to listen to music. Or paint a painting when you want to.*

Perceptions of freedom and mobility were identified by Molony et al. [27, p. 510] as ingredients for high levels of at-homeness. Privacy, being able to do things for oneself, and being able to care for oneself were considered to be important factors by residents too [27, p. 511]. van Hoof et al. [30] also identified the freedom of placement as important, for instance, having access to a taxi service. Lewinson et al. [26, p. 752] found that scheduling transportation was a problem to residents. Residents described that as "feeling trapped in the facility." In the study by van Hoof et al. [16], some of the residents were unsure whether they were allowed to stay in the present room or whether they needed to move within the nursing home. These participants said that they were unsure whether they would ever develop a sense of home.

In relation to decorating their own rooms, residents should be allowed to hang things on the walls and be allowed to drill holes [16]. According to Falk et al. [21], being in charge is a dimension of attachment to place. Being allowed to independently decide whom to include and to exclude is important too. Inviting a coresident to one's private room is equivalent to that of inviting someone into one's home [21]. Residents should have the ability to find pride in managing even the smallest chores by themselves.

> *George's private bedroom in the rest home wing provided him with little sense of sanctuary, especially as he was still unable to prevent other residents entering at will. [12, p. 7]*

Cooney [15, pp. 192-193] continued by stating that participants who "created" their own space usually considered the facility their home. Their comments suggested a feeling of "ownership" of their space.

Whether participants' move to long-term care was voluntary or involuntary was a determining factor in whether they found a home or not [12, 15]. Klaassens and Meijering [25] found that residents should be allowed to do as they wished, and there should be a shift away from risk avoidance to risk management. Being able to lock one's own door improves the sense of control and not "being locked up." In the study by van Dijck-Heinen et al. [2], the rules of nursing homes

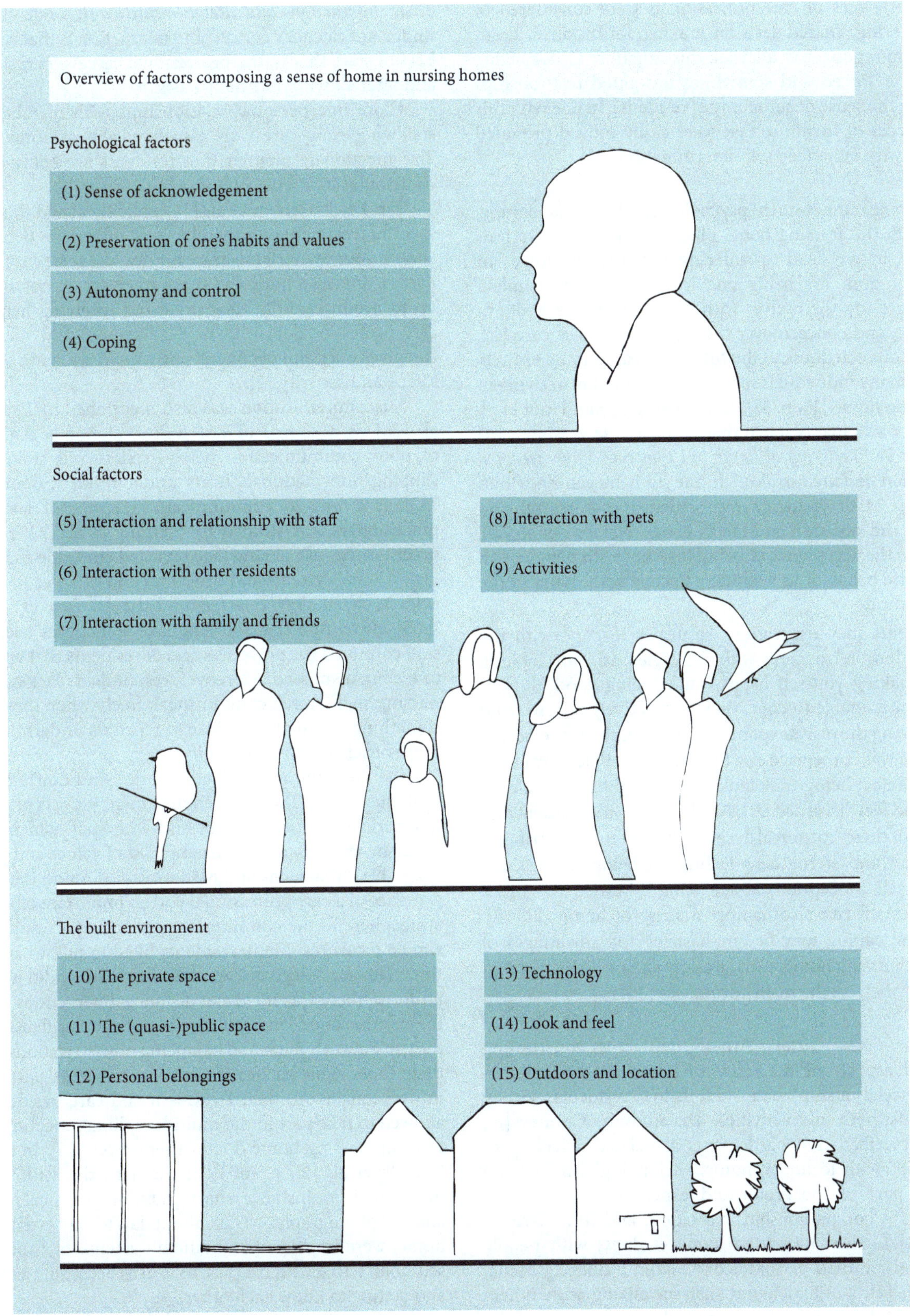

FIGURE 2: Overview of factors composing a sense of home in nursing homes.

and the practices of care professionals were considered to be too steering. Shared decision-making, for instance, about medication regime, can alleviate this situation. Group living can lead to forced and sometimes unwanted relationships breaching the sense of autonomy of residents. In line with this factor, pieces of furniture that were easily moved provided residents with enhanced self-determination [24].

3.1.4. Coping. The fourth psychological factor is coping. First of all, the nursing home placement itself is a serious life event. It may lead to suffering and grieving losses or feelings of guilt for being unable to prevent placement, second guessing themselves with regard to the necessity of placement, and concern over the circumstances of care [29, p. 496]. Connectedness to the future appeared to be entirely severe as many individuals spoke with resignation of dying in the nursing home [19, p. 35]. In the study by van Hoof et al. [30, p. 6], participants stated that "*living in the nursing home will never be like living at home but that they have accepted the situation and are satisfied.*" In the study by van Zadelhoff et al. [31, p. 2493], residents were settled, at ease, restful, and accepting the situation and life as it was. Nakrem et al. [28, p. 220] see the acceptance of being together with people with problematic behavior as a strategy to cope with living in the nursing home.

Residents may use various strategies to cope with the move to long-term care, with strategies as "not looking back," "making yourself happy," and "being good" [15]. If residents are unable to cope, they may actively refrain from personalizing the private room, which strengthens the notion that home was someplace else for them [21]. One may either accept or reject being frail, look on the bright side of life, or give up and feel discarded [21]. In addition, some residents are ashamed of their "corporeal decay," which in turn contributes to isolation and strengthens feelings of being an outsider. Negative self-conceptions about being a burden to others, including staff, can also hamper a sense of home [21, 28]. Part of the coping may be emphasizing the advantages of living in a nursing home, such as safety and receiving prompt emergency help as the main advantages [28].

3.2. Theme: Social Factors. Among the factors constituting the social aspects of the sense of home are the interaction and relationship with staff, fellow residents, family and friends, pets, and activities. The study by Cooney [15, p. 192] described that participants associated a feeling of "belonging" with feeling at home. "Belonging" was defined as being part of the group and experienced as a sense of solidarity, companionship, relaxation, and fun. Carboni [19, p. 34] further added that connectedness with people was severely limited or completely lost in a nursing home. Falk et al. [21, p. 1003] found that socializing with others made residents aware of their physical appearance, and the opportunity to dress up and to have one's hair set was important to maintain continuity of sense of self-identity and personal values. In the following section, these relationships, interaction, and activities are described in greater detail.

3.2.1. Interaction and Relationship with Staff. The most important category concerning interaction is that with members of staff, that is, the professional caregivers residents see and interact with on a daily basis.

Close interpersonal relationships with members of the staff who "really cared" are associated with at-homeness [27]. The affectionate manner that residents are being cared for contributes to a sense of home [30].

van Dijck-Heinen et al. [2] explicitly stated that a disrespectful treatment by a member of staff and not being able to choose your own friends were hindrances to a sense of home. Participants also indicated that caregivers do not always live up to promises. Still, they preferred receiving help from a care professional instead of via technological solutions. A caregiver is a point of contact and provides a sense of privacy, safety, and security [2].

Miscommunication was also mentioned by Lewinson et al. [26] as a source of not feeling at home. An example of poor communication between staff and residents was slipping informational sheets under resident doors [26, p. 752] as a way to communicate. The use of language of practitioners was studied by Fleming et al. [22, p. 9]. The practitioners' use of language revealed embeddedness within institutional systems and processes and this was particularly evident when they referred to patients. Falk et al. [21, p. 1005] also wrote that the language sometimes used by the staff connoted the powerlessness of residents that was related to feeling dismissed. Moreover, respondents lacking trust in nursing staff felt reluctant to speak freely when they thought something was wrong. A fear of reprisals undermined their sense of self-worth and dignity.

The literature revealed several do's and don'ts related to staff interaction. The social environment is a mix of residents' interactions with each other and with staff, which is influenced by wider issues, for example, staff values and practices [15, p. 194]. Klaassens and Meijering [25] found that that the presence of a care professional had an important effect on the atmosphere in the communal room and as a result of some simple measures. Many residents liked to talk to and spend time with the caregivers. As staff in this study did not wear a uniform, there was no visual distance. Interactions reshaped the relationships between caregivers and residents, closing the gap between them and balancing power relations, making them more equal parties. To increase residents' participation in decisions about their treatment and care, residents were allowed to take part in the multidisciplinary meetings and to visit the nursing home doctor themselves [25]. In the study by Falk et al. [21, p. 1003], doing activities with staff was mentioned. For instance, sharing autobiographical memories and old photographs, to talk about day-to-day events and in-home, were important to maintain a sense of continuity of self-connecting with the past, as well as becoming acquainted and getting to know each other.

In the study by Nakrem et al. [28, p. 222], the residents referred to the staff as "kind," "pleasant," and "clever," and many thought that the staff cared for them on a personal level. At the same time though, staff did not know the residents' names and staff felt that they did not have the energy to get to know them. Moreover, residents said that it was strenuous to repeatedly explain to new caregivers how to do the procedures. The quality of the staff was judged by their interest or motivation for doing something extra for the residents. Some nurses only did tasks that were expected of them and they were not able to give emotional support. In the study by Hauge and Heggen [23, p. 464], the "*residents were eager to answer questions and to discuss everyday matters with the staff. This sometimes ended up in cheerful discussions with laughter and smiles – what we have called golden moments.*"

In order to experience these "golden moments," there are numerous aspects related to staff that need to be fulfilled. According to Robinson et al. [29, p. 497], a lack of adequate staff to provide attentive, individualized care is detrimental to the sense of home. Nursing homes may become "more like a hospital," and staff may be overloaded in terms of the number of residents they care for. In the same study, also family participants noticed that the quality of the home was significantly influenced by the workload, the personality and strengths of the professional caregiver, and the fit between the resident and the setting of care. In the study by Nakrem et al. [28, p. 221], the residents thought that the staff were too busy to be able to provide attentive care.

> *Many felt and that they could not ask for more help because there was always someone else that needed to be prioritized. [28, p. 221]*

This notion is also shared by practitioners, who were concerned about the lack of staff to provide sufficient care to their residents [22, p. 9] or who indicated that they would like to pay more attention to each individual resident [31, p. 2495]. In the latter study, conducted in small scale group accommodation, staff also indicated that it is important to know how the residents used to live and their personal biography. In this way, staff have a better understanding of residents' behavior and this improves the interaction. Staff are more perceptive and talk more about their private life than in a regular setting. They spend a part of their free time organizing and joining activities, which makes the connection with residents more intimate than in a regular setting [31, p. 2496]. Falk et al. [21] concluded that the dignity of the residents was violated when nursing staff made them wait for help or ignored their wishes. On this topic, Cooney [15, p. 194] made a remark at the level of individual staff members; three key factors impacted on residents' experience, that is, the "availability," "reliability," and "flexibility" of staff. It was important to participants that staff were physically and emotionally accessible to them.

Therefore, ideally, staff should be able to balance stability and predictability with flexible routines that matched the individual needs of the resident [29, p. 498].

Apart from issues related to the organization of the work, there are also some personal staff characteristics believed to contribute to relational connection with the residents, such as well-developed observation skills, personal interest in each resident, a sense of humor, ability to take things in their stride, attention to details, caring, kindness, and respect for the residents as persons [29, p. 498]. The individual staff member needs to be multitalented, have time to devote to their relationships with both residents and families, and be able to make informed decisions about the most effective manner of delivering individualized care [29, p. 504]. de Veer and Kerkstra [20, p. 432] stated that showing interest in the resident, providing a quick response to a request for help, and a friendly attitude were important.

Apart from the direct relationship between staff and residents, also the staff's attention for family is of great value. This is confirmed in studies by Robinson et al. [29, p. 500], which highlights the importance of a family-centered approach to care where there is strong recognition that illness is a family affair even when the ill member resides outside the family home. In the study by van Zadelhoff et al. [31, p. 2495], it was found that family feels that nursing staff can spend more time with individual residents in a relaxed way. Robinson et al. [29, p. 498] stated that staff may become acknowledged as the residents' second families. The "real relatives" believed it was a staff responsibility to take a stand and be firm in inviting, encouraging, or leading the resident to engage in healthful daily activities. While supporting the belief that residents should not be forced, they did not believe the only alternative was letting the resident do what they preferred when it was clearly not in their best interest [29, p. 503]. Transparent communication between staff and relatives, therefore, is of great importance to balance mutual expectations.

An agreement on the use of keys also appears to be important in the relationship and respect of privacy and dignity between staff and residents. Although the nursing staff had keys in the study by Falk et al. [21, p. 1003], the locked door symbolized privacy. The staff was welcome when the respondents needed assistance. A locked door symbolized that no one was welcome to enter, and a breach of that rule was experienced as infringement.

Nakrem et al. [28, p. 221] raised the issue of the interaction with staff during mealtimes. Residents were disappointed that the consumption and quality of the meals and food were "institutional" and not homelike. As the staff did not have time to sit down with the residents during meals, they served ready-made sandwiches to save time. However, the residents felt they could not help themselves in the unit kitchen, mainly because the area was perceived as controlled by the staff. In the study by Klaassens and Meijering [25, p. 97], staff would also eat or drink coffee with the residents, besides cooking, which highly contributed to the homelike feeling. Therefore, using meals together seems to be important.

Reciprocity in care relationships is an important aspect of relating with staff. Bland [12, p. 8] found that there was no role for residents, other than being the passive and grateful recipients of care. Experiencing symmetric power relations to the nursing staff was an important dimension of feeling valued and was experienced as reliant and well inclined, which contributed to sense of self-worth [21, p. 1004]. This could be organized through having respondents to join homelike activities, such as setting the table and folding linen [31]. Residents could help in the preparation of meals in the kitchen. This creates domestic circumstances and feelings, and residents make a positive contribution. Lewinson et al. [26, p. 752] stated that residents believed they should be involved by sharing their unique talents and hobbies with other residents.

3.2.2. Interaction with Other Residents. Social relationships with and between fellow residents are very important to feeling at home in the nursing home [2, 27]. In the study by van Hoof et al. [30], a number of residents valued the dining atmosphere, especially in relation to being seated around a table together. van Zadelhoff et al. [31] found that residents are gathered together in the living room during the day. They talk with one another, drink coffee, or read a magazine. According to Cooney [15], the social environment was a mix of residents' interactions with each other and with staff. Klaassens and Meijering [25], too, stated that the residents shared their daily life with other residents. The participants in their study typically described their fellow residents as acquaintances rather than friends, though a small number of residents said that there were some fellow residents with whom they got along. The researchers' observations showed that not much interaction occurred between the residents during their study. de Veer and Kerkstra [20] also found that residents may feel disturbed, instead of being friends with, by other residents. Nakrem et al. [28] stated that spending time with the other residents was both an opportunity to be socially active and a source of irritation. In this study, an unbalanced mix of gender in the unit had made social relationships more superficial and some residents experienced that differences in interests sometimes resulted in disagreements. For instance, being the only cognitively intact resident in a unit could make it impossible to talk with the other residents [12, p. 7].

3.2.3. Interaction with Family and Friends. According to Molony et al. [27, p. 509], closeness and involvement with family are associated with at-homeness in a nursing home environment. In the study by van Hoof et al. [30, p. 6], a number of participants indicated that they valued their contact with relatives as most positive, in particular having close contacts and being visited on a regular basis. Robinson et al. [29, p. 496] found that family members were considered the best caregivers for persons with dementia. Both Lewinson et al. [26] and Bland [12] spoke of the importance of visits by friends and relatives, who should be incorporated into planned activities, and of occasional visits back home. Both van Dijck-Heinen et al. [2] and Bland [12] made remarks about living together with a spouse. In the Dutch study [2], the residents stated that it should be possible to move into a nursing home with a partner. In the study from New Zealand, having to live apart from a spouse was a source of concern. van Zadelhoff et al. [31, pp. 2494-2495] found that relatives felt more involved in the group life in the context of small scale nursing homes than in a traditional nursing home. In small scale nursing homes, relatives were treated as group members instead of visitors. Furthermore, family frequently joined dinner and drinks. Despite their importance for the well-being of residents, relatives sometimes experienced tensions concerning the expected responsibilities and about their roles in relation to staff members [31].

3.2.4. Interaction with Pets. Interaction with pets may complement the interaction with other human beings and may be a great source of distraction and joy during the day. Pets provide opportunities to engage when other people are not available. van Hoof et al. [30], for instance, found in their study that in one of the living rooms in a gerontopsychiatric ward there was a wild crow, eating from a net of peanuts hanging in front of the window. Residents considered these wild birds as pets. An animal gives a sense of consolation and warmth and makes a resident feel less lonely [2]. In the study by Fleming et al. [22], social engagement was raised by several participants and included engaging pets and even dolls.

3.2.5. Activities. Activities are essential to make it through the day and provide meaning to life. Activities can be conducted alone or with members of staff, relatives, fellow residents, and others. Some residents engaged in activities arranged by the community, which help them preserve their continuity with the past and society, as well as reaching beyond the institution [21, p. 1004]. Lewinson et al. [26] found that the inability to get out of the facility more frequently to enjoy a variety of community venues was a common complaint. At the facility itself, residents were able to engage in social activities that included bingo, group exercise classes, cookouts, book club discussions, and other planned events. But at the same time, residents reported that activity planning problems inhibited feeling at home. Other activities mentioned by van Hoof et al. [30] were a cooking club, arts and crafts such as paint workshops, and reminiscence activities conducted in the activity space. Several studies found that activities and stimulation should be appropriate to the residents' needs, skills, education level, and abilities, including the need for customized activities or more private activities with relatives [2, 15, 22]. Outings, for instance, with spouses, girlfriends, or children, are also important activities [2, 25, 27]. In the case of small scale group accommodation [25, 29, 31], scheduled activities have been incorporated into daily life, which enhanced satisfaction and evoked a sense of homeliness. Residents actively engaged in meaningful activities, for instance, domestic tasks such as cooking. Participants who for some reason were unable to participate or who found that the activities did not suit them were forced to fall back on their own resources [15, p. 192], having to organize their own activities and not being able to join in group activities.

3.3. Theme: The Built Environment. Factors constituting the theme built environment include the private space and the (quasi-)public space, personal belongings, technology, look and feel, and the outdoors and location.

3.3.1. The Private Space. The private space, whether it is a single-person room or a room shared with other residents, has an impact on the sense of home. In the study by Nakrem et al. [28, p. 220], "home" was associated with having a private room in the nursing home. A shared bedroom was unacceptable for most residents in this study. The desire for a private room may have a foundation in having opportunities to be on one's own, wishing for privacy, and having personal belongings around oneself [15, p. 192]. Central to nesting and the creation of attachment to place was spending time in one's room or apartment and being engaged in domestic chores [21]. Both findings by Klaassens and Meijering [25] and de Veer and Kerkstra [20] stressed the need for being on your own and withdraw to the own room, the opportunity to create your own environment. The need for privacy seems to be a main driver for having a private room. Private rooms govern the opportunity to talk with others in private or to withdraw from the communal living areas [16, 20, 25, p. 432]. The spontaneous opening of doors of private rooms is one of the actions hindering having privacy [2]. In this study, residents indicated that having a private room with private sanitary facilities was a must reported by all participants. Another desire in this study was to have a separate bedroom or recess for sleeping [2, 16].

Residents also indicated that having social interaction with the neighbors or coresidents should be facilitated through the design of the building [2]. Some of the residents asked for more spacious rooms, in particular the shower and kitchen areas. Also many residents in the study by Jonsson et al. [24, p. 28] felt that their private rooms were overfurnished and they wanted a larger space. van Hoof et al. [16] found that residents with larger apartments indicated that they could have visitors when they wanted. There was also the wish for having multiple rooms, a spare room that can be used when guests are staying for the night, a room for tools, or a work corner with a desk. In contrast, Klaassens and Meijering [25] found that the majority of the residents had no problem with the small size of the room.

Sanitary facilities are often mentioned as being important for residents, their comfort, and their feeling at home. The study by Robinson et al. [29] found that a private space including large private bathrooms with showers impeded a sense of home, because showers were unused as tub bathing was preferred by most residents. The private bathroom is also mentioned in other studies [22, 25, 30]. The bathroom can be a source of joy, if people can access it without difficulties, and they can wash and shower themselves. When having to share a bathroom with another resident, this may result in a lack of control around the use of the toilet. In the study by Fleming et al. [22], there were some differences in opinion on the necessity of ensuring privacy through having an ensuite or shared bathroom and a single bedroom or shared bedroom.

3.3.2. The (Quasi-)Public Space. Many recommendations were made regarding the design of the public space, that is, the indoor space that resident shares with others. As some residents claim sections of this public space as their own, in this paper we describe this set of factors as quasi-public space. Hauge and Heggen [23], for instance, stated that the living room reflected unclear and somewhat inconsistent expectations. The boundaries between the public and private spheres are ambiguous and thereby differ from the comparatively sharp boundaries characterizing a home.

In general, smaller residential density, including family-style dining, increased perceptions of belonging [27, p. 512]. In many facilities, residents may have their own place around the (dining) table [30, p. 6]. The spatial layout in shared spaces with lounge furniture and dining tables may create an inviting atmosphere to share a cup of coffee and some talk with nursing staff and coresidents [21, p. 1003]. Also the study of Fleming et al. [22, p. 6] mentioned that residents should have to get out of their private room in order to engage with others.

Sometimes the communal space can also give rise to distraction and confusion though. Klaassens and Meijering [25] stated that residents may be easily distracted by other residents and by staff in communal rooms. Hauge and Heggen [23, p. 464] came up with set of findings that relate to the living room of nursing homes. Interior symbols in the living room, such as family photographs, carpets, and tablecloths, should be clear and consistent and make the room feel like a living room instead of a waiting room. A similar description of nursing homes not feeling like home was also given by Carboni [19, p. 35]. The living room was a difficult setting for engaging in private conversation with ten to twelve listeners sitting around all the time. Maintaining a certain degree of privacy, therefore, required the residents to leave the living room and go into their own rooms or the corridor. The same conclusion was drawn by van Zadelhoff et al. [31, p. 2494], who found that, to some residents, it is important to have the possibility to retire to one's room or withdraw.

Some other aspects of the public space were found to be important. Robinson et al. [29, p. 502] stressed the need for a place to walk. The lack of such opportunities could lead to increased physical deterioration. An ideal design put forward by one participant in the study by Fleming et al. [22] would be a circle so that people would not arrive at a dead end. van Hoof et al. [16] further added that it is important that residents are able to reach all parts of a space from a wheelchair. Fleming et al. [22] found that wide corridors and wide doorways were seen as vital for easy access for those with wheelchairs.

3.3.3. Personal Belongings. Personal belongings seem essential elements in the development and maintenance of a sense of home [2, 15, 16, 19, 22, 23, 25, 30]. Creating attachment to place consisted of two dimensions: nesting and being in charge. Personal belongings help to create attachment to place in terms of in nesting and being in charge. Personalizing the environment, making room for personal belongings with furniture, and memorabilia can transform a private room to a place of recognition and familiarity that symbolized and strengthened one's self-identity, distilled from a lifetime of memories, experiences, and meanings attached to them [21, p. 1002]. Lewinson et al. [26, p. 750] stated that being able to bring personal histories into the space through beloved items and cherished furniture may contribute to feeling home. Many photographs contained items with emotional connections to previous homes. Jonsson et al. [24] found that certain pieces of furniture in their private rooms were only meant to accommodate significant others such as family or guests and therefore considered important. In addition, individual and unique pieces of furniture were a source of delight and were able to evoke memories [24].

van Hoof et al. [16, 30] researched the importance of personal possessions and found that there is a wide array of pieces of furniture or personal belongings that are present in the rooms of the residents. Small items such as drawings of grandchildren meant a lot to the participants, because they represented memories of loved ones [30, p. 6]. Among the items that were deemed most important were pictures, paintings, and pieces of furniture [16]. Personal belongings reflect the emotional value they bring to the individual. In addition, paintings have a particular decorative value and make the room more homelike. Some of the pieces of furniture were brought along at the time of admission for practical reasons, such as lift chairs. Often, there is an emotional value attached to the pieces of furniture, because they remind people of their former home or because they were purchased together with a partner [16]. Also, residents value the freedom in the choice and positioning of furniture in order to make the room cozier. To some of the residents, the personal belongings do not (yet) contribute to a sense of home, because the new living situation is rather overwhelming [16].

3.3.4. Technology. The small category of technology describes the facilitating role that modern (communication) technologies can play in relation to improving the ease of life and being in charge and, in an indirect manner, could facilitate a sense of home. According to the findings by de Veer and Kerkstra [20], easy access to one's personal (i.e., patient) data contributed to feeling at home, and technology may play a role in this procedure. According to the study by van Dijck-Heinen et al. [2], technological solutions, which are already used by the participants, are of a different league compared to assistive technologies used by care professionals. These technological solutions are necessary for mobility or to ask for help after a fall incident. Some technologies which were already in use are considered to be acceptable, whereas future developments were approached with skepticism. Fleming et al. [22] stated that there is a need to approach the use of technology, so that it is understandable and acceptable to the person regardless of one's cognitive ability. In the field study by van Hoof et al. [16], the researchers found that the television sets were considered the most valued item in the private room. It provided the residents with a link to the outside world and distraction.

3.3.5. Look and Feel. The factors constituting "look and feel" relate to architecture, interior design, and the general maintenance. In the study by Robinson et al. [29] and Fleming et al. [22], the authors stated that, in order to be counted as home, the facility needed to both look and feel like home or have a homely feel. The building should be "homey," more organized, and more welcoming of family members [29].

Satisfaction was negatively influenced by concerns about the physical design, as well as cleanliness. Cleaning tools and products, kept inside the private room, had a certain meaning in the study by van Hoof et al. [30]; namely, there was a sense that the room was kept clean and tidy. In addition, flowers may contribute to a homely atmosphere [30]. The appreciation for cleanliness and decorations was also acknowledged by Lewinson et al. [26, p. 750].

The decor, color, warmth, and light of the facility were also important to residents in the study by Cooney [15, p. 194]. A homelike environment may also be created through putting residents' artwork on display. Participants did not report the same ease or contentment in settings that were not "homely" [15, p. 194]. van Dijck-Heinen et al. [2] further stated that a sense of home connected with warmth and coziness. Some of the residents mentioned daylight access, color, and a "fresh" appearance without smelly odors as being important. A hospital-like environment is something all residents participating in the study wanted to avoid. Furthermore, buildings with long corridors and "nooks and crannies" were deemed unsafe.

Fleming et al. [22] also stressed the engagement with the senses, by mentioning ventilation and a window nearby as well as music in order to provide comfort right at the end of life. Some residents may require an environment that is free of noise or free of excessive visual stimuli.

Finally, Jonsson et al. [24] stated that a physical environment that makes activities accessible and promotes pleasure and stimulation of all the senses with lighting and support of visual perception is especially important for those with limited mobility. Also, the physical comfort was a major aspect stated by the residents in the shared rooms. Chairs that did not fit the body shape were a major problem. A homelike appearance in the shared rooms was preferred to encourage a sense of home for the residents. Descriptions of furniture-related factors with homelike characteristics included an old style and wood as a material. Institutional environments with neutralized, single hue interiors without contrasts and natural lacquered wood furniture were not desirable.

3.3.6. Outdoors and Location. The outdoor environment constitutes the outdoor space belonging to the own premises and the neighborhood at large. In the study by de Veer and Kerkstra [20, p. 432], there was a significant relationship with the degree of urbanization. Nursing homes located in large or very large cities had a higher proportion of residents not feeling at home in the nursing home. Nursing homes located in the own home town or the old neighborhood were preferred [2]. The presence of loved ones and children plays a role in this preference. Inaccessibility or loss of familiar places that provided the memories of past experiences is considered a negative factor in developing a sense of home [19]. Residents may also have a desire for going to shops and stores in the direct neighborhood for making small purchases [30].

Robinson et al. [29] provided an example of the important role of the outdoor environment, as participants expressed their concerns about the lack of trees and walkways outdoors. For them, "it was home-like indoors but not so outdoors" [29, p. 500]. Landscaping should be done with care. In the study by Robinson et al. [29], solid fencing that blocked a view was a reason for dissatisfaction. Many family members expressed dissatisfaction with the lack of connection to nature and the absence of a garden. In the study by van Hoof et al. [30], the green environment, in which the nursing home was located, was appreciated. This did not mean that all residents could appreciate the landscape by going outside, but in such cases the view of nature was considered to be attractive and pretty. Using outside spaces to facilitate engagement with the senses was seen as very important by caregivers [22]. Residents expressed a desire to go outside the facility more often in the study by Klaassens and Meijering [25]. Having a view in itself was also important to residents. Residents did not make a distinction between the types of view from the room [30]. Any type of view was appreciated, whether it was a park, traffic, a playground with children, a lively street, or a building [2, 30]. Residents value balconies and the views from the room [16].

4. Discussion

4.1. Main Findings. This is the first systematic review to identify factors that influence the sense of home of nursing home residents from their own perspective. Seventeen articles based on qualitative, quantitative, or mixed methods were identified. The majority of the data was based on qualitative research investigating factors of the sense of home among nursing home residents. Results show that the sense of home is influenced by 15 factors, divided into three themes: (1) psychological factors (including the sense of acknowledgement, preservation of one's habits and values, autonomy and control, and coping); (2) social factors (including relationships and interaction with staff, residents, family and friends, and pets) and activities; and (3) the built environment (including the private space and the (quasi-)public space, personal belongings, technology, the look and feel, and the outdoors and location) (Figure 2). Factors that were mentioned most often in the literature were the interaction with staff, autonomy and control, activities, the spaces, and role of personal belongings.

The three themes identified in this study were consistent with the results of previous work by Oswald and Wahl [32], who categorized factors constituting the sense of home into the following three groups: physical, social, and individual factors. These themes also emerged in research by Felix et al. [33] on the everyday lived experience of the house in The Netherlands, which was conducted with community-dwelling older people. The results also support earlier findings by Percival [34] on the uses and meanings of domestic spaces in the daily lives of older people in the United Kingdom. In this British study, older people require adequate, accessible, and personalized domestic spaces in order to facilitate three objectives, namely, routines, responsibilities, and reflection. The study by Róin [35] found that home as a concept has different meanings for different older people, depending on various conditions. Groger [36] found that the respondents' ability to consider a nursing home a "home" was related primarily to the criteria they used to define "home." Other indicators that emerged from her study included the circumstances of nursing home placement, previous experience with nursing homes, and the degree of continuity achieved after placement. It seems that older people residing in the community and in nursing homes broadly have the same needs. However, they may face different boundary conditions in the extent to which they are autonomous in their choices and actions. In this view, coping styles and being able to deal with living in a nursing home in general are important. Residents who are not open to the new situation or environment may never be able to feel at home in a nursing home [14]. Mortenson et al. [37] studied the impact novel surveillance technologies would have on the everyday experience of home in community-dwelling older people. They concluded that new technologies may alter the perceptions of home as surveillance technologies increase the permeability of the home by extending the power of observation into what was previously regarded as an intimate and private space. In the near future, novel care technologies may also pose an unknown influence to the development of a sense of home in the nursing home, which deserves attention in future studies and practice.

The main challenge for future work is how to move from specifying themes to the identification and development of feasible and replicable evidence-based interventions that contribute to the sense of home. Based on the themes and factors identified in this study, scales and questionnaires could be developed as a first step to objectively measure the aspects of a sense of home that nursing home residents experience. No studies, to our knowledge, have investigated these aspects in residents of nursing homes on a large scale. Regarding the gathering of objective evidence of at-homeness, there is a need for conducting larger, longitudinal studies using a reliable and valid measure of at-homeness such as the Experience of Home Scale [38]. We need to examine predictors and sequelae of at-homeness in both small group homes that incorporate architectural qualities of home as well as social and care-related interventions [27]. For instance, the U.S. model of the so-called Green House nursing homes [39], which are created to be a "real home," yet lacks clarity on the mediating role of the perceived or lived experience of at-homeness on the outcomes. In many Dutch small group homes, homelikeness is propagated, whereas the sense of home may be more fitting and appropriate construct to consider. As the sense of home encompasses social, psychological, and architectural aspects, it remains to be determined whether these aspects should be addressed, in terms of interventions, separately or holistically. Preliminary work shows that certain aspects of Dutch small group homes are successful in providing a homelike atmosphere, such as privacy, own choice, and emphasizing autonomy [40]. Nursing staff and healthcare managers can create a sense of personal freedom in which residents can decorate their rooms according to personal preferences. In order to measure the impact of improvement efforts, there are more tools available within the domain of nursing sciences compared to the domain of architectural studies to measure effects. Future research should address all these aspects and measure their effectiveness. As for coping styles, this is an area not studied extensively in the context of nursing home residents [41, 42].

The factors identified in this study relate to the sense of home of nursing home residents. However, this review also elaborated further on aspects that have an indirect relationship to the sense of home. These factors were taken into account for two reasons. First, the additional information in this review provides important guidance for practice. An example of this is the text about family involvement and large apartments to receive visitors. Second, these additional aspects possibly mediate associations with the sense of some, for example, the need to feel known and valued as an individual. Some studies describe that identity of residents is the strongest when their sense of their own value and uniqueness and other people's actions that communicated their worth matched. The concept of dignity seems very relevant here, and it is not only just a part of a psychological theme, but also interactional and part of a larger social theme. All kinds of engagement identified in this study, for instance, the engagement with one's senses and spiritual engagement, highlight the interaction within and across themes.

Some of the factors identified in this study, for instance, the sense of acknowledgement, describe that the identity of residents was the strongest when their sense of their own value and uniqueness and other people's actions that communicated their worth matched. The concept of dignity seems very relevant here, and it is not only just a part of a psychological theme, but also interactional and part of a larger social theme. All kinds of engagement identified in this study, for instance, the engagement with one's senses and spiritual engagement, highlight the interaction within and across themes.

Apart from these interrelationships, there are also tensions between factors. There may be tensions between resident preferences and family preferences, in relation to autonomy and control on the one hand and continuity of family relationships on the other hand [31]. There may also be tensions that emerge when health and functional disability limit the ability to engage in behaviors, activities, rituals, or social interactions that limit the ability to preserve continuation of old life. Not all nursing home organizations seem to be able to come up with adequate solutions in order to try to create a sense of home. In future studies, the prioritization of needs should be studied in order to gain a better understanding of such tensions and how these tensions can be resolved.

4.2. Strengths and Limitations. This review's strengths lie in its extensive search strategy, covering databases in the fields of social sciences, health care, and architecture. This systematic and multidisciplinary approach is also reflected in the extraction of factors from qualitative research, which was done by two independent reviewers from different backgrounds (psychology and engineering) and verified by several researchers with a background in medicine, health studies, architecture, and applied gerontology. Another strength is the inclusion of all types of available evidence, regardless of the type of research method (qualitative, quantitative, or mixed methods). The qualitative data included in this study was rich and yielded many factors and illustrative quotes.

Some limitations have to be acknowledged. First, moderating or mediating relationships between factors were not investigated in this review due to lack of available data. However, this review is one of the few studies that investigated the sense of home in a holistic manner, including both the social and care environments, as well as the architecture and interior design of the nursing home. Another limitation to this study is that studies were not appraised in terms of their methodological strength. Results of the included studies were treated equally. Finally, the studies included in this review gathered data from Western countries from three continents (North America, Australasia, and Europe). The results may reflect the sense of home as it is experiences in Western contexts, and the findings could, therefore, be different if studies from Asia would have been available.

4.3. Implications for Practice. This review has identified 15 major and minor factors influencing the sense of home of nursing home residents. Most findings can be directly implemented into practice. Care professionals, for instance, can pay attention to their actions and attitudes towards the sense of home of nursing home residents. In addition, managers and policy makers are offered practical guidance on how to improve facility-related aspects that influence the sense of home, for example, the built environment. The findings of this study need to be viewed in the context of policy and practice. In every country, policies related to nursing home administration and financing, as well as care practices, differ, and so do national building codes, methods of construction, and architectural preferences. Nevertheless, this review forms a basis for future studies which should help identify the exact needs of residents, within a national context or within certain financial constraints.

Attitudes and Social Interaction. Nursing staff could start engaging with the residents and stimulate them in having social interaction with others and taking parts in activities which are meaningful and make the best use of remaining capabilities. Relatives should be welcomed to give a helping hand and should also feel at home to some degree. This requires a different set of skills of nursing staff other than being qualified to provide care, for instance, empathetic, social, and communicative competences.

The Built Environment. The general attitude of a facility should be welcoming, not only on a social engagement level, but also in relation to being free in redesigning and decorating the private rooms and even the communal living rooms or corridors. Being able to decorate a room enables residents to turn the nursing home space into a private room which has a connection to the previous life. Residents, who wish to decorate their room, paint it in a different color, or put up artwork, should not be confronted with strict rules but should be invited to make changes and engage in a dialogue (supported by a loved one) to mutually explore the boundaries of their actions. Architects should consider such needs when designing, retrofitting, or transforming nursing homes, for instance, by providing sufficient space for personal belongings.

The Outdoor Environment. Gardens and neighborhoods should be available to residents who are still able to enjoy a fitting degree of freedom. They form an integrated part of life in a nursing home. Despite these recommendations, one needs to be aware that the development of a sense of home depends on a large number of factors that may vary for each individual. One solution to raise awareness among professional caregivers could be the provision of factsheets containing hints for improving the factors identified in this study. Education and training may be other instruments to improve the living conditions in nursing homes.

5. Conclusions and Recommendations

This study has shown that the sense of home of nursing home residents is influenced by a multitude of psychological and social factors, as well as the built environment of nursing homes. Further research is needed to determine if and how the factors in this review are interrelated, if there are differences in perspectives between the various stakeholders involved, and how the factors can be implemented in practice as viable solutions to improve the sense of home. The built environment is an import theme which should be considered when trying to improve the sense of home of nursing home residents. These environmental factors are not always addressed in practice, as they are not considered a core item in the provision of health care. Therefore, it should be stimulated to have architects, designers, and care professionals work together in the creation of optimal designs of nursing home environments. In relationship to the social and psychological factors, a person-centered approach in nursing home care seems important, and this person-centeredness should also include the relatives of the residents. The quality of the interaction with care staff and the activities that are being conducted deserve more attention in daily practice and offer a means for improving the sense of home. Finally, we recommend addressing the interaction between the psychological, social, and environmental components of living in a nursing home in a holistic manner. To date, there is insufficient evidence on how to stimulate this interaction. In the end, the sense of home is centered on balancing these three aspects. In practice, the emphasis is either on quality of care and interaction or on the quality of the built environment. A better way forward may lie in stimulating empathic care professionals in how to use the building and its interior design to the full advantage of their professional task and the residents.

Competing Interests

The authors declare that they have no competing interests.

Acknowledgments

The RAAK (Regional Attention and Action for Knowledge Circulation) scheme, which is managed by the Foundation Innovation Alliance (Stichting Innovatie Alliantie (SIA)) with funding from the Dutch Ministry of Education, Culture and Science (OCW), is thanked for its financial support (SIA Project number 2014-01-05P, *Project Het verpleeghuis van de toekomst is (een) thuis*). RAAK aims to improve knowledge exchange between SMEs and universities of applied sciences in The Netherlands. The authors would like to thank all participants of the sessions for their willingness to volunteer and share their views: BrabantZorg, Vitalis WoonZorg Groep, Savant Zorg, and Archipel Zorggroep. Mrs. Margreet Vossen (Fontys University of Applied Sciences) is acknowledged for the managerial support. Dr. S. M. G. Zwakhalen and Professor J. P. H. Hamers are thanked for their critical input during the literature review.

References

[1] E. van Zadelhoff and H. Verbeek, *Morgen Mag ik Naar het Verpleeghuis! Toekomstvisie op Zorg voor Mensen met Dementie*, Boom-Lemma, The Hague, The Netherlands, 2012 (Dutch).

[2] C. J. M. L. van Dijck-Heinen, E. J. M. Wouters, B. M. Janssen, and J. van Hoof, "The environmental design of residential care facilities: a sense of home through the eyes of nursing home residents," *International Journal for Innovative Research in Science & Technology*, vol. 1, no. 4, pp. 57–69, 2014.

[3] G. Bloemendal, M. Duijnstee, and J. C. M. Hattinga Verschure, *Thuis in het Verpleeghuis. Werken-Wonen-Bezoeken*, Uitgeverij Intro, Nijkerk, The Netherlands, 1985 (Dutch).

[4] S. Schüssler, C. Lohrmann, and A. Marengoni, "Change in care dependency and nursing care problems in nursing home residents with and without dementia: a 2-year panel study," *PLoS ONE*, vol. 10, no. 10, Article ID e0141653, 2015.

[5] J. van Hoof, M. H. Wetzels, A. M. C. Dooremalen et al., "Technological and architectural solutions for Dutch nursing homes: results of a multidisciplinary mind mapping session with professional stakeholders," *Technology in Society*, vol. 36, no. 1, pp. 1–12, 2014.

[6] J. van Hoof, A. M. C. Dooremalen, M. H. Wetzels et al., "Exploring technological and architectural solutions for nursing home residents, care professionals and technical staff: focus groups with professional stakeholders," *International Journal for Innovative Research in Science & Technology*, vol. 1, no. 3, pp. 90–105, 2014.

[7] J. van Hoof, M. H. Wetzels, A. M. Dooremalen et al., "The essential elements for a nursing home according to stakeholders from healthcare and technology. Perspectives from multiple simultaneous monodisciplinary workshops," *Journal of Housing for the Elderly*, vol. 28, no. 4, pp. 329–356, 2014.

[8] C. Gillsjö, D. Schwartz-Barcott, and I. Von Post, "Home: the place the older adult can not imagine living without," *BMC Geriatrics*, vol. 11, article 10, 2011.

[9] H. W. Wahl, "Environmental influences on aging and behavior," in *Handbook of the Psychology of Aging*, J. E. Birren and K. W. Schaie, Eds., pp. 215–237, Elsevier, San Diego, Calif, USA, 5th edition, 2011.

[10] I. Van Steenwinkel, S. Baumers, and A. Heylighen, "Home in later life: a framework for the architecture of home environments," *Home Cultures*, vol. 9, no. 2, pp. 195–217, 2012.

[11] I. Van Steenwinkel, C. Van Audenhove, and A. Heylighen, "Mary's little worlds: changing person-space relationships when living with dementia," *Qualitative Health Research*, vol. 24, no. 8, pp. 1023–1032, 2014.

[12] M. Bland, "The challenge of feeling 'at home' in residential aged care in New Zealand," *Nursing Praxis in New Zealand*, vol. 21, no. 3, pp. 4–12, 2005.

[13] R. A. Kane, A. L. Caplan, E. K. Urv-Wong, I. C. Freeman, M. A. Aroskar, and M. Finch, "Everyday matters in the lives of nursing home residents: wish for and perception of choice and control," *Journal of the American Geriatrics Society*, vol. 45, no. 9, pp. 1086–1093, 1997.

[14] S. L. Molony, "The meaning of home: a qualitative meta-synthesis," *Research in Gerontological Nursing*, vol. 3, no. 4, pp. 291–307, 2010.

[15] A. Cooney, "'Finding home': a grounded theory on how older people 'find home' in Long-term care settings," *International Journal of Older People Nursing*, vol. 7, no. 3, pp. 188–199, 2012.

[16] J. van Hoof, M. L. Janssen, C. M. C. Heesakkers et al., "The importance of personal possessions for the development of a sense of home of nursing home residents," *Journal of Housing for the Elderly*, vol. 30, no. 1, pp. 35–51, 2016.

[17] J. van Hoof and E. J. M. Wouters, Eds., *Het Verpleeghuis van de Toekomst Is (Een) Thuis*, Bohn Stafleu van Loghum, Houten, The Netherlands, 2014 (Dutch).

[18] J. W. Duyvendak, "Thuisvoelen. Een korte introductie op drie artikelen," *Sociologie*, vol. 5, no. 2, pp. 257–260, 2009 (Dutch).

[19] J. T. Carboni, "Homelessness among the institutionalized elderly," *Journal of Gerontological Nursing*, vol. 16, no. 7, pp. 32–37, 1990.

[20] A. J. E. de Veer and A. Kerkstra, "Feeling at home in nursing homes," *Journal of Advanced Nursing*, vol. 35, no. 3, pp. 427–434, 2001.

[21] H. Falk, H. Wijk, L.-O. Persson, and K. Falk, "A sense of home in residential care," *Scandinavian Journal of Caring Sciences*, vol. 27, no. 4, pp. 999–1009, 2013.

[22] R. Fleming, F. Kelly, and G. Stillfried, "'I want to feel at home': establishing what aspects of environmental design are important to people with dementia nearing the end of life Palliative care in other conditions," *BMC Palliative Care*, vol. 14, no. 1, article 26, 2015.

[23] S. Hauge and K. Heggen, "The nursing home as a home: a field study of residents' daily life in the common living rooms," *Journal of Clinical Nursing*, vol. 17, no. 4, pp. 460–467, 2008.

[24] O. Jonsson, B. Östlund, A. Warell, and E. Dalholm Hornyánszky, "Furniture in Swedish nursing homes: a design perspective on perceived meanings within the physical environment," *Journal of Interior Design*, vol. 39, no. 2, pp. 17–35, 2014.

[25] M. Klaassens and L. Meijering, "Experiences of home and institution in a secured nursing home ward in the Netherlands: a participatory intervention study," *Journal of Aging Studies*, vol. 34, no. 3, pp. 92–102, 2015.

[26] T. Lewinson, V. Robinson-Dooley, and K. W. Grant, "Exploring 'home' through residents' lenses: assisted living facility residents identify homelike characteristics using photovoice," *Journal of Gerontological Social Work*, vol. 55, no. 8, pp. 745–756, 2012.

[27] S. L. Molony, L. K. Evans, S. Jeon, J. Rabig, and L. A. Straka, "Trajectories of at-homeness and health in usual care and small house nursing homes," *Gerontologist*, vol. 51, no. 4, pp. 504–515, 2011.

[28] S. Nakrem, A. G. Vinsnes, G. E. Harkless, B. Paulsen, and A. Seim, "Ambiguities: residents' experience of 'nursing home as my home,'" *International Journal of Older People Nursing*, vol. 8, no. 3, pp. 216–225, 2013.

[29] C. A. Robinson, R. C. Reid, and H. A. Cooke, "A home away from home: the meaning of home according to families of residents with dementia," *Dementia*, vol. 9, no. 4, pp. 490–508, 2010.

[30] J. van Hoof, M. M. Verhagen, E. J. M. Wouters, H. R. Marston, M. D. Rijnaard, and B. M. Janssen, "Picture your nursing home: exploring the sense of home of older residents through photography," *Journal of Aging Research*, vol. 2015, Article ID 312931, 11 pages, 2015.

[31] E. van Zadelhoff, H. Verbeek, G. Widdershoven, E. van Rossum, and T. Abma, "Good care in group home living for people with dementia. Experiences of residents, family and nursing staff," *Journal of Clinical Nursing*, vol. 20, no. 17-18, pp. 2490–2500, 2011.

[32] F. Oswald and H. W. Wahl, "Dimensions of the meaning of home," in *Home and Identity in Late Life: International Perspectives*, G. D. Rowles and H. Chaudhury, Eds., pp. 21–46, Springer, New York, NY, USA, 2005.

[33] E. Felix, H. de Haan, L. Vaandrager, and M. Koelen, "Beyond thresholds: the everyday lived experience of the house by older people," *Journal of Housing for the Elderly*, vol. 29, no. 4, pp. 329–347, 2015.

[34] J. Percival, "Domestic spaces: uses and meanings in the daily lives of older people," *Ageing & Society*, vol. 22, no. 6, pp. 729–749, 2002.

[35] Á. Róin, "The multifaceted notion of home: exploring the meaning of home among elderly people living in the Faroe Islands," *Journal of Rural Studies*, vol. 39, pp. 22–31, 2015.

[36] L. Groger, "A nursing home can be a home," *Journal of Aging Studies*, vol. 9, no. 2, pp. 137–153, 1995.

[37] W. B. Mortenson, A. Sixsmith, and R. Beringer, "No place like home? Surveillance and what home means in old age," *Canadian Journal on Aging*, vol. 35, no. 1, pp. 103–114, 2016.

[38] S. L. Molony, D. Dillon McDonald, and C. Palmisano-Mills, "Psychometric testing of an instrument to measure the experience of home," *Research in Nursing & Health*, vol. 30, no. 5, pp. 518–530, 2007.

[39] L. W. Cohen, S. Zimmerman, D. Reed et al., "The green house model of nursing home care in design and implementation," *Health Services Research*, vol. 51, supplement 1, pp. 352–377, 2016.

[40] H. Verbeek, S. M. G. Zwakhalen, E. van Rossum, G. I. J. M. Kempen, and J. P. H. Hamers, "Small-scale, homelike facilities in dementia care: a process evaluation into the experiences of family caregivers and nursing staff," *International Journal of Nursing Studies*, vol. 49, no. 1, pp. 21–29, 2012.

[41] W. J. Puentes, "Coping styles, stress levels, and the occurrence of spontaneous simple reminiscence in older adult nursing home residents," *Issues in Mental Health Nursing*, vol. 22, no. 1, pp. 51–61, 2001.

[42] B. P. O'Connor and R. J. Vallerand, "Motivation, self-determination, and person-environment fit as predictors of psychological adjustment among nursing home residents," *Psychology and Aging*, vol. 9, no. 2, pp. 189–194, 1994.

22

Death Anxiety, Reliability, Validity, and Factorial Structure of the Farsi Form of the Arabic Scale of Death Anxiety in Iranian Old-Aged Persons

Mahboubeh Dadfar,[1] David Lester,[2] and Fazel Bahrami[3]

[1] *School of Behavioral Sciences and Mental Health, Tehran Institute of Psychiatry, Iran University of Medical Sciences, International Campus, Tehran, Iran*
[2] *Department of Psychology, Stockton University, Galloway, NJ, USA*
[3] *Department of Islamic Theology and Department of Counseling, University of Social Welfare and Rehabilitation Sciences, Tehran, Iran*

Correspondence should be addressed to Fazel Bahrami; bahrami.fazel@yahoo.com

Academic Editor: F. R. Ferraro

The present study is aimed at examining the level of death anxiety and the sex-related differences among old-aged Iranian individuals sample to compare the old-aged persons with young college students and to explore the psychometric properties of the Arabic Scale of Death Anxiety (ASDA) factors in old-aged sample. A sample of 146 volunteer Iranian individuals took part in the study. The mean ages were 68.58 (SD = 7.10), men 68.81 (SD = 7.44) and women 68.28 (SD = 6.76), respectively. The mean score of the ASDA was 51.09 (SD = 20.19). Cronbach's alpha of the ASDA was found to be high (0.94); and Spearman-Brown coefficient was 0.92. Women had a significantly higher mean total score on the ASDA. Old-aged individuals had a significantly higher mean ASDA total score than younger college students (M age = 25.77). The factor analysis of the ASDA items yielded three factors accounting for 67.88% of the total variance labeled (F1) fear of dead people and tombs; (F2) fear of lethal disease and postmortem events; and (F3) death fear. These factors were highly replicable with previous factors extracted from a middle-aged Kuwaiti sample. On the basis of the present results, there are the following three general conclusions: death anxiety is not significantly correlated with age; the sex-related differences on death anxiety are striking in the Iranian samples; and the ASDA has a highly replicable factor structure among two Iranian and Arab countries.

1. Introduction

Death anxiety is a multifaceted construct. It was defined and described the different ways in which it is manifested [1–3]. Death anxiety has been conceptualized as fear of death of oneself; fear of death of others; fear of dying of self; and fear of the dying of others [4–7]. Many factors influence death anxiety such as age, sex, culture, religion, physical health, and mental health [2]. Aging is a stage in developmental psychology and associated with various medical problems, loss of loved ones, and deteriorating cognitive abilities. Old-aged individuals being nearer to the end of life may experience death anxiety or death fear [8, 9].

Cultural variations in conceptualizations of death can determine death anxiety in different ages [10–12]. Many researches showed that death anxiety exists among different cultures including Iranian culture [8, 13–15]. Missler et al. revealed that Dutch elderly people who were in an assisted living facility had higher levels of fear for others and of the dying process than of fear of the unknown. The fear for important others correlated with poor somatic health; and fear of the dying process correlated with low self-esteem, small goal in life, and poor mental well-being [16]. For most of old-aged individuals who encounter death of their spouses, death anxiety increases in them. For example, Momtaz et al., on a national cross-sectional survey in Malaysian middle-aged and older couples, reported that women (52%) had significantly higher spousal death anxiety compared to men (45%). Caregiving issues for older men and financial security for older women could predict increasing spousal death anxiety [17].

Death anxiety impacts behavior and life and death decisions [18, 19], and one study found that depression and severity of illness positive correlated with death anxiety [20]. One study showed that death anxiety could be a determining factor of health promoting behaviors both in young and older adults [21]. Abdel-Khalek and Lester found that somatic symptoms were associated with death anxiety, on the Arabic Scale of Death Anxiety (ASDA) and the Collett-Lester Fear of Death Scale (CLFDS); the Kuwaiti young adults with good somatic health were anxious about death compared with American young adults [22].

The ASDA has been used in various populations, for example, health professionals [23], drug dependents [24], psychiatric patients, healthy individuals [25], college students [3], and middle-aged individuals [26], to investigate the factors related to death anxiety.

In spite of the fact that death anxiety is one of the issues related to health, well-being, and welfare of elderly persons in the societies, the little studies have focused on it among the elder population. In the present study it is hypothesized that (a) Iranian old-aged women would have higher death anxiety, (b) death anxiety levels would differ between Iranian young adults and older adults, and (c) and (d) the Farsi form of the Arabic Scale of Death Anxiety (ASDA) has good psychometric properties of factors among Iranian old-aged individuals.

2. Methods

2.1. Participants. The study was a cross-sectional, descriptive study. A sample of 146 volunteer Iranian old-aged individuals took part in the study. They were selected by convenient sampling. The elders had come to the neighborhood parks for leisure, recreation, and the activities done for enjoyment when they were not working. The study is limited to the old persons located in Tehran city. The range of age was 60–90 years, with mean ages 68.58 (SD = 7.10), male being 68.81 (SD = 7.44) and female being 68.28 (SD = 6.76), respectively. 80 (58%) were male and 58 (42%) female. The majority of them were married (n = 107; 75%) and had an education level of diploma (n = 56; 39%).

2.2. Measures. Demographic characteristics sheet of the sample includes age, gender, education status, and marital status. The Arabic Scale of Death Anxiety (ASDA) was developed by Abdel-Khalek, and it is one of the scales for measuring death anxiety [27]. The ASDA has been validated in the Arabic countries of Egypt, Kuwait, and Syria [26–28], the Western countries [29], and the Asian countries of Turkey [3]. It has 20 items, and each item is answered on a five-point intensity scale anchored by no (1) and very much (5) [28].

Abdel-Khalek and Al-Kandari reported that Cronbach's alpha of the ASDA was high (0.93), and the ASDA yielded three factors disease in Kuwaiti middle-aged individuals labeled (F1) fear of dead people and tombs; (F2) fear of postmortem events; and (F3) fear of lethal disease [26]. Sarıçiçek Aydoğan et al. found Cronbach's alpha for Turkish version of the ASDA was 0.86, for each item was from 0.85 (for items (11) and (12)) to 0.90 (for item (20)), the Guttman coefficient was 0.86, and the ASDA was highly associated with the DAS (r = 0.68). They obtained five factors in the sample of Turkish college students, accounting for 65.6% of the total variance and labeled (F1) fear provoked by visual stimuli related to death; (F2) fear of physical and psychological pain related to death; (F3) fear of other situations reminding of death; (F4) fear of postmortem events; and (F5) fear of the act of dying [3].

3. Results

The Pearson correlations between the total score of the ASDA and age was 0.012 (no significance); sex −.443 (p > .01); education −.155 (no significant); and marital status .302 (p > .01).

3.1. Reliability of the ASDA. For old-aged individuals' sample, the Cronbach alpha was 0.94, the split-half reliability was 0.86, the Spearman-Brown coefficient was 0.92, and the Guttman coefficient was 0.92. The intercorrelations between the items ranged from 0.15 to 0.79, and the item-total correlations ranged from 0.60 to 0.80 in the sample.

The mean score of the ASDA was 51.09 (SD = 20.19), for women 62.36 (SD = 17.00) and men 44.33 (SD = 18.93). Old-aged women had a significantly higher mean ASDA total score than men (t = 5.75, p < .001). The mean scores of the ASDA items were from 1.67 (SD = 1.10) for item (12) "I dread walking in graveyards" to 3.58 (1.49) for item (6) "I worry that death deprives me of someone dear to me." Old-aged women had significantly higher mean scores in all of the ASDA items than men (Table 1).

The mean score of the ASDA for elders was 51.09 (SD = 20.19) and for college students 41.40 (SD = 12.73). Old-aged individuals had a significantly higher mean ASDA total score than younger college students (t = −5.86 and p < .001) (Table 2).

3.2. Factor Analysis of the ASDA. The criteria for the factor analysis were evaluated using the Kaiser-Meyer-Olkin Measure of Sampling Adequacy (KMO) and the Bartlett Test of Sphericity. The KMO was 0.919, indicating the adequacy of the sample of college students, and the Bartlett Test of Sphericity was 2.203E3 (df = 190 and p < .001) indicating that the factor analysis was justified in the elders sample. Three components with eigenvalues greater than one were retained in the sample of elders as reported in Table 3.

Factor 1 (8 items) explained 49.71% of the observed variance and was labeled "fear of lethal disease and death." It included the following items: "I fear looking at the dead," "I am afraid of looking at a corpse," "witnessing the burial procedure terrifies me," "I dread walking in graveyards," "I am preoccupied with thinking about what will happen after death," "I get upset by witnessing a funeral," "the sight of

TABLE 1: Mean and standard deviation of the Arabic Death Anxiety Scale items in Iranian elders.

(ASDA) items	M (SD) Total	M (SD) Women	M (SD) Men	t	p
(1) I fear death whenever I because ill.	2.41 (1.45)	2.89 (1.44)	2.12 (1.39)	3.16	.002
(2) I fear looking at the dead.	1.95 (1.26)	2.50 (1.48)	1.63 (.97)	4.11	.000
(3) I fear visiting graves.	2.01 (1.39)	2.65 (1.58)	1.62 (1.09)	4.51	.000
(4) The possibility of having a surgical operation terrifies me.	2.58 (1.49)	3.29 (1.33)	2.11 (1.41)	4.95	.000
(5) I am afraid of suffering heart attack.	3.07 (1.45)	3.77 (1.10)	2.62 (1.47)	4.99	.000
(6) I worry that death deprives me of someone dear to me.	3.58 (1.49)	4.12 (1.07)	3.30 (1.60)	3.38	.001
(7) I am apprehensive of unknown things after death.	2.79 (1.57)	3.43 (1.35)	2.40 (1.57)	4.02	.000
(8) I am afraid of looking at a corpse.	1.90 (1.29)	2.34 (1.52)	1.65 (1.05)	3.15	.002
(9) I fear the torture of the grave.	2.99 (1.55)	3.75 (1.32)	2.57 (1.51)	4.76	.000
(10) I fear getting a serious disease.	3.32 (1.45)	3.98 (1.08)	2.93 (1.50)	4.51	.000
(11) Witnessing the burial procedure terrifies me.	1.97 (1.35)	2.37 (1.53)	1.67 (1.12)	3.11	.002
(12) I dread walking in graveyards.	1.67 (1.10)	2.01 (1.31)	1.46 (.88)	2.95	.004
(13) I am preoccupied with thinking about what will happen after death.	2.57 (1.51)	3.22 (1.45)	2.20 (1.42)	4.13	.000
(14) I am afraid of sleeping and not waking up again.	2.34 (1.59)	2.93 (1.75)	1.93 (1.31)	3.80	.000
(15) The pain accompanying death terrifies me.	3.19 (1.43)	3.75 (1.04)	2.85 (1.55)	3.84	.000
(16) I get upset by witnessing a funeral.	2.08 (1.33)	2.48 (1.42)	1.87 (1.23)	2.66	.009
(17) The sight of a dying person frightens me.	2.45 (1.40)	3.13 (1.35)	2.10 (1.27)	4.58	.000
(18) Talking about death upsets me.	2.14 (1.36)	2.63 (1.43)	1.87 (1.26)	3.30	.001
(19) I am afraid of getting cancer.	3.47 (1.54)	4.03 (1.12)	3.16 (1.68)	3.42	.001
(20) I fear death.	2.51 (1.60)	3.00 (1.62)	2.21 (1.52)	2.91	.004
Total score of the ASDA	51.09 (20.19)	62.36 (17.00)	44.33 (18.93)	5.75	.000

TABLE 2: Mean and standard deviation of the Arabic Death Anxiety Scale in Iranian elders ($N = 146$) and college students ($N = 252$).

Arabic Scale of Death Anxiety (ASDA)	Elders M (SD)	College students M (SD)	t	p
	51.09 (20.19)	41.40 (12.73)	−5.86	.000

a dying person frightens me," and "talking about death upsets me."

Factor 2 (8 items) explained 11.95% of the observed variance and was labeled "fear of lethal disease and postmortem events" and included the following items: "the possibility of having a surgical operation terrifies me," "I am afraid of suffering heart attack," "I worry that death deprives me of someone dear to me," "I am apprehensive of unknown things after death," "I fear getting a serious disease," "I am preoccupied with thinking about what will happen after death," "the pain accompanying death terrifies me," and "I am afraid of getting cancer."

Factor 3 (4 items) explained 6.20% of the observed variance and was labeled "death fear". It included the following items: "I fear death whenever I because ill," "I fear visiting graves," "I am afraid of sleeping and not waking up again," and "I fear death".

4. Discussion and Conclusion

The first hypothesis was confirmed. The study showed that female Iranian elders had a significantly higher mean ASDA total score compare to men. The gender and age results in this Iranian sample are similar to that in some Western, Arabic, and Indian samples. For example Neimeyer and Fortner found that women had higher death anxiety than men [30]. Suhail and Akram showed that Pakistani Muslims women had higher death anxiety than men [31]. Abdel-Khalek using the ASDA declared that Egyptian women in clinical and nonclinical groups had higher mean scores than men [25]. Another study showed that there were strong sex differences in the DAS scores of men and women [11]. Abdel-Khalek and Al-Kandari found Kuwaiti middle-aged women had a significantly higher mean ASDA total score also on 17 out of 20 items of the scale [26]. On the Death Anxiety Survey Schedule from an Indian perspective, Madnawat and Kachhawa indicated that women were significantly more anxious about the word of death [32]. Abdel-Khalek et al. found that, on the ASDA, Egyptian, Kuwaiti, Lebanese, Syrian, Spanish, and American women (no English women) had significant higher mean scores than men [29]. Missler et al. reported that women compared to men had more fear of the death of loved ones and of the consequences of their own death on these loved ones [16]. Singh reported that women as compared with men had more death anxiety [33]. Thabet et al. found that Palestinian women had more death anxiety than men [34]. Our results were not similar to findings of Fortner and Neimeyer that reported gender did not predict death anxiety in elderly people but death anxiety was higher in young female adults [35]; Wu et al. showed that gender does not affect death anxiety in Chinese elderly people [36]; Chuin and Choo found that Malaysian

TABLE 3: Factor loadings of the Farsi version of the Arabic Scale of Death Anxiety (ASDA) in Iranian elders ($N = 146$).

(ASDA) items	Component 1	2	3
(1) I fear death whenever I because ill.			**.707**
(2) I fear looking at the dead.	**.754**		
(3) I fear visiting graves.			**.777**
(4) The possibility of having a surgical operation terrifies me.		**.610**	
(5) I am afraid of suffering heart attack.		**.782**	
(6) I worry that death deprives me of someone dear to me.		**.631**	
(7) I am apprehensive of unknown things after death.		**.506**	
(8) I am afraid of looking at a corpse.	**.788**		
(9) I fear the torture of the grave.			
(10) I fear getting a serious disease.		**.862**	
(11) Witnessing the burial procedure terrifies me.	**.799**		
(12) I dread walking in graveyards.	**.692**		
(13) I am preoccupied with thinking about what will happen after death.	**.509**	.517	
(14) I am afraid of sleeping and not waking up again.			**.696**
(15) The pain accompanying death terrifies me.		**.749**	
(16) I get upset by witnessing a funeral.	**.854**		
(17) The sight of a dying person frightens me.	**.769**		
(18) Talking about death upsets me.	**.766**		
(19) I am afraid of getting cancer.		**.888**	
(20) I fear death.			**.652**
Eigen value	9.94	2.39	1.24
% of variance	49.71	11.95	6.20
% of total variance	67.88		

Factor 1 (items: (2), (8), (11), (12), (13), (16), (17), and (18)): fear of dead people and tombs.
Factor 2 (items: (4), (5), (6), (7), (10), (13), (15), and (19)): fear of lethal disease and postmortem events.
Factor 3 (items: (1), (3), (14), and (20)): death fear.

women had lower death anxiety [37]; and Mimrot indicated that gender had no impact on death anxiety; and there was no significant difference between Indian old age men and women in death anxiety scores [38]. Rasmussen and Johnson found female undergraduate college students had higher levels of death anxiety than males [39]. On the Death Anxiety Scale (DAS), Death Depression Scale (DDS), and Death Obsession Scale (DOS), Bahrami et al. reported that Iranian Muslim female older adults had higher death distress than men but no significant difference [8]. Overall, it seems that Iranian elder women were more expressive of their death anxiety, and elder men were more in denial of their death anxiety. Schumaker et al. indicated that causes of higher death anxiety in women include encouraging to pursue success and attain accomplishments for men in many cultures, more readily admitting troubling feelings in women, and different connotations and implications for men and women [40]. Chuin and Choo indicated that men like women have death anxiety but suppress it or deny it [37]; also process of socialization [25], emotional evaluation of death by women, and cognitive evaluation of death by men can justify lower death anxiety in men [41].

The second hypothesis was affirmed. Our findings showed that old-aged individuals had a significantly higher mean ASDA total score than younger college students. Suhail and Akram showed that Pakistani Muslim elders had higher death anxiety [31]. Mimrot found that Indian old age people had high death anxiety. Some studies reported findings inconsistent with our results [38]. Keller et al. reported that middle age and late-middle age individuals were significantly less anxious in regard to evaluation of death in general than older and younger persons. Old age individuals had the least anxiety toward death anxiety related to self [42]. Studies of Feifel and Nagy; Maiden and Walker; Walker and Maiden, cited in Chuin and Choo, declared that age was not related to death fear and age did not impact death anxiety as elders were no more likely to fear death compared to younger persons [37]. Singh reported that younger persons as compared with older persons had more death anxiety [33]. Goebel and Boeck, cited in Mimrot, reported low death anxiety in late adulthood; and age was not a significant factor in determining the degree of death anxiety in late adulthood [38]. Rasmussen and Brems indicated that psychosocial maturity was a stronger predictor of death anxiety than age; and both age and psychosocial maturity were significantly inversely related to death anxiety [43]. Abdel-Khalek and Al-Kandari found that Kuwaiti middle-aged individuals had a significantly lower mean ASDA total score than younger college students [26]. Chuin and Choo revealed that death anxiety levels did not differ between Malaysian young adults and older adults [37].

There was a linear increase in death anxiety along with the advance in age [44]. Goebel and Boeck, cited in Mimrot, found no relationship between death anxiety and age [38]. One study found that individuals with physical and mental health problems are more sensitive to death anxiety [41]. Another study showed that Indian old age people living in the family had high death anxiety. There was a difference between Indian old age people living in family and old age institutionalized people in death anxiety; and old age people living in the family had high death anxiety [38]. One study indicated that elders living in the more dangerous situations had higher death anxiety than those living in less dangerous situations [33]. Overall, death anxiety levels change according to used tools for death anxiety, place of living, and lifestyle of old-aged persons, and are also related to experiences that elders had during their lives.

Mimrot concluded that ego integrity or an accomplishment and fulfillment of personal sense, founded in religion or some other related measures, is probably the greatest factor in death anxiety [38]. Our finding may reflect cultural differences in death anxiety. Also our study did not support Erikson's theory because the Iranian old-aged sample could not be viewed in the ego integrity stage of Erikson's theory and they experienced high death anxiety. It is probable that an old person can equilibrate for psychosocial maturity in Rasmussen-Brens's theory with ego integrity Erikson's theory, so we can consider supporting Erikson's studies in Iranian old-aged persons.

The third hypothesis of the present study was to explore the reliability, validity, and descriptive statistics of the Farsi version of Abdel-Khalek's ASDA in the Iranian samples of elders. The hypothesis was proved. The results indicate that the ASDA has high internal consistency, split-half, and Spearman-Brown reliabilities (ranging from 0.86 to 0.94) in the sample. The principal components analysis identified three components of the ASDA in Iranian elders as follows: "fear of dead people and tombs," "fear of lethal disease and postmortem events," and "death fear." These factors were highly replicable with previous high internal consistency and factors extracted from a Kuwaiti college student sample and a Kuwaiti middle-aged sample [26]. Abdel-Khalek obtained four components in an Egyptian sample, labeled "fear of dead people and tombs," "fear of postmortem events," "fear of lethal disease," and "death preoccupation." The first two factors were almost completely identical in three Arab countries [28]. Sarıçiçek Aydoğan et al. obtained five factors in a Turkish college students sample, labeled "fear provoked by visual stimuli related to death," "fear of physical and psychological pain related to death," "fear of other situations reminding death," "fear of postmortem events," and "fear from the act of dying" [3]. There were some similarities in specific factors between the previous results and the present findings.

In the present study, mean score of the ASDA was 51.09 (SD = 20.19). In study of Chuin and Choo mean score of the DAS was 7.35 (SD = 3.49) in middle adulthood and elders [37]; and, in study of Bahrami et al. (2014), mean score of the DAS was 7.48 (SD = 3.32) in Iranian elders [8]. The ASDA items receiving the highest mean score in the present sample of old ages were as follows: item (5) "I am afraid of suffering heart attack" (3.07), item (6) "I worry that death deprives me of someone dear to me" (3.58), item (15) "The pain accompanying death terrifies me" (3.19), item (10) "I fear getting a serious disease" (3.32), and item (19) "I am afraid of getting cancer" (3.47).

Religious attitudes are one of the correlates of death anxiety in aging. One study found that religiousness buffered against the death and dying anxiety in American late adulthoods [45]. Several studies investigated the relationship between religiosity and death anxiety [46, 47]. Rasmussen and Johnson showed that spirituality had a significant negative relationship with death anxiety [39]. Chuin and Choo showed that religious individuals did not have lower death anxiety [37]. Dadfar et al. found that there was no significant association between religious spiritual well-being and death anxiety total scores among Iranian Muslim elders [9]. In view of Pyne, relationship between religiosity and death fear is consistent with rational choice theory [48].

Our present findings showed that death anxiety has no significant correlation with age; the sex-related differences on death anxiety are striking in the Iranian samples; and the ASDA has a highly replicable factor structure. These results are similar to findings of Abdel-Khalek and Al-Kandari of the volunteer Kuwaiti middle-aged individuals [26]. Therefore, we conclude that the ASDA is useful for assessing death anxiety in Iranian elders in clinical and nonclinical samples.

The present results must be viewed within the limitations imposed by the data. Despite the good psychometric characteristics of the ASDA, the recruitment of the sample was not random but rather one of convenience. The sample was related to the population who live in Tehran, the capital of Iran and Tehran Province, in the north of the country, with a population of around 9 million in the city and 16 million in the wider metropolitan area. It is known that population who live in Tehran may differ from other regions in the country of Iran. Religious spiritual attitudes can predict death anxiety in old-aged individuals, but they were not assessed in our study. However, the ASDA may be useful in research on death anxiety among Iranian old-aged and middle-aged persons, and it is hoped that this study will stimulate further cross-cultural research on the ASDA in the elders.

Future research should be differentiated between the concept of death and the process of dying. Constructing validity of the ASDA with the other scales, using Multidimensional Fear of Death Scale (MFODS), Death Attitude Profile-Revised (DAPR), longitudinal and qualitative studies, comparing old age people living in institutions with old people living in the family, improving the quality of life and health care services for elderly, and investigating death anxiety and factorial structure of the ASDA on the Iranian middle-aged population, physical patients, addicted patients, and the assessing of components and correlates of demographic, psychological, social, religious spiritual, and subcultural of death anxiety in future studies are recommended.

Competing Interests

No conflict of interests was declared by the authors.

References

[1] D. I. Templer, "The contruction and validation of a Death Anxiety Scale," *The Journal of General Psychology*, vol. 82, no. 2, pp. 165–177, 1970.

[2] M. Dadfar and D. Lester, "Death concern and death obsession in iranian nurses," *Psychological Reports*, vol. 116, no. 3, pp. 704–709, 2015.

[3] A. Sarıçiçek Aydoğan, Ş. Gülseren, Ö. Öztürk Sarıkaya, and Ç. Özen, "Reliability and validity of the Turkish version of Abdel-Khalek's Death Anxiety Scale among college students," *Archive of Neuropsychiatry*, no. 52, pp. 371–375, 2015.

[4] D. Lester, "The Collett-Lester fear of death scale," in *Death Anxiety Handbook: Research, Instrumentation and Application*, R. A. Neimeyer, Ed., pp. 45–60, Taylor & Francis, New York, NY, USA, 1994.

[5] D. Lester, "The factorial structure of the revised collett-lester fear of death scale," *Death Studies*, vol. 28, no. 8, pp. 795–798, 2004.

[6] D. Lester and A. M. Abdel-Khalek, "The collett-lester fear of death scale: a correction," *Death Studies*, no. 27, pp. 81–85, 2003.

[7] M. Dadfar, D. Lester, M. K. Atef Vahid, A. A. Asgharnejad Farid, and B. Birashk, *Death Distress in Nurses: Psychoeducational Interventions*, Mir-Mah Publications, Tehran, Iran, 2015.

[8] F. Bahrami, M. Dadfar, D. Lester, and A. M. Abdel-Khalek, "Death distress in Iranian older adult," *Advances in Environmental Biology*, vol. 8, no. 12, pp. 56–62, 2014.

[9] M. Dadfar, F. Bahrami, F. Sheybani Noghabi, and M. Askari, "Relationship between religious spiritual well-being and death anxiety in Iranian elders," *International Journal of Medical Research & Health Sciences (IJMRHS)*, vol. 5, no. 6, pp. 283–287, 2016.

[10] J. T. Gire, "How death imitates life: cultural influences on conceptions of death and dying," in *Online Readings in Psychology and Culture (Unit 14, Chapter 2)*, W. J. Lonner, D. L. Dinnel, S. A. Hayes, and D. N. Sattler, Eds., Center for Cross-Cultural Research, Western Washington University, Bellingham, Wash, USA, 2002.

[11] D. Lester, D. I. Templer, and A. Abdel-Khalek, "A cross-cultural comparison of death anxiety: a brief note," *Omega*, vol. 54, no. 3, pp. 255–260, 2006-2007.

[12] M. Maxfield, B. Kluck, J. Greenberg et al., "Age-related differences in responses to thoughts of one's own death: mortality salience and judgments of moral transgressions," *Psychology Aging*, vol. 22, no. 2, pp. 341–353, 2013.

[13] M. Dadfar, D. Lester, A. A. Asgharnejad Farid, M. K. Atef Vahid, and B. Birashk, "Death depression in Iranian nurses," *Advances in Environmental Biology*, vol. 8, no. 13, pp. 218–222, 2014.

[14] M. Dadfar, D. Lester, A. A. Asgharnizad Farid, M. K. Atef Vahid, and B. Birashk, "Reasons for fearing death in Iranian nurses," *Global Journal on Advances in Pure and Applied Sciences*, no. 4, pp. 335–341, 2014.

[15] M. Dadfar, A. A. Asgharnejad Farid, D. Lester, M. K. Atef Vahid, and B. Birashk, "Effectiveness of death education program by methods of didactic, experimental, and 8A model on the reduction of death distress among nurses," *International Journal of Medical Research & Health Sciences*, vol. 5, no. 7, pp. 60–71, 2016.

[16] M. Missler, M. Stroebe, L. Geurtsen, M. Mastenbroek, S. Chmoun, and K. Van Der Houwen, "Exploring death anxiety among elderly people: a literature review and empirical investigation," *Omega*, vol. 64, no. 4, pp. 357–379, 2011.

[17] Y. A. Momtaz, Sh. A. Haron, R. Ibrahim, and T. A. Hamid, "Spousal death anxiety in old age: gender perspective," *Omega*, vol. 72, no. 1, pp. 69–80, 2015.

[18] M. Dadfar and D. Lester, *Death Education Program: A Practical Guide for Healthcare Professionals*, Mir-Mah, Tehran, Iran, 2014.

[19] M. Dadfar and D. Lester, "Fear of death in Iranian nurses," *The Neuroscience Journal of Shefaye Khatam*, vol. 2, no. 3, supplement 1, p. 62, 2014.

[20] M. Anvar, A. Javadpour, and S. M. Zadeh, "Assessing death anxiety and its correlates among severe medically ill in- patients," *Shiraz E Medical Journal*, vol. 13, no. 3, pp. 122–127, 2012.

[21] M. Ghorbanalipoor, A. Borjali, F. Sohrabi, and M. R. Falsafinejad, "Effect of death anxiety and age on health promoting behaviors," *The Journal of Urmia University of Medical Sciences*, vol. 21, no. 1, pp. 286–292, 2010.

[22] A. M. Abdel-Khalek and D. Lester, "Death anxiety as related to somatic symptoms in two cultures," *Psychological Reports*, vol. 105, no. 2, pp. 409–410, 2009.

[23] F. Ayyad, "Death distress among two samples of lower and higher stress in health care professionals," *Psychological Reports*, vol. 113, no. 1, pp. 1332–1341, 2013.

[24] F. Daradkeh and H. F. Moselhy, "Death anxiety (Thanatophobia) among drug dependents in an Arabic psychiatric hospital," *The American Journal of Drug and Alcohol Abuse*, vol. 37, no. 3, pp. 184–188, 2011.

[25] A. M. Abdel-Khalek, "Death anxiety in clinical and non-clinical groups," *Death Studies*, vol. 29, no. 3, pp. 251–259, 2005.

[26] A. M. Abdel-Khalek and Y. Al-Kandari, "Death anxiety in Kuwaiti middle-aged personnel," *Omega*, vol. 55, no. 4, pp. 297–310, 2007.

[27] A. M. Abdel-Khalek, "A general factor of death distress in seven clinical and non-clinical groups," *Death Studies*, vol. 28, no. 9, pp. 889–898, 2004.

[28] A. M. Abdel-Khalek, "The Arabic Scale of Death Anxiety (ASDA): its development, validation, and results in three Arab countries," *Death Studies*, vol. 28, no. 5, pp. 435–457, 2004.

[29] A. Abdel-Khalek, D. Lester, J. Maltby, and J. Tomás-Sábado, "The Arabic scale of death anxiety: some results from East and West," *Omega*, vol. 59, no. 1, pp. 39–50, 2009.

[30] R. A. Neimeyer and B. V. Fortner, "Death anxiety in the elderly," in *Encyclopaedia of Aging*, G. Maddox, Ed., pp. 252–253, Springer, New York, NY, USA, 2nd edition, 1995.

[31] K. Suhail and S. Akram, "Correlates of death anxiety in Pakistan," *Death Studies*, vol. 26, no. 1, pp. 39–50, 2002.

[32] A. V. S. Madnawat and P. S. Kachhawa, "Age, gender, and living circumstances: discriminating older adults on death anxiety," *Death Studies*, vol. 31, no. 8, pp. 763–769, 2007.

[33] R. S. Singh, "Death anxiety among aged Manipuris, India," *ZENITH International Journal of Multidisciplinary Research*, vol. 3, no. 1, pp. 209–216, 2013.

[34] A. A. Thabet, A. A. Tawahina, E. E. Sarraj, and P. Vostanis, "Death anxiety, PTSD, trauma, grief, and mental health of Palestinian victims of war on Gaza," *Health Care Current Reviews*, vol. 112, pp. 1–8, 2013.

[35] B. V. Fortner and R. A. Neimeyer, "Death anxiety in older adults: a quantitative review," *Death Studies*, vol. 23, no. 5, pp. 387–411, 1999.

[36] A. M. S. Wu, C. S. K. Tang, and T. C. Y. Kwok, "Death anxiety among Chinese elderly people in Hong Kong," *Journal of Aging and Health*, vol. 14, no. 1, pp. 42–56, 2002.

[37] C. L. Chuin and Y. C. Choo, "Age, gender, and religiosity as related to death anxiety," *Sunway Academic Journal*, no. 6, pp. 1–16, 2010.

[38] B. H. Mimrot, "A comparative study of death anxiety of old persons," *Indian Streams Research Journal*, vol. I, no. 7, 2011.

[39] C. H. Rasmussen and M. E. Johnson, "Spirituality and religiosity: relative relationships to death anxiety," *Omega; Journal of Death and Dying*, vol. 29, no. 4, pp. 313–318, 1994.

[40] J. F. Schumaker, R. A. Barraclough, and L. M. Vagg, "Death anxiety in Malaysian and Australian university students," *The Journal of Social Psychology*, vol. 128, no. 1, pp. 41–47, 1988.

[41] S. J. DePaola, M. Griffin, J. R. Young, and R. A. Neimeyer, "Death anxiety and attitudes toward the elderly among older adults: the role of gender and ethnicity," *Death Studies*, vol. 27, no. 4, pp. 335–354, 2003.

[42] J. W. Keller, D. Sherry, and C. Piotrowski, "Perspectives on death: a developmental study," *The Journal of Psychology*, vol. 116, no. 1, pp. 137–142, 1984.

[43] C. A. Rasmussen and C. Brems, "The relationship of death anxiety with age and psychosocial maturity," *The Journal of Psychology*, vol. 130, no. 2, pp. 141–144, 1996.

[44] K. D. Wagner and R. P. Lorion, "Correlates of death anxiety in elderly persons," *Journal of Clinical Psychology*, vol. 40, no. 5, pp. 1235–1241, 1984.

[45] P. Wink and J. Scott, "Does religiousness buffer against the fear of death and dying in late adulthood? Findings from a longitudinal study," *Journals of Gerontology—Series B Psychological Sciences and Social Sciences*, vol. 60, no. 4, pp. P207–P214, 2005.

[46] D. Lester and A. M. Abdel-Khalek, "Religiosity and death anxiety using non-Western scales," *Psychological Reports*, vol. 103, no. 3, pp. 652–722, 2008.

[47] Y.-H. Wen, "Religiosity and death anxiety," *The Journal of Human Resource and Adult Learning*, vol. 6, no. 2, pp. 31–37, 2010.

[48] D. Pyne, A model of religion and death, 2008, http://www.sciencedirect.com/science/article/pii/1053535709001140.

23

Validity of the German Version of the Continuous-Scale Physical Functional Performance 10 Test

Irene Härdi,[1] Stephanie A. Bridenbaugh,[1] M. Elaine Cress,[2] and Reto W. Kressig[1]

[1] *University Center for Medicine of Aging and Rehabilitation, Felix Platter-Hospital, Basel Mobility Center, Basel, Switzerland*
[2] *Department of Kinesiology, Institute of Gerontology, University of Georgia, Athens, GA, USA*

Correspondence should be addressed to Irene Hardi; irene.haerdi@fps-basel.ch

Academic Editor: Barbara Shukitt-Hale

Background. The Continuous-Scale Physical Functional Performance 10 Test (CS-PFP 10) quantitatively assesses physical functional performance in older adults who have a broad range of physical functional ability. This study assessed the validity and reliability of the CS-PFP 10 German version. *Methods.* Forward-translations and backtranslations as well as cultural adaptions of the test were conducted. Participants were German-speaking Swiss community-dwelling adults aged 64 and older. Concurrent validity was assessed using Pearson correlation coefficients between CS-PFP 10 and gait velocity, Timed Up and Go Test, hand grip strength, SF-36 physical function domain, and Freiburger Physical Activity Questionnaire. Internal consistency was calculated by Cronbach's alpha. *Results.* Backtranslation and cultural adaptions were accepted by the CS-PFP 10 developer. CS-PFP 10 total score and subscores (upper body strength, upper body flexibility, lower body strength, balance and coordination, and endurance) correlated significantly with all measures of physical function tested. Internal consistency was high (Cronbach's alpha 0.95–0.98). *Conclusion.* The CS-PFP 10 German version is valid and reliable for measuring physical functional performance in German-speaking Swiss community-dwelling older adults. Quantifying physical function is essential for clinical practice and research and provides meaningful insight into physical functional performance of older adults. This trial is registered with ClinicalTrials.gov NCT01539200.

1. Introduction

The ability to perform activities of daily living such as walking, dressing, or carrying objects is crucial for functional independence. Physical functional limitations in older adults are often strong predictors for disability, nursing home admission, and death [1]. Maintenance of functional independence is a primary goal of older adults, their care providers, and the health-care system. The first step in preventing functional decline is to determine current physical functional performance and beginning deficits [2]. A variety of functional measures exists, from self-reported questionnaires to performance-based assessments of selected tasks [3]. Instruments such as the "Short Physical Performance Battery" [4] or the "Physical Performance Test" [5] measure mobility and balance in older adults but they only provide a partial view of functional performance with little insight into the extent to which the individual is actually restricted in performing everyday activities. Many physical performance measures have floor or ceiling effects [6] which restrict their applicability to a certain range of physical functional performance. Tests of physical functional performance applicable to frail populations often lack meaningful outcomes when used in healthy, vigorous older adults because of an instrument's ceiling effects. Although clinical experience in the evaluation of function is valuable and important, subjective measures of performance can bias scoring and interpretation as well as limit the comparability of results. The quantification of physical function is a crucial addition to clinical practice and clinical research, particularly in providing objective measures and measures of changes over time. It is greatly beneficial to be able to use the same assessment tool in people with a broad range of physical functional ability so that it is applicable for frail, vulnerable, and vigorous populations.

The Continuous-Scale Physical Functional Performance Test (CS-PFP) was developed in the United States by

Professor Elaine Cress (MEC) to accurately, precisely, and objectively assess functional performance in older adults across a broad spectrum of abilities [7]. The English version of the CS-PFP and its short version, the Continuous-Scale Physical Functional Performance 10 Test (CS-PFP 10), are standardized, validated, reliable, and objective measures of physical function in everyday tasks in ambulatory older adults [8]. The CS-PFP 10 addresses a wide range of activities that are important for independence in older adults using 10 common tasks such as picking up something from the floor, transferring laundry from the washer to the dryer, and climbing stairs [7, 8]. From the perspective of evidence-based research, it is essential to have the instrument of interest available in the native language of those being tested and that this instrument undergoes the process of validation to become a widely accepted tool for assessing physical function in older adults with higher physical ability. Furthermore, in order to allow cross-cultural comparisons of study outcomes, the instruments must not only be well-translated, linguistically speaking, but also adapted culturally to maintain the content validity of the instrument [9].

The aims of this study were to describe the translation process as well as the site set-up of the CS-PFP 10 laboratory in a German-speaking region of Switzerland. Furthermore, the study aimed to investigate the concurrent validity and the internal reliability of the German version of the CS-PFP 10 in a sample of community-dwelling, self-reported healthy, older adults.

2. Methods

2.1. Study Design and Population. The present study (validation of the German version of the CS-PFP 10) was part of a randomized placebo-controlled parallel group trial. The main study investigated the effects of 6-month once daily oral whey-protein supplementation in combination with a once weekly Jaques-Dalcroze Eurhythmics training (multicomponent music-based group exercise) on functionality, probability of independence, and/or functional reserve among community-dwelling seniors compared to the effects of 6-month Jaques-Dalcroze Eurhythmics training alone (study abbreviation "NUDAL," ClinicalTrials.gov identifier NCT01539200). Community-dwelling older adults were recruited through information and recruitment events in regional senior centers as well as advertisements in local newspapers and in the local radio of the Canton Basel City. The training sessions took place at different senior centers throughout the Canton Basel City. The baseline data was collected between February 2012 and May 2013. The baseline data used for this substudy was extracted from the entire database of the main study. The study—the main study as well as the present substudy—was approved by the local ethics committee. Written informed consent was given by each participant before study participation.

Inclusion criteria were as follows: (I) community-dwelling males and females, (II) age $\geq$ 64 years, (III) being able to walk unassisted for 15 meters, and (IV) Mini Mental State Examination (MMSE) score $\geq$ 24 points. Exclusion criteria were as follows: (I) serum 25(OH) vitamin D $>$ 100 nmol/L from the blood sampling at baseline, (II) current regular (defined as >3x/week) use of high protein oral nutritional supplements, (III) milk protein allergy, (IV) lactose intolerance, (V) severe visual impairment (corrected near vision $<$ 0.2 in both eyes), (VI) severe neurological, orthopedic, rheumatologic, or psychiatric illness causing inability to understand or follow task instructions or to walk 15 meters without assistance, and (VII) terminal illness with life expectancy less than 12 months, as determined by a physician.

2.2. Procedures. All tests were performed at the Basel Mobility Center or at the Clinical Trial Unit at the University Hospital Basel by trained research assistants or the study physician. Baseline testing consisted of two test batteries which occurred on two separate days maximum 14 days apart. The first test battery included the informed consent, Mini Mental State Examination, the Freiburger Physical Activity Questionnaire, and 36-item Short-Form General Health Survey (SF-36) version 1. The second test battery included the demographic and health data, physical examination, and the functional measurements—hand grip strength, Timed Up and Go Test, gait analysis, and CS-PFP 10.

2.3. Development of the German CS-PFP 10. The translation and cross-cultural adaptation of the original English version of the CS-PFP 10 into German were performed in two respects. First, the test instructions were translated from English to German. Second, the CS-PFP 10 site set-up was culturally adapted, using typically Swiss household items and products (see Site Set-Up).

2.3.1. Test Instructions. The translation of the CS-PFP 10 from English to German was done by one medical doctor (native language American English, fluent German speaker) who was familiar with the objectives of the test. The backtranslation from German to English was done by a different researcher (native language American English, fluent German speaker) who had no prior knowledge of the instrument, was blind to the original version of the CS-PFP 10 instructions, and yet was familiar with health-related topics. MEC, the developer of the CS-PFP 10, examined the backtranslation and approved the test instructions.

2.3.2. Site Set-Up. The site set-up was done in accordance with the "Specification of Measurement by Task" document available on the CS-PFP website (http://www.drelainecress.com/). The CS-PFP 10 consists of 10 everyday tasks and, therefore, requires diverse equipment. To fulfill the requirements of the set-up guidelines, most of the equipment was purchased in the USA, for example, Posey® safety belts, pylons, cooking pots (task 1), jackets (task 2; white hip-length lab jackets are used at our site), and tote bags (task 9), or was constructed just for our laboratory, for example, stair platform (task 8 and 9) that fulfills the stair tread height and depth requirements. However, with approval by MEC, some of the household appliances, accessories, and products were typical of the local culture. For the floor sweep (task 5), a horsehair broom and a hand brush with a short-handled

Table 1: Continuous-Scale Physical Functional Performance 10 Test—tasks and measurements.

	Measurements
Low effort tasks:	
(1) Kitchen pot carry	Time, weight
(2) Put on/take off jacket	Time
(3) Scarves pickup	Time
(4) Maximal reach	Distance
Medium effort tasks:	
(5) Floor sweep	Time
(6) Laundry loading/unloading	Time
(7) Sit down and get up from the floor	Time
Hard effort tasks:	
(8) Stair climbing	Time
(9) Grocery carrying and walking	Time, weight
(10) 6-minute walk	Distance

dustpan was used instead of a broom with synthetic fibers and a long handled dustpan. For the first part of sixth task, the laundry loading task, a top-loading washing machine was replaced by a front-loading washing machine. The grocery items (task 9) were purchased in the Swiss chain grocery stores Coop and/or Migros so that the food and household products were easily recognized by our study participants. These accepted changes to the site set-up protocol made the devices and food products recognizable for the older adults being tested, which made the simulated tasks (such as grocery shopping or sweeping the floor) more realistic. One exception, approved by MEC, was that the sand bags (task 1) were filled with lead granulates; however, the weight and the number of sandbags remained in accordance with the site set-up guidelines.

2.4. Functional Measurements and Questionnaires

2.4.1. CS-PFP 10. The Continuous-Scale Physical Functional Performance 10 Test was developed to quantify information about physical functionality of older adults performing everyday tasks. The test consists of 10 tasks which are carried out under standard conditions and in a predetermined order of increasing intensity and difficulty (see Table 1). A detailed description of the tasks has been reported elsewhere [7]. For each task, the objective values of "time," "weight," or "distance" are measured. The participants are asked to perform each task safely and comfortably but as quickly as possible and with maximal effort. The execution of the task itself is determined by the participants' judgment. The participants are guided by a test administrator throughout the whole test. The instructions, the timing, and other measurements of the tasks and the data entry are standardized. To ensure safety, a Posey safety belt was placed around each patient's waist for easy grasp by the test administrator to prevent a fall.

The measured results are manually entered in the assessment tool software. The software converts the raw data into a scaled score between zero and 100 and provides a total score of the CS-PFP 10, as well as five subscores—upper body strength (UBS), lower body strength (LBS), upper body flexibility (UBF), balance and coordination (B&C), and endurance (END). The total score is the average of all variables. A higher score indicates a higher level of functioning. The CS-PFP value of 57 points or higher is predictive of a physical reserve and independent living status [10]. The original CS-PFP 10 (English version) is a valid, reliable, and sensitive measure with no floor or ceiling effects [7, 8, 11].

2.4.2. Gait Assessment. The spatiotemporal parameters of gait were collected with the GAITRite® system (GAITRite Platinum, CIR System, Sparta, NJ, USA, Version 4.7), a 10-meter-long electronic walkway with integrated pressure sensors [12]. The walking trials were performed according to the European guidelines for spatial-temporal gait analysis [13]. The gait analysis for the NUDAL study consisted of six different walking tasks, whereas walking at habitual, self-selected walking speed (referred to as normal walking in this text) represented the first and second task. Results of both normal walking speed tasks were averaged to be used for analysis. Details regarding the description of the gait analysis at the Basel Mobility Center have been reported elsewhere [14]. Before testing, a trained evaluator gave standardized verbal instructions regarding the test procedure. In order to measure steady-state gait, the patients initiated and terminated each walk 1.25 m before and after the 10 m walkway allowing sufficient distance to accelerate and decelerate. No practice trials were performed. To ensure safety, a Posey safety belt was placed around each patient's waist for easy grasp by the trained evaluator who walked behind the patients during all trials. The patients performed all trials wearing their own footwear. A video camera was used during the gait analysis to allow detailed review. General conditions of the described gait assessment were also reported in a previous article of the principal author [15]. Gait velocity (cm/s) during normal walking (average of two trials) was the parameter of interest for this substudy.

2.4.3. Timed Up and Go Test. Basic mobility was assessed with the Timed Up and Go Test (TUG) [16]. The TUG measures the time in seconds that it takes an individual to rise from a chair with armrests, walk three meters at the person's habitual, self-selected speed, turn, walk back, and sit down again. Older adults who require 14 seconds or longer to complete the task have a high risk for falls [17].

2.4.4. Hand Grip Strength. Hand grip strength was measured in the dominant hand with a GRIP-A T.K.K. 5001 Grip Strength Dynamometer®. The participants performed the test while sitting comfortably with shoulder adducted and neutrally rotated, the elbow flexed to 90 degrees, forearm and wrist in neutral position [18]. The participants were instructed to perform a maximal isometric contraction. The test was repeated after 10 seconds and the higher value (kg) was recorded for data analysis [19]. Reference values for hand grip strength are commonly presented according to age, gender, and side specificity. The average normal value for females aged 70–74 years has been reported to be 24.2 kg for the right-hand side [20].

2.4.5. Freiburger Physical Activity Questionnaire. This self-report questionnaire assesses levels of basic physical activity (e.g., gardening, climbing stairs), leisure time physical activity (e.g., dancing, bowling), and sports activity (e.g., jogging, swimming) in the previous week or in the previous month. Significant test-retest reliability was reported for the summed physical activity level ($r = 0.56$), in people between the ages of 18 and 78 years. Cross-correlation with maximum oxygen uptake revealed a significant correlation coefficient of $r = 0.42$ [21]. For the present study the short version of the questionnaire was used [22] and the parameter of interest was the overall activity (total time in hours per week).

2.4.6. SF-36. Self-perceived physical function was assessed using the validated 36-item Short-Form Health Survey (SF-36) version 1 [23]. The questionnaire consists of 36 questions, is self-administered, and assesses quality of life and well-being in eight multi-item scales regarding physical functioning and perception of physical role, vitality, general and mental health, perception of emotional role, social functioning, and bodily pain. For the present study only the physical function domain (SF-36 PF), which consists of 10 items, was assessed. Each item is scaled between 0 and 100 with higher scores reflecting higher self-perceived function.

2.5. Clinical Evaluation and Assessments. Clinical assessment included the demographic and health data as well as a physical examination. The following data was used for the present study: age, sex, height, weight, falls (defined as unintentionally coming to rest on the ground or other surfaces [24]) in the preceding 12 months (single-item question), fear of falling (single-item question), and relevant medical problems.

2.6. Statistical Analysis. Characteristics of baseline assessment, functional measurements, and questionnaires were summarized descriptively using either means and standard deviations or frequencies and percentages, as appropriate.

The concurrent validation, a subtype of criterion-related validity, of the German version of the CS-PFP 10 was assessed by examining correlation between the CS-PFP 10 (total score and its subscores) and the gait velocity, TUG, hand grip strength, Freiburger Physical Activity Questionnaire, and the SF-36 physical function domain. Correlation was performed using the Pearson correlation coefficient. A correlation value greater than 0.50 indicates a large relationship, a value between 0.50 and 0.30 indicates a moderate relationship, and a value between 0.30 and 0.1 indicates a small relationship [25]. Probability values less than 0.05 were considered statistically significant.

Internal reliability of the German version of the CS-PFP 10 was evaluated by calculating Cronbach's alpha coefficient [26] for each subscore and the total score. Ceiling and floor effects of the CS-PFP 10 and its subscores were determined by reaching the minimum or maximum score.

Analyses were conducted using the SPSS version 22.0 (IBM Corp., Armonk, NY) software program for Windows.

TABLE 2: Participant characteristics at baseline.

Variable	Total sample ($N = 109$)
Age (years)	74.1 ± 6.4
Gender	
Female	91 (83.5)
Male	18 (16.5)
MMSE score (points)	28.2 ± 1.6
Previous fall in the last 12 months	
None	34 (31.2)
1 or more	75 (68.8)
Fear of falling	
Yes	18 (16.5)
No	91 (83.5)
Height (cm)	165.9 ± 7.3
Weight (kg)	72.7 ± 15.4
BMI (kg/m^2)	26.3 ± 4.7

Notes. Values are mean ± standard deviation or frequencies and percentage; MMSE = Mini Mental State Examination; BMI = Body Mass Index.

3. Results

3.1. Development of the German Version of the CS-PFP 10. The translation and backtranslation of the instructions proceeded without difficulties. All participants understood the test and task instructions. For the CS-PFP 10 site set-up, all equipment fulfilled the prescribed guidelines. Either they were purchased in the USA to have the same style and sizes used in the original CS-PFP laboratory or culturally specific Swiss items were used, as approved by MEC and described in the Methods.

The developer of the original CS-PFP 10 version (MEC) visited our CS-PFP 10 site at the Basel Mobility Center in Basel and approved the backtranslation of the test instructions, the set-up of the CS-PFP 10 laboratory, and the cultural adaptions. No alterations were necessary. The Basel Mobility Center is a certified CS-PFP 10 site. Stephanie A. Bridenbaugh (coauthor) is a certified CS-PFP test administrator and a CS-PFP test trainer.

3.2. Descriptive Characteristics of Study Population and Measurements. Table 2 provides the characteristics of the 109 participants included in this substudy. The mean age of the community-dwelling participants was 74.1 ± 6.4 years with an age range of 64–89, and 91 (83.5%) were women.

On average, the participants completed the CS-PFP 10 in approximately 50 minutes. No participants fell or were injured during testing. The mean CS-PFP 10 total score was 44.1 ± 16.2 points, ranging from 9.1 to 84.7 points (Table 3). The performance of task seven "sit down and get up from the floor" was declined by 6 participants (5.5%). Reasons stated were problems with herniated disc ($n = 1$) and concerns about their ability to kneel ($n = 5$; osteoarthritis in knees ($n = 1$), subjective inability after knee or hip surgery ($n = 4$)). For those who declined or were unable to perform this function, a score of zero was entered for this task. All other tasks were carried out by the participants. In total, 87 participants

TABLE 3: Descriptive data of the measurements.

Variable	Minimum	Maximum	Mean	SD
CS-PFP 10 TOT	9.1	84.7	44.1	16.2
CS-PFP 10 UBS	12.4	97.8	46.4	18.7
CS-PFP 10 LBS	6.5	82.3	36.3	16.8
CS-PFP 10 UBF	18.7	83.4	56.0	13.0
CS-PFP 10 B&C	6.9	86.2	44.5	17.1
CS-PFP 10 END	9.1	87.5	45.8	16.8
Gait velocity	56.3	177.5	117.6	22.2
TUG	7.0	20.0	10.9	2.5
Hand grip strength	10.0	47.0	24.9	7.2
Freiburger PA	0.0	35.1	10.1	7.2
SF-36 PF	30.0	100.0	84.7	18.3

Notes. SD = standard deviation, CS-PFP 10 TOT = CS-PFP 10 total score, CS-PFP 10 UBS = CS-PFP 10 upper body strength score, CS-PFP 10 LBS = CS-PFP 10 lower body strength score, CS-PFP 10 UBF = CS-PFP 10 upper body flexibility score, CS-PFP 10 B&C = CS-PFP 10 balance and coordination score, CS-PFP 10 END = CS-PFP 10 endurance score, Freiburger PA = Freiburger Physical Activity Questionnaire, TUG = Timed Up and Go Test, and SF-36 PF = 36-item Short-Form General Health Survey, Physical Function subscore.

(79.8%) had a total score below the threshold score of 57 points, indicating low physical function for carrying out daily activities independently.

No ceiling or floor effects were observed because no participants obtained the highest (100 points) or lowest (0 points) score.

3.3. Validity and Reliability of the German CS-PFP 10

3.3.1. Concurrent Validity. Pearson's product moment correlation coefficients between the CS-PFP 10 total score and subscores and gait velocity, TUG time, hand grip strength, Freiburger Physical Activity Questionnaire results, and SF-36 PF scores are provided in Table 4. The CS-PFP 10 total score as well as the subscores correlated significantly with each of the concurrent validation measures. Scatter plots of the correlations are presented in Figure 1. The total scores' correlations with gait velocity, TUG time, and SF-36 PF score were with the highest magnitude ($r = 0.71$, -0.73, and 0.56, resp.), indicating a large correlation. The total score showed moderate-to-small correlations with the hand grip strength and the Freiburger Physical Activity Questionnaire results ($r = 0.45$ and 0.27, resp.). The CS-PFP 10 subscores' correlations with the other measures were also in the predicted direction and magnitude; for example, the Timed Up and Go Test time correlated highly with the CS-PFP balance and coordination score ($r = -0.73$) and moderately with the CS-PFP upper body flexibility ($r = -0.49$).

3.3.2. Internal Reliability. Internal consistency for the five subscores and total score of the CS-PFP 10 are provided in Table 5. Internal consistency (Cronbach's alpha) for the total score was $\alpha = 0.95$. For the subscores, the coefficient ranged between $\alpha = 0.95$ and 0.98, reaching high reliability for all subscores and the total score.

4. Discussion

In this study, we translated the CS-PFP 10 into German and set up the test laboratory in accordance with the guidelines with some approved (MEC) cultural adaptions. To our knowledge, this is the first time that a German version of the CS-PFP 10 has been validated.

Although physical function is a component of many functional performance assessments (e.g., Timed Up and Go Test [16], 6-minute walk test [27, 28], and Short Physical Performance Battery [4]), these tools often assess only a single task or a small aspect of functional performance and cannot sufficiently determine physical function in older adults who have beginning, subtle functional limitations. It is particularly advantageous to have one standardized, validated, reliable assessment that can be used in frail, vulnerable, and vigorous older adults. In everyday life, physical performance involves more than, for example, rising from a chair, turning around a pylon, and sitting down again, as tested in the TUG [16]. The CS-PFP 10 was developed to assess a broad range of physical functional performance of common, everyday tasks important to functional independence in older adults [7]. This test has been developed for English-speaking people living in the USA, yet there is a need for such functional, objective assessments that can be used in non-English-speaking countries, are well-translated, are adapted to the culture, and are validated to allow comparability of data [9].

Concurrent validity and internal consistency were investigated for the German version of the CS-PFP 10 in this study. The CS-PFP 10 is significantly related to concurrent measures of physical function (gait velocity, TUG, and hand grip strength) as well as self-reported measures (SF-36 physical functioning, Freiburger Physical Activity Questionnaire). The high correlations between the CS-PFP 10 total score and the gait velocity ($r = 0.71$) and with TUG times ($r = -0.73$) confirm the concurrent construct validity of the CS-PFP 10 for evaluating elements of walking ability and general mobility in older adults. The CS-PFP 10 endurance score showed the highest correlation with gait velocity ($r = 0.72$) and TUG times ($r = 0.74$), whereas the CS-PFP 10 upper body flexibility score showed the lowest correlation with these two measures of physical function ($r = 0.55$ and -0.49, resp.), as expected. The third performance-based measure, hand grip strength, showed low-to-moderate correlations with the CS-PFP 10 (values range between $r = 0.22$ and 0.47), except for the CS-PFP 10 upper body strength score ($r = 0.60$). This result seems plausible since the hand grip strength test measures a specific construct which targets most closely the construct of upper body strength. To our knowledge, there are no validity studies that compare the CS-PFP 10 with these measures of physical function. In relation to self-reported measures, the CS-PFP 10 total score highly correlated to the SF-36 physical functioning domain ($r = 0.56$). Cress et al. [7] reported a correlation coefficient of $r = 0.75$ between the CS-PFP 10 total score and the SF-36 physical function domain. The lower correlation coefficient in our study could be explained by two possible factors that affect the size of correlations. It is known from statistics that the

TABLE 4: Pearson's product moment correlation.

	Gait velocity	TUG	Hand grip strength	Freiburger PA	SF-36 PF
CS-PFP 10 TOT	0.71^{**}	-0.73^{**}	0.45^{**}	0.27^{**}	0.56^{**}
CS-PFP 10 UBS	0.60^{**}	-0.63^{**}	0.60^{**}	0.21^{**}	0.58^{**}
CS-PFP 10 LBS	0.69^{**}	-0.71^{**}	0.47^{**}	0.28^{**}	0.58^{**}
CS-PFP 10 UBF	0.55^{**}	-0.49^{**}	0.22^{*}	0.17^{**}	0.30^{**}
CS-PFP 10 B&C	0.70^{**}	-0.73^{**}	0.39^{**}	0.25^{**}	0.51^{**}
CS-PFP 10 END	0.72^{**}	-0.74^{**}	0.40^{**}	0.26^{**}	0.55^{**}

Notes. All correlations are statistically significant with $^{**}p < 0.01$ or $^{*}p < 0.05$; $n = 109$ except for SF-36 physical function, where only $n = 105$ were available; CS-PFP 10 TOT = CS-PFP 10 total score; CS-PFP 10 UBS = CS-PFP 10 upper body strength score; CS-PFP 10 LBS = CS-PFP 10 lower body strength score; CS-PFP 10 UBF = CS-PFP 10 upper body flexibility score; CS-PFP 10 B&C = CS-PFP 10 balance and coordination score; CS-PFP 10 END = CS-PFP 10 endurance score; Freiburger PA = Freiburger Physical Activity Questionnaire; TUG = Timed Up and Go Test; SF-36 PF = 36-item Short-Form General Health Survey, Physical Function subscore.

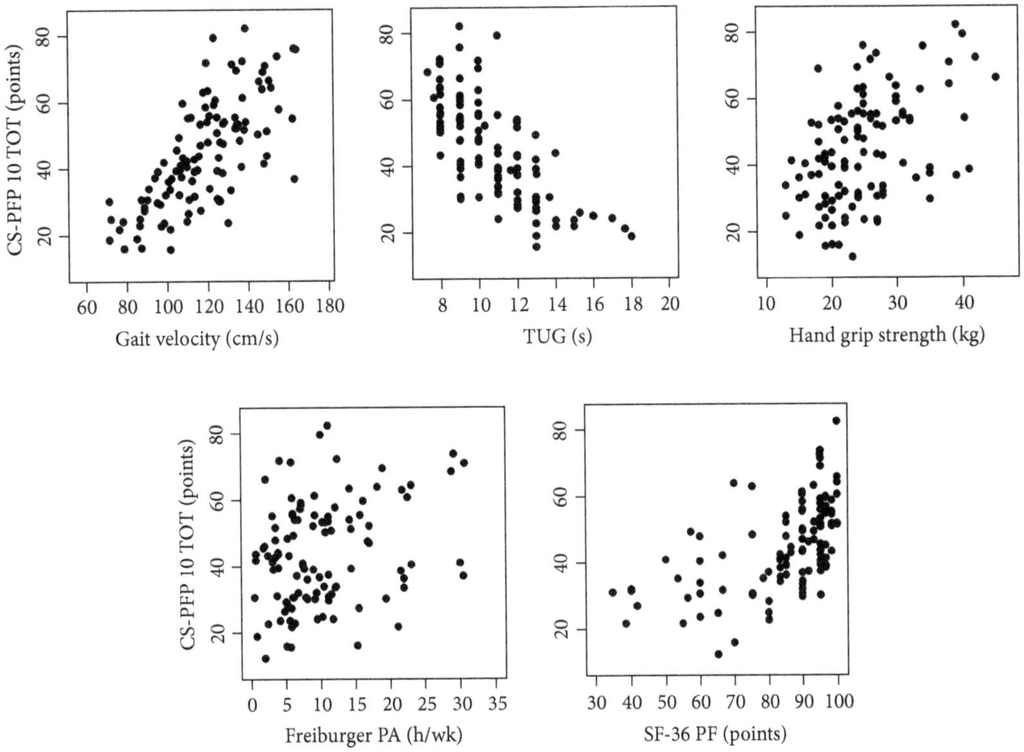

FIGURE 1: Scatter plots of the CS-PFP 10 total score and the concurrent validity measures.

TABLE 5: Cronbach's alpha.

	α
CS-PFP 10 TOT	0.95
CS-PFP 10 UBS	0.97
CS-PFP 10 LBS	0.95
CS-PFP 10 UBF	0.98
CS-PFP 10 B&C	0.95
CS-PFP 10 END	0.95

CS-PFP 10 TOT = CS-PFP 10 total score, CS-PFP 10 UBS = CS-PFP 10 upper body strength score, CS-PFP 10 LBS = CS-PFP 10 lower body strength score, CS-PFP 10 UBF = CS-PFP 10 upper body flexibility score, CS-PFP 10 B&C = CS-PFP 10 balance and coordination score, and CS-PFP 10 END = CS-PFP 10 endurance score.

value of r is affected by the amount of variability in the data [29]. In other words, the greater the range of scores in both variables, the greater the correlation between these variables. This factor is likely to be overlapped by the characteristics of the sample that can affect the size of r. In the present study, only community-dwellers were included; meanwhile, in the study of Cress et al. [7], community-dwellers as well as residents of a long-term care facility (including those who required assistance and those who did not) participated. Another possible reason for the lower value might be the fact that we used the CS-PFP short version of the test. Although there was a discrepancy in the amount of the correlation coefficient found, the high correlations support the similarity of the constructs.

Our study demonstrated excellent internal consistency of the translated version. Internal consistency reflects the extent to which items measure the same characteristics [30]. Cronbach's alpha coefficient of $\alpha = 0.95$ of the total score found in this study was comparable with the result of the validation study of the original version [7]. The coefficients of the single subscores in this study ranged between $\alpha = 0.95$ and 0.98 compared to the lower coefficients demonstrated in the original validation study (between $\alpha = 0.74$ and 0.87). Discrepancies found can be explained by the differing test versions. The original validation study [7] was conducted with the 16-task CS-PFP test, whereas the present study was done with its short version of 10 tasks.

No floor or ceiling effects were observed in this study population. The CS-PFP 10 is targeted to assess abilities within a functional range and requires the participants to be ambulatory. In ambulatory individuals no floor effects have been seen. Since tasks are administered from easiest to most difficult, maximal information is gathered in a person who may not be able to complete all tasks. On the other hand, ceiling effects have not been observed even in the healthy adult populations showing that the CS-PFP 10 has the property of measuring functional performance among older adults with a wide range of physical ability. Due to this strength, the CS-PFP 10 is well suited to demonstrate change in physical function in exercise intervention studies [11, 31, 32] as well as in various disease conditions including Parkinson's disease [33], heart disease [34, 35], and fibromyalgia [36].

The CS-PFP 10 was recommended in a systematic review from 2012 [3] regarding geriatric screening and assessment as well as for scientific and research purposes in community-dwelling older adults. In contrast to the measurement of gait velocity, the CS-PFP 10 is more complex in use and requires significant space, which may restrict the fields of application. However, the clinical benefits of the CS-PFP 10 lie in the performance-based quantification of a broad spectrum of physical everyday functions which can provide, for example, general practitioners a more profound insight in the physical abilities of their older patients. Also, the tests subscores allow a more detailed localization of functional deficits that helps therapists target deficits from the beginning and quantify therapy success.

This study was conducted as part of a randomized placebo-controlled parallel group trial with healthy older adults. All participants understood and easily followed the test instructions. The time taken to complete the test was in average 50 minutes. However, only concurrent validity and internal reliability was tested in this substudy. Further study will be needed to test intrarater and interrater reliability as well as predictive validity of this assessment in German-speaking older adults.

5. Conclusion

The study reports the translation of the CS-PFP 10 into German and the site set-up in accordance with the CS-PFP 10 guidelines and the local cultural settings. Concurrent validity and internal reliability were established. In addition to the original version of the CS-PFP 10, this German version can be used to quantify physical functional performance in older adults who are primarily nondisabled and might exhibit ceiling effects for traditionally used functional performance measures.

Conflicts of Interest

The authors declare that there are no competing interests regarding the publication of this manuscript.

Acknowledgments

The authors would like to thank Dr. Stefanie von Felten and Sabine Schädelin from the Clinical Trial Unit of the University Hospital Basel for their collaboration with the statistical analyses. They also thank Sarah Reinhard and Ladina Guidon for helpful ideas and assistance during the writing process.

References

[1] T. M. Gill, "Assessment of function and disability in longitudinal studies," *Journal of the American Geriatrics Society*, vol. 58, pp. S308–S312, 2010.

[2] M. E. Cress, "Quantifying physical functional performance in older adults," *Muscle and Nerve*, vol. 20, no. 5, pp. S17–S20, 1997.

[3] E. Freiberger, P. De Vreede, D. Schoene et al., "Performance-based physical function in older community-dwelling persons: a systematic review of instruments," *Age and Ageing*, vol. 41, no. 6, pp. 712–721, 2012.

[4] J. M. Guralnik, E. M. Simonsick, L. Ferrucci et al., "A short physical performance battery assessing lower extremity function: association with self-reported disability and prediction of mortality and nursing home admission," *Journals of Gerontology*, vol. 49, no. 2, pp. M85–M94, 1994.

[5] D. B. Reuben, "An objective measure of physical function of elderly outpatients: the physical performance test," *Journal of the American Geriatrics Society*, vol. 38, no. 10, pp. 1105–1112, 1990.

[6] E. M. Simonsick, A. B. Newman, M. C. Nevitt et al., "Measuring higher level physical function in well-functioning older adults: expanding familiar approaches in the health ABC study," *Journals of Gerontology—Series A: Biological Sciences and Medical Sciences*, vol. 56, no. 10, pp. M644–M649, 2001.

[7] M. E. Cress, D. M. Buchner, K. A. Questad, P. C. Esselman, B. J. DeLateur, and R. S. Schwartz, "Continuous-scale physical functional performance in healthy older adults: A validation study," *Archives of Physical Medicine and Rehabilitation*, vol. 77, no. 12, pp. 1243–1250, 1996.

[8] M. E. Cress, J. K. Petrella, T. L. Moore, and M. L. Schenkman, "Continuous-scale physical functional performance test: validity, reliability, and sensitivity of data for the short version," *Physical Therapy*, vol. 85, no. 4, pp. 323–335, 2005.

[9] F. Guillemin, C. Bombardier, and D. Beaton, "Cross-cultural adaptation of health-related quality of life measures: literature review and proposed guidelines," *Journal of Clinical Epidemiology*, vol. 46, no. 12, pp. 1417–1432, 1993.

[10] M. E. Cress and M. Meyer, "Maximal voluntary and functional performance levels needed for independence in adults aged 65 to 97 years," *Physical Therapy*, vol. 83, no. 1, pp. 37–48, 2003.

[11] M. E. Cress, D. M. Buchner, K. A. Questad, P. C. Esselman, B. J. deLateur, and R. S. Schwartz, "Exercise: effects on physical functional performance in independent older adults," *Journals of Gerontology, Series A: Biological Sciences and Medical Sciences*, vol. 54, no. 5, pp. M242–M248, 1999.

[12] B. Bilney, M. Morris, and K. Webster, "Concurrent related validity of the GAITRite walkway system for quantification of

the spatial and temporal parameters of gait," *Gait and Posture*, vol. 17, no. 1, pp. 68–74, 2003.

[13] R. W. Kressig, O. Beauchet, J. Anders et al., "Guidelines for clinical applications of spatio-temporal gait analysis in older adults," *Aging Clinical and Experimental Research*, vol. 18, no. 2, pp. 174–176, 2006.

[14] S. A. Bridenbaugh and R. W. Kressig, "Laboratory review: the role of gfait analysis in seniors' mobility and fall prevention," *Gerontology*, vol. 57, no. 3, pp. 256–264, 2011.

[15] I. Härdi, S. A. Bridenbaugh, Y. J. Gschwind, and R. W. Kressig, "The effect of three different types of walking aids on spatiotemporal gait parameters in community-dwelling older adults," *Aging Clinical and Experimental Research*, vol. 26, no. 2, pp. 221–228, 2014.

[16] D. Podsiadlo and S. Richardson, "The timed "Up & Go": a test of basic functional mobility for frail elderly persons," *Journal of the American Geriatrics Society*, vol. 39, no. 2, pp. 142–148, 1991.

[17] A. Shumway-Cook, S. Brauer, and M. Woollacott, "Predicting the probability for falls in community-dwelling older adults using the timed up & go test," *Physical Therapy*, vol. 80, no. 9, pp. 896–903, 2000.

[18] E. E. Fess, "Clinical Assessment Recommendations," J. S. Casanova, Ed., vol. 8, pp. 625–627, American Society of Hand Therapists, Chicago, Ill, USA, 2nd edition, 1983.

[19] E. Innes, "Handgrip strength testing: a review of the literature," *Australian Occupational Therapy Journal*, vol. 46, no. 3, pp. 120–140, 1999.

[20] R. W. Bohannon, A. Peolsson, N. Massy-Westropp, J. Desrosiers, and J. Bear-Lehman, "Reference values for adult grip strength measured with a Jamar dynamometer: a descriptive meta-analysis," *Physiotherapy*, vol. 92, no. 1, pp. 11–15, 2006.

[21] I. Frey, A. Berg, D. K. Grathwohl, and J. Keul, "Freiburger questionnaire on physical activity - design, validation and application," *Sozial- und Praventivmedizin*, vol. 44, no. 2, pp. 55–64, 1999.

[22] I. Frey and A. Berg, "Erfassung der körperlichen Aktivität in Klinik und Praxis," in *Körperliche Aktivität in Prävention und Therapie: Evidenzbasierter Leitfaden für Klinik und Praxis*, G. Samitz and G. Mensink, Eds., pp. 81–86, Hans Marseille Verlag GmbH, München, Germany, 2002.

[23] J. E. Ware and C. D. Sherbourne, "The MOS 36-item short-form health survey (SF-36): I. Conceptual framework and item selection," *Medical Care*, vol. 30, no. 6, pp. 473–483, 1992.

[24] S. E. Lamb, E. C. Jørstad-Stein, K. Hauer, and C. Becker, "Development of a common outcome data set for fall injury prevention trials: the prevention of falls network Europe consensus," *Journal of the American Geriatrics Society*, vol. 53, no. 9, pp. 1618–1622, 2005.

[25] N. Döring and J. Bortz, "Forschungsmethoden und Evaluation in den Sozial- und Humanwissenschaften," p. 1063, Springer-Verlag, 2015.

[26] L. J. Cronbach, "Coefficient alpha and the internal structure of tests," *Psychometrika*, vol. 16, no. 3, pp. 297–334, 1951.

[27] P. L. Enright, "The six-minute walk test," *Respiratory Care*, vol. 48, no. 8, pp. 783–785, 2003.

[28] T. Troosters, R. Gosselink, and M. Decramer, "Six-minute walk test: a valuable test, when properly standardized," *Physical Therapy*, vol. 82, no. 8, pp. 826-827, Aug 2002.

[29] L. D. Goodwin and N. L. Leech, "Understanding correlation: factors that affect the size of r," *The Journal of Experimental Education*, vol. 74, no. 3, pp. 249–266, 2006.

[30] D. L. Streiner, G. R. Norman, and J. Cairney, *Health Measurement Scales. A Practical Guide to Their Development and Use*, Oxford University Press, New York, NY, USA, 4th edition, 2014.

[31] T. A. Miszko, M. E. Cress, J. M. Slade, C. J. Covey, S. K. Agrawal, and C. E. Doerr, "Effect of Strength and Power Training on Physical Function in Community-Dwelling Older Adults," *The Journals of Gerontology Series A: Biological Sciences and Medical Sciences*, vol. 58, no. 2, pp. M171–M175, 2003.

[32] T. L. Moore-Harrison, E. M. Speer, F. T. Johnson, and M. E. Cress, "The effects of aerobic training and nutrition education on functional performance in low socioeconomic older adults," *Journal of Geriatric Physical Therapy*, vol. 31, no. 1, pp. 18–23, 2008.

[33] M. Schenkman, D. A. Hall, A. E. Baron, R. S. Schwartz, P. Mettler, and W. M. Kohrt, "Exercise for people in early- or mid-stage parkinson disease: a 16-month randomized controlled trial," *Physical Therapy*, vol. 92, no. 11, pp. 1395–1410, 2012.

[34] P. A. Savage, A. O. Shaw, M. S. Miller et al., "Effect of resistance training on physical disability in chronic heart failure," *Medicine and Science in Sports and Exercise*, vol. 43, no. 8, pp. 1379–1386, 2011.

[35] R. A. Gary, M. E. Cress, M. K. Higgins, A. L. Smith, and S. B. Dunbar, "Combined aerobic and resistance exercise program improves task performance in patients with heart failure," *Archives of Physical Medicine and Rehabilitation*, vol. 92, no. 9, pp. 1371-1381, 2011.

[36] J. D. Kingsley, L. B. Panton, T. Toole, P. Sirithienthad, R. Mathis, and V. McMillan, "The effects of a 12-week strength-training program on strength and functionality in women with fibromyalgia," *Archives of Physical Medicine and Rehabilitation*, vol. 86, no. 9, pp. 1713-1721, 2005.

Permissions

All chapters in this book were first published in JAR, by Hindawi Publishing Corporation; hereby published with permission under the Creative Commons Attribution License or equivalent. Every chapter published in this book has been scrutinized by our experts. Their significance has been extensively debated. The topics covered herein carry significant findings which will fuel the growth of the discipline. They may even be implemented as practical applications or may be referred to as a beginning point for another development.

The contributors of this book come from diverse backgrounds, making this book a truly international effort. This book will bring forth new frontiers with its revolutionizing research information and detailed analysis of the nascent developments around the world.

We would like to thank all the contributing authors for lending their expertise to make the book truly unique. They have played a crucial role in the development of this book. Without their invaluable contributions this book wouldn't have been possible. They have made vital efforts to compile up to date information on the varied aspects of this subject to make this book a valuable addition to the collection of many professionals and students.

This book was conceptualized with the vision of imparting up-to-date information and advanced data in this field. To ensure the same, a matchless editorial board was set up. Every individual on the board went through rigorous rounds of assessment to prove their worth. After which they invested a large part of their time researching and compiling the most relevant data for our readers.

The editorial board has been involved in producing this book since its inception. They have spent rigorous hours researching and exploring the diverse topics which have resulted in the successful publishing of this book. They have passed on their knowledge of decades through this book. To expedite this challenging task, the publisher supported the team at every step. A small team of assistant editors was also appointed to further simplify the editing procedure and attain best results for the readers.

Apart from the editorial board, the designing team has also invested a significant amount of their time in understanding the subject and creating the most relevant covers. They scrutinized every image to scout for the most suitable representation of the subject and create an appropriate cover for the book.

The publishing team has been an ardent support to the editorial, designing and production team. Their endless efforts to recruit the best for this project, has resulted in the accomplishment of this book. They are a veteran in the field of academics and their pool of knowledge is as vast as their experience in printing. Their expertise and guidance has proved useful at every step. Their uncompromising quality standards have made this book an exceptional effort. Their encouragement from time to time has been an inspiration for everyone.

The publisher and the editorial board hope that this book will prove to be a valuable piece of knowledge for researchers, students, practitioners and scholars across the globe.

List of Contributors

Wei-Chen Lee
Health Policy & Management, Program on Health Workforce Analysis and Policy, School of Rural Public Health, Texas A&M Health Science Center, College Station, TX 77843-1266, USA

Marcia G. Ory
Health Promotion & Community Health Sciences, Program on Healthy Aging, School of Rural Public Health, Texas A&M Health Science Center, College Station, TX 77843-1266, USA

Howard B. Degenholtz, Abby L. Resnick, Natalie Bulger and Lichun Chia
University of Pittsburgh, 130 DeSoto Street, Pittsburgh, PA 15261, USA

E. M. Macri
Centre for Hip Health and Mobility, University of British Columbia, Vancouver, BC, Canada V5Z 1M9

J. A. Lewis and N. A. de Morton
Department of Physiotherapy, Monash University, Melbourne, VIC 3800, Australia

K. M. Khan and M. C. Ashe
Centre for Hip Health and Mobility, University of British Columbia, Vancouver, BC, Canada V5Z 1M9
Department of Family Practice, University of British Columbia, Vancouver, BC, Canada V6T 1Z4

Koren L. Fisher
Department of Kinesiology, California State University, Fullerton 800 N. State College Boulevard, Fullerton, CA 92831, USA

Karen E. Chad
Department of Kinesiology, University of Saskatchewan, 87 Campus Drive, Saskatoon, SK, Canada S7N 5B2

Elizabeth L. Harrison
School of Physical Therapy, University of Saskatchewan, 1121 College Drive, Saskatoon, SK, Canada S7N 0W3

Bruce A. Reeder
Department of Community Health and Epidemiology, University of Saskatchewan, Health Science Building, 107 Wiggins Road, Saskatoon, SK, Canada S7N 5E5

Nazmi Sar
Department of Economics, University of Saskatchewan, Arts 815, 9 Campus Drive, Saskatoon, SK, Canada S7N 5A5

Ingeborg Nilsson
Department of Community Medicine and Rehabilitation, Occupational Therapy, Umeå University, 901 87 Umeå, Sweden
Umeå University, Ageing and Living Conditions Program, 901 87 Umeå, Sweden

Fredrica Nyqvist and Mikael Nygård
Faculty of Education and Welfare Studies, Social Policy Unit, Åbo Akademi University, 651 01 Vasa, Finland

Yngve Gustafson
Department of Community Medicine and Rehabilitation, Geriatric Medicine, Umeå University, 901 87 Umeå, Sweden

Stephen Thielke
Department of Psychiatry, University of Washington, Seattle, WA 98195, USA
Geriatrics Research, Education, and Clinical Center, Puget Sound VA Medical Center and Psychiatry and Behavioral Sciences, University of Washington, Seattle, WA 98195, USA

Paula Diehr
Departments of Biostastitics and Health Services, University of Washington, Seattle, WA 98195, USA

Emerson Sebastião, Kelechi Ibe-Lamberts, Julie Bobitt, Andiara Schwingel and Wojtek Chodzko-Zajko
Aging and Diversity Lab, Department of Kinesiology and Community Health, University of Illinois, 209 Louise Freer Hall, 906 S Goodwin Avenue, Urbana, IL 61801, USA

Dario Riva and Manuel Momenté
International Society of Proprioception and Posture, Turin, Italy

Flavio Rocca
Proprioception Center, Via Valgioie 85-87, 10146 Turin, Italy

Carlo Mamo
Epidemiology Unit, Local Health Unit TO3, Piemonte Region, Grugliasco, Italy

Mara Fanì
Sanitary District 2, Local Health Unit TO1, Piemonte Region, Turin, Italy

Marianna Fratta and Patrizia Saccavin
Department of Functional Rehabilitation, Local Health Unit TO1, Piemonte Region, Turin, Italy

Kimberly J. Alvarez and Thelma J. Mielenz
Department of Epidemiology, Mailman School of Public Health, Columbia University, 722 West 168th Street, New York, NY 10032, USA

Shannen Kirchner, Serena Chu and Sarah Smith
College of Physicians and Surgeons, Columbia University, New York, NY 10032, USA

Wendy Winnick-Baskin
Atria Senior Living, Louisville, KY 40202, USA

Julie Hicks Patrick
Department of Psychology, West Virginia University, Morgantown, WV 26506-6040, USA

Jenessa C. Steele
Department of Psychology, West Virginia University, Morgantown, WV 26506-6040, USA
Department of Psychology, Radford University, Radford, VA 24141, USA

S. Melinda Spencer
Department of Psychology, West Virginia University, Morgantown, WV 26506-6040, USA
Department of Health Promotion Education and Behavior, University of South Carolina, Columbia, SC 2920, USA

K. M. Rice and C. Gillette
Center for Diagnostic Nano systems and Robert C. Byrd Biotechnology Science Center, Marshall University, Room 241D, 1700 3rd Avenue, Huntington, WV 25755-1090, USA

J. C. Fannin
Department of Pharmacology, Physiology and Toxicology, Joan C. Edwards School of Medicine, Marshall University, Huntington, WV, USA

E. R. Blough
Department of Pharmacy Practice, Administration, and Research, School of Pharmacy, Marshall University, Huntington, WV, USA
Department of Pharmaceutical Sciences and Research, School of Pharmacy, Marshall University, Huntington, WV, USA

Shekhar K. Gadkaree, Daniel Q. Sun, Carol Li, Frank R. Linand and Yuri Agrawal
Department of Otolaryngology-Head & Neck Surgery, Johns Hopkins University School of Medicine, Baltimore, MD, USA

Luigi Ferrucci and Eleanor M. Simonsick
National Institute on Aging, National Institutes of Health, Baltimore, MD, USA

Sepali Guruge and Birpreet Birpreet
School of Nursing, Ryerson University, 350 Victoria Street, Toronto, ON, Canada M5B 2K3

Joan A. Samuels-Dennis
School of Health Science, Humber College ITAL, 205 Humber College Boulevard, Toronto, ON, Canada M9W5L7

Christopher J. Dondzila
Department of Health, Exercise, and Sport Science, The Citadel, Deas Hall, Room 113, 171 Moultrie Street, Charleston, SC29409, USA

Ann M. Swartz, Kevin G. Keenan and Scott J. Strath
Department of Kinesiology, The University of Wisconsin-Milwaukee, Enderis Hall, 2400 East Hartford, Milwaukee, WI 53201, USA
Center for Aging and Translational Research, The University of Wisconsin Milwaukee, NWQ-B, Room 1427, Milwaukee, WI, USA

Amy E. Harley
Zilber School of Public Health, The University of Wisconsin-Milwaukee, Zilber School of Public Health Building, Room 409, 1240North 10th Street, Milwaukee, WI 53205, USA

Razia Azen
Department of Educational Psychology, The University of Wisconsin-Milwaukee, Enderis Hall, Room 769, 2400 East Hartford, Milwaukee, WI 53201, USA

Liza Stathokostas, Robert M. D. Little and Donald H. Paterson
Canadian Centre for Activity and Aging, School of Kinesiology, The University of Western Ontario, London, 3M Centre 2225, ON, Canada N6A 3K7

A. A. Vandervoort
School of Physical Therapy, Elborn College 1400, The University of Western Ontario, London, ON, Canada N6A 3K7

Supawadee Putthinoi and Suchitporn Lersilp
Department of Occupational Therapy, Faculty of Associated Medical Sciences, Chiang Mai University, 110 Intawaroroj Rd., Sripoom Subdistrict, Meung, Chiang Mai 50200, Thailand

Nopasit Chakpitak
Chiang Mai University International College, Chiang Mai University, 239 Huaykaew Rd., Chiang Mai 50200, Thailand

Christina Bermeitinger and Cathleen Kappes
University of Hildesheim, Hildesheim, Germany

Wenbin Liang and Tanya Chikritzhs
National Drug Research Institute, Curtin University, Perth, WA 6845, Australia

Donna Kritz-Silverstein and Elizabeth Barrett-Connor
Department of Family Medicine and Public Health, University of California San Diego, La Jolla, CA 92093-0628, USA

Ericha G. Anthony
Department of Family Medicine and Public Health, University of California San Diego, La Jolla, CA 92093-0628, USA
Graduate School of Public Health, San Diego State University, San Diego, CA 92182, USA

M. D. Rijnaard, J. van Hoof, W. Pocornie and E. J. M. Wouters
Fontys University of Applied Sciences, Institute of Allied Health Professions, Dominee Theodor Fliednerstraat 2, 5631 BN Eindhoven, Netherlands
Fontys University of Applied Sciences, Fontys EGT-Centre for Health Care and Technology, Dominee Theodor Fliednerstraat 2, 5631 BN Eindhoven, Netherlands

B. M. Janssen
Fontys University of Applied Sciences, Fontys School of People and Health Studies, Dominee Theodor Fliednerstraat 2, 5631 BN Eindhoven, Netherlands

H. Verbeek and H. C. Beerens
Department of Health Services Research, Maastricht University, Duboisdomein 30, 6229 GT Maastricht, Netherlands

A. Eijkelenboom
EGM Architecten, Wilgenbos 20, 3311 JX Dordrecht, Netherlands

S. L. Molony
Quinnipiac University School of Nursing, North Haven Campus, Office MNH 470P, 275 Mount Carmel Avenue, Hamden, CT 06518-1908, USA

Mahboubeh Dadfar
School of Behavioral Sciences and Mental Health, Tehran Institute of Psychiatry, Iran University of Medical Sciences, International Campus, Tehran, Iran

David Lester
Department of Psychology, Stockton University, Galloway, NJ, USA

Fazel Bahrami
Department of Islamic Theology and Department of Counseling, University of Social Welfare and Rehabilitation Sciences, Tehran, Iran

Irene Härdi, Stephanie A. Bridenbaugh and Reto W. Kressig
University Center for Medicine of Aging and Rehabilitation, Felix Platter-Hospital, Basel Mobility Center, Basel, Switzerland

M. Elaine Cress
Department of Kinesiology, Institute of Gerontology, University of Georgia, Athens, GA, USA

Index

www.ingramcontent.com/pod-product-compliance
Lightning Source LLC
LaVergne TN
LVHW060526210926
848485LV00005B/1152
9781639270002